Not Fit to Stay

Not Fit to Stay

*Public Health Panics and
South Asian Exclusion*

Sarah Isabel Wallace

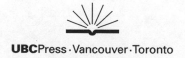

UBCPress · Vancouver · Toronto

25 24 23 22 21 20 19 18 17   5 4 3 2 1

Printed in Canada on FSC-certified ancient-forest-free paper (100% post-consumer recycled) that is processed chlorine- and acid-free.

Library and Archives Canada Cataloguing in Publication
Wallace, Sarah Isabel, author

  Not fit to stay : public health panics and South Asian exclusion / Sarah Isabel Wallace.

Includes bibliographical references and index.
Issued in print and electronic formats.
ISBN 978-0-7748-3218-2 (hardback). – ISBN 978-0-7748-3219-9 (pbk.)
ISBN 978-0-7748-3220-5 (pdf). – ISBN 978-0-7748-3221-2 (epub)
ISBN 978-0-7748-3222-9 (mobi)

1. South Asians – Health and hygiene – Pacific Coast (North America) – History – 20th century. 2. Immigrants – Health and hygiene – Pacific Coast (North America) – History – 20th century. 3. Public health – Political aspects – Pacific Coast (North America) – History – 20th century. 4. Public health – Social aspects – Pacific Coast (North America) – History – 20th century. 5. Racism – Pacific Coast (North America) – History – 20th century. 6. Marginality, Social – Pacific Coast (North America) – History – 20th century. 7. Pacific Coast (North America) – Ethnic relations – History – 20th century. 8. Pacific Coast (North America) – Emigration and immigration – History – 20th century. I. Title.

RA446.5.P32W34 2017   362.1097909'041   C2016-906292-9
                                                     C2016-906293-7

Canadä

UBC Press gratefully acknowledges the financial support for our publishing program of the Government of Canada (through the Canada Book Fund), the Canada Council for the Arts, and the British Columbia Arts Council.

This book has been published with the help of a grant from the Canadian Federation for the Humanities and Social Sciences, through the Awards to Scholarly Publications Program, using funds provided by the Social Sciences and Humanities Research Council of Canada.

Printed and bound in Canada by Friesens
Set in NewBaskerville and Galliard by Apex CoVantage, LLC
Copy editor: Matthew Kudelka
Cover designer: Jessica Sullivan

UBC Press
The University of British Columbia
2029 West Mall
Vancouver, BC V6T 1Z2
www.ubcpress.ca

Contents

Figures and Tables

Acknowledgments

First of all, I would like to thank God for watching over me while I prepared this manuscript.

I would like to thank my editor Darcy Cullen and my anonymous reviewers for their help and guidance. I also wish to thank Dr. Jeffrey Brison and Dr. Barrington Walker of Queen's University for their assistance, and Dr. Patricia Roy for her invaluable suggestions and editing. I would also like to thank Dr. Galen Roger Perras for kindly agreeing to read early drafts of this book and for providing me with guidance with my archival research.

I wish to thank the Senator Frank Carrel Foundation and the Social Sciences and Humanities Research Council for helping fund this project.

I would like to thank the many individuals who agreed to be interviewed for this project, in British Columbia, California, and Ottawa. Many others generously welcomed me into their *gurdwaras* and their homes. I would especially like to thank Dalwinder Gill of Ottawa, the Johal family of Vancouver, and the India Cultural Centre of Canada.

I would also like to acknowledge my beloved grandfather, Dr. John K. Hampshire [1914-2007], who encouraged me to pursue higher education, and my mother, Christine Wallace, for proofreading this manuscript and for being my trusty research assistant in San Francisco. Finally, I would like to offer special thanks to my wonderful husband, Joshua Laviolette, for supporting and encouraging me in countless ways.

Not Fit to Stay

Introduction

A RUMOUR RIPPLED ACROSS Washington State in the fall of 1907. The *Blaine Review* first broke the story that the newly arrived South Asian labourers working in local mills had been responsible for an outbreak of spinal meningitis the previous spring. Methodist bishop James Mills Thoburn, who had recently returned home from India after nearly thirty years, asserted that "Hindoo immigration to the coast was responsible for a great deal of the plague, cerebro-spinal meningitis and other diseases that have been sweeping the country," as South Asians were "leaving India in the hopes of escaping the plague, the germs of which they carry with them." He warned that "great trouble would result" unless Americans excluded the newcomers.[1] While Thoburn's assertions had no basis in fact, the connection he drew between South Asians and contagious disease offered local residents an attractive rationale for opposing South Asian immigration.

Between 1899, when South Asians began migrating to North America, and 1917, when the United States legislated Indian exclusion, more than 13,000 South Asian immigrants entered British Columbia and the US Pacific coast states to work and to establish communities. Typically referred to as "Hindus" or "Hindoos" by government officers, the press, and members of the general public, almost all were male Sikh labourers from the northern Indian province of Punjab. As Sikhs, most wore turbans and some or all of the other five dress requirements of males in this mono-theistic religion – uncut hair and beard, a comb worn under the turban, a special, loose-fitting cotton underwear garment, a small steel sword strapped on the hip, and a steel bangle (bracelet) on the wrist.[2] The vast majority settled in BC and California, although some moved to the logging and agricultural zones throughout Washington State and Oregon. As South Asians arrived on the coast in ever-increasing numbers, local labour leaders, politicians, and community groups perceived them as labour competition and as threats to "white" (mainly western European) culture and society. Despite a steady need for unskilled labour along the Pacific coast, and the general reliability of Indian workers, regional trade unions and politicians lobbied successfully to bar most South Asians from Canada in 1908, and from the United States in 1910.

Beginning in 1906 in BC and in 1907 in Washington State, Oregon, and California, South Asians encountered escalating hostility. The opponents of South Asian immigration, who viewed the new arrivals as "uncivilized" and "undesirable" members of a racial minority and as physically unsuited to the Pacific Northwest's climate, almost immediately adopted the argument that immigrants from India suffered from medical conditions and diseases that could be specifically attributed to their race. This idea was initially a subset of a broader argument that South Asians could not assimilate because they had a lower standard of living, followed caste prejudices, and spoke a different language. Quickly, however, the disease argument took on a life of its own and came to dominate the tide of opposition to the South Asian presence along the coast. The timing of this opposition was critical: the first wave of South Asian migrants to BC coincided with a massive public outcry against immigrants from Japan (evident especially in the 1907 Vancouver riot).[3] To appease labour groups without utterly excluding Japanese immigrants, Canada's federal government under Wilfrid Laurier effectively barred South Asians from the country. The initial South Asian arrival in the Pacific coast states coincided with the reappearance of meningitis and especially bubonic plague in the region, and this cemented Americans' association between the new arrivals and disease.[4]

This book analyzes the many ways in which the issue of public health shaped official and popular responses to first wave South Asian immigrants in Canada and the United States. It also examines how these racially based responses led to the exclusion of South Asians from the continent. In Canada, the 1908 legislation excluding Indians from the country was the direct result of a vociferous two-year campaign in BC built on precepts of South Asian racial "otherness"; shortly thereafter, a similar movement in the Pacific coast states brought about American exclusion of South Asians. At its heart, this book argues that while South Asians were widely categorized as "Asians" by policy-makers, sociologists, and racial theorists, their physical appearance, social customs, religion, and especially their association with disease set them apart from (and in many cases below) other races in the evolving racial hierarchy of the Canadian and American west;

as a consequence, they became medical scapegoats in Pacific coast communities.[5] All of this both challenges and expands on traditional interpretations that focus almost exclusively on Chinese and Japanese immigrants in discussions about nativist perceptions of Asians as inferior, backward, and diseased.

The coast's widespread anti-Indian sentiment was based in part on a well-exploited but empirically unsupported argument that South Asians were unsanitary and suffered from racially attributable medical conditions that impaired their productivity and/or endangered community health. Since the late nineteenth century, many Americans had believed that the cost of meeting the nation's constant need for immigrants was social deterioration through economic recession, overcrowding, and (especially) labour competition. John Higham's now-classic text on American nativism defines it as both a conscious perpetuation of native cultural characteristics and an economic and socio-political policy promoting the welfare of established residents over those of immigrants. Nativism, as a "complex of ideas," manifested itself in several ways, including the application of natural science and Galtonian theory in immigration policy. Howard Markel and Alexandra Stern add that this new approach to immigration embraced "the ubiquitous racializing and 'othering' discourses of the Progressive Era" – discourses that workers mobilized in an attempt to safeguard their jobs.[6] Specific ethnic groups, including Asians, Jews, Italians, and Eastern Europeans, became special targets of what Alan Kraut refers to as "medicalized nativism," which arises when "the justification for excluding members of a particular group includes charges that they constitute a health menace and may endanger their hosts." Although some members of a given immigrant population may indeed carry and transmit disease, the "association with disease in the minds of the native born" stigmatizes all members of that immigrant population: each newcomer is reduced from "a whole and usual person to a tainted, discounted one."[7]

In addition, India's colonial status planted discourse on the "Hindu" issue at the crossroads of medicalized nativism, eugenics, and colonial theory. In this context, charges of racial and genetic inferiority often spilled over into other, more sensational areas – for example, South Asians were associated with sexual deviance and criminality. While many immigration gatekeepers were genuinely concerned that South Asians threatened public health and morality, others realized that this concern was ungrounded. Many who fell within the latter group nevertheless employed the disease argument as a veil or guise for objections to South Asian immigration based on racial or labour reasons. In BC, as in the Pacific coast states, Asians encountered widespread (albeit varying) levels of resistance and hostility to their presence. This variance of opinion persisted at the medical, bureaucratic, and political levels, as well as within the press and civil society, but since there was widespread popular acceptance of the disease argument, it soon became an important thread interwoven with the racial, social, political, and economic arguments for South Asian exclusion.

The vast majority of first wave South Asians in both BC and the Pacific coast states came from a similar socio-economic background in India. They had left the Punjab at roughly the same time and for the same economic opportunities, and they took similar types of logging, railway, and agricultural work on both sides of the Canada–US border. Thus, I will be treating their migration to North America as one movement, not as two. As South Asians arrived on the continent, first at BC ports and later in Washington State (through BC or by sea), in Oregon, and finally in northern California, local populaces on both sides of the border perceived them as one unified group. This perception ensured that the local reception of individual South Asians was essentially the same along the Pacific coast, although there were some key differences between Indian immigrant experiences in Canada and the United States. A major anti-Asian riot in Vancouver prompted the Canadian government to legislate South Asian exclusion in early 1908, yet a specifically anti-Indian riot in northern Washington State did not compel US officials to do the same at that time. The political reasons for these disparate official reactions to the riots will be discussed in Chapters 2 and 5. The Canadian arguments that South Asians were unsuited to the Pacific coast climate, and that as a group they were especially susceptible to tuberculosis, gained less currency in the United States than in Canada. Moreover, the Canadian treatment of South Asian immigration overall was partly influenced – although by no means determined – by the fact that Canada and India were both part of the British Empire.

While recognizing these important differences, this book also demonstrates the significant similarities between the South Asian experiences in BC and the Pacific coast states. The disease argument transcended the 49th Parallel and was taken up (although sometimes contested) by physicians and other health workers, government officials, labour organizations, politicians, members of the press, and others. Furthermore, by 1910, the US Department of Commerce and Labor's Immigration Service's (IS) policy of executive restriction – a term first coined by Joan Jensen to mean a stringent, often questionable interpretation of immigration legislation – ensured that most South Asians were effectively barred from the United States only two years later than in Canada.[8] IS agents and Canadian immigration officers often corresponded and even met face to face to discuss policy alignment on the "Hindu issue," especially during the early stages of South Asian immigration in 1906, and then later after the Americans encountered hookworm (ancylostomiasis) among South Asians at the Angel Island quarantine station in California in 1910. Exclusionist literature and activities by the San Francisco–based Asiatic Exclusion League (AEL) often crossed the border – as a prime example, AEL members participated in and even helped organize the 1907 Vancouver riot. A guiding precept of the AEL and of the major labour organizations representing the interests of white workers – the Canadian Trades and Labour Congress (TLC) in BC, and the American Federation of Labour (AFL) in the Pacific coast states – was that South Asians threatened the public health, morality, and society of the entire Pacific coast.

The South Asian response to exclusionist campaigning was also transnational. Especially after 1907, South Asians often travelled across the border, by legal or illegal means, to find work, participate in community gatherings, or organize and engage in protests over their treatment on the continent. Also, anti-imperial revolutionary ideologies and materials routinely circulated among South Asians on both side of the border, especially in the years directly preceding the First World War, when some migrants used transnational platforms to challenge the disease argument.[9] All of this highlights the need for a Canadian–American study of first wave South Asian immigration.

Using the theoretical lenses of nativism, race theory, post-colonial theory, Orientalism, Diaspora theory, and scientific racism, I compare and contrast the Canadian and American treatment of South Asians in British Columbia and the Pacific coast states in the first two decades of South Asian settlement in North America. In this examination of race, labour, and especially public health, I show that official and popular efforts to exclude Indians for health reasons were, at least in some cases, motivated by concerns about South Asians settling down in white communities and participating in the workforce rather than by a genuine desire to protect public health. Bringing immigrant subjectivity to the forefront as much as possible, I discuss the experiences of this racialized group, whom white populations perceived and treated as "others" separate from other Asians, and, in Canada, as members of the British Empire but not equal citizens. In so doing, I address the imbalance in scholarship that historian Tony Ballantyne points out has traditionally favoured post-1970s Sikh migration at the expense of "the struggles and successes" of first wave Indian migrants, whose stories "are too frequently glossed over" or "are merely treated as a prelude to the recent histories of community formation."[10]

A significant breadth of historiography has explored important elements of the South Asian immigration question – especially the government surveillance of independence activists in North America and organized labour's response to the entry of "Hindu" workers.[11] Recent work has also investigated issues relating to sexuality within the broader framework of South Asian immigration and settlement.[12] These key topics in the history of Indian immigration and settlement serve as important building blocks to my narrative but are never its sole focus. Instead, I address the many instances when municipal, provincial, state, and federal politicians, bureaucrats, medical doctors, labour leaders, press editors, and others argued that South Asians presented a public health threat because of their purported racial predilection to have and spread disease, to live in unsanitary conditions, and to engage in abhorrent cultural practices and immoral behaviour. Scientific racism, the theoretical backbone of the Eugenics movement, is generally defined as any ostensibly scientific and medical explanations, approaches, or findings used to validate racial stereotypes and ethnic categorizations.[13] Whether or not the anxiety behind these anti-Indian arguments was genuine, all of this fostered a particular form of scientific racism that was heightened when Canada's Immigration Branch of the Department of the Interior (hereafter the Immigration Branch) and the American IS exaggerated their concerns over the health, hygiene, and supposedly inherited racial characteristics of this ethnic group.

In exploring the "Hindu disease" thesis in its broader context, this book seeks a middle ground between the narrative-driven teleological accounts that have long fallen out of favour among social historians, and postmodern structuralist literature that foregrounds theme and theory at the expense of both time and the possibility of causality.[14] Thus the following chapters are organized roughly by chronological order, but within each chapter, events are discussed and interpreted thematically. K.N. Panikkar, a scholar of the post-colonial history of India, convincingly asserts that an approach is needed that recognizes the meaning that actors (such as

Indian colonial subjects) gave to the events of their time and that broadly recognizes how these actors influenced societal, political, and/or economic outcomes.[15] This book thus pursues a balance between Immanuel Kant and Michel Foucault's assertions that events cannot be seen as causal factors leading to specific outcomes within a grand narrative frame, and G.W.F. Hegel's defence of teleology as a useful mechanism for understanding how and why events and actions can shape certain outcomes.[16] In other words, I strive to avoid both the trap of historical progress and the argument that the struggles of first wave immigrants were necessary for the broad acceptance of South Asians in North America today, while still recognizing the significance of those struggles and their connections to the events that followed them.

The following pages offer a similar balance between methodologies on migration. Adam McKeown, Tony Ballantyne, and other scholars of migration adopt a transnational approach that moves beyond national borders and seeks out social, cultural, and economic transactions between geographically separated communities. This approach is "international" in that it studies the connections between two or more countries or diasporas and, in the case of Ballantyne, emphasizes the shared experiences and enduring connections among migrants throughout the British Empire. George M. Fredrickson and others instead compare "cross-national" commonalities and disparities between two or more groups of related or similar peoples who have migrated to different countries. For example, Stanley Elkins has made the now classic argument that African slaves experienced slavery differently in American and Spanish territories because of the diverging religious and political views of their overseers; thus, the distinctions between slavery in the American South and the Caribbean require a distinctly nationally based approach for studying the experiences of the involuntary migrants of those territories.[17]

Kevin Kenny convincingly argues that neither methodological approach is adequate. A purely transnational study often fails to capture the ongoing control and influence of various nation-states and the evolution of "nationally specific ethnicities that sharply differentiate an ostensibly unitary 'people' ... across time and space." National comparisons ignore the complex interactions among migrants, the consequences of their resettlement around the globe, their engagement in the domestic politics of their country of origin, and, perhaps most importantly, the germination and expansion of a shared culture, literature, and politics that ties groups together despite their geographic separation. Indeed, Paul Kramer agrees that the "nation state as historical 'container' was and is both a function of and a participant in nation-building programs, and insufficient for tracking and resolving the threads that bind a tangled world." Kenny thus calls for a history of migration that includes both the "transnational" and the "cross-national" so as to situate migration and settlement within a broader global milieu.[18]

The following pages on the South Asian diaspora in western North America will thus integrate information about the reasons for its establishment – what Kenny would call its transnational "origin, articulation, and temporality" – and its various national consequences.[19] In this book, "transnational" primarily refers to the social and cultural transactions that transcended the 49th Parallel, but I also employ the term to describe the enduring connections between migrants and the Indian Subcontinent. Here the terms "nation" and "state" hold two meanings. First, they designate "Canada," the "United States," and other populations separated by political boundaries. In analyzing the South Asian experience in these countries, I affirm Erika Lee's method of examining how exclusion "at its bottom fringes" was enforced and contested in each national case."[20] Second, moving beyond political borders, "nation" and "state" also refer to the religious and cultural identities in India that distinguish Sikh from Hindu and Muslim, and Punjabi from Bengali; these distinctions remained important after the group's settlement in North America.[21]

Chapter 1 examines the arrival of first wave South Asian immigrants on the Pacific coast between 1904 and 1907. Despite a labour shortage throughout most of the region, by 1906 Vancouver civic officials were seeking Dominion intervention to stop the increase in South Asian immigration, a request echoed by the province's federal Members of Parliament, Dominion immigration agents stationed at Pacific coast ports, and the Superintendent of Immigration himself. Rising tensions between federal and municipal officials culminated in a well-publicized crisis on Vancouver's waterfront, which was resolved only days before city residents turned their attention to the dramatic allegation that South Asians had committed a horrific crime against a white woman. When the Canadian government stalled on the Indian issue, exclusionists mobilized the "disease" theory – along with the argument that South Asians were uniquely unsuited to BC's climate – to agitate for South Asian exclusion. The chapter then turns to the Pacific coast states, where South Asians began to arrive only months after landing in Canada. Seizing on recent theories of scientific determinism and Orientalist conceptions of Asian exoticism, immorality, and disease, American opponents of South Asian immigration, like their counterparts in Canada, began to associate Indians with bubonic plague, tuberculosis, and "poor physique."

Opening with the causes and consequences of two major riots in Bellingham and Vancouver in September 1907, Chapter 2 details the beginning of Canada's executive restriction of South Asians in that month, as Immigration Branch executives tasked Dominion medical examiners at BC ports with finding reasons to keep out as many of the prospective immigrants as possible. Vancouver municipal reports about the unsanitary living conditions of South Asians further hardened public opinion against the newcomers, and Immigration Branch officials used these conditions and the broader "Hindu disease" and climate arguments to lobby for legislative exclusion. South of the 49th Parallel, the coincidence of the initial South Asian arrival with the reappearance of meningitis and especially bubonic plague offered a timely justification for exclusion. Meanwhile, because of the strong popular resentment against their presence, IS inspectors on the Pacific coast began to exclude South Asians either for a supposed lack of physical unfitness or for being likely to become a public charge (LPC).

Chapter 3 begins by examining the intent of the 1908 "continuous journey" legislation and the Dominion government's unsuccessful attempts to influence Britain and India to limit South Asian immigration to Canada. The outcome of a plan to deport BC's South Asians to a tropical colony forced officials to reconsider the still popular "climate" argument, and opponents of the South Asian presence in Canada further revitalized the "disease" theory. The chapter then shows the mixed results of US executive restriction between 1908 and 1910, as officials struggled to bar South Asians after two successive US presidents refused to introduce exclusionary legislation. Employing the South Asian reputation for disease that resonated through most sectors of American Pacific coast society, US officials diagnosed some South Asian arrivals at Pacific coast ports with "poor physique." This assertion, and the related contention that South Asians threatened public health, was difficult to prove.

Opening with the initial impact of the 1910 discovery that South Asians arriving at San Francisco were carrying hookworm, Chapter 4 explores how this finding affected the admission of new arrivals from India to that port. As it turned out, San Francisco was the last US Pacific port to enact executive restriction. The hookworm discovery would influence the closing of a key loophole in the US executive exclusion of South Asians. Turning to Canada, the chapter then demonstrates how Canadian immigration officials mobilized the American hookworm discovery to screen the small number of South Asians arriving at BC ports after 1911 and to prepare for a major challenge to legislative exclusion in 1914.

Chapter 5 begins by showing how a rising star in Canada's Immigration Branch influenced a key decision on the continuous journey provision in 1912. Echoing BC popular opinion and testimony delivered during a 1913 provincial study on labour issues, federal officials used health- and eugenics-based arguments to rationalize the government's treatment of the passengers of the SS *Komagata Maru* at Vancouver in 1914. Watching events at Vancouver's harbour in the summer of 1914, American opponents of South Asian immigration warned that Canada's *Komagata Maru* incident might set a precedent for others from India to increase their efforts to migrate to the continent; for this reason, US officials reporting from Canada emphasized the urgent need for exclusionary legislation. That same year, exclusionist participants in the "Hindu Immigration Hearings" in Washington, DC, used public health arguments to lobby a bipartisan government committee for South Asian legislative exclusion. The chapter concludes with a discussion of how these same issues later resurfaced in the congressional push for American legislative exclusion.

After exploring the continuing anti-Indian sentiment within Canada's Immigration Branch during and immediately after the First World War, Chapter 6 discusses the outcome of the Dominion's opposition party leader's investigation into introducing the South Asian franchise in 1922. The focus then shifts to the South Asians' quest for the franchise in the United States. Several of them had become citizens in the first two decades of the century, but in 1923 a major court decision revoked their citizenship and decreed that South Asians could no longer become citizens. I explain how the US federal government maintained this policy by resorting to the argument that South Asians could not assimilate because of their health practices and morality, and how the perpetuation of these same arguments in the Pacific coast states and especially in California legitimized and affirmed America's legislative exclusion of South Asians.

The concluding chapter revisits key themes and concepts addressed in earlier chapters, and briefly describes the transition to an Indian immigration quota system in both countries in the period immediately following the Second World War. The chapter further suggests areas for a future study with a wider, comparative focus on all Asian immigrant groups, and especially the widespread conception that "Oriental" diseases threatened non-Asian public health in the first half of the twentieth century.

1

"Leprosy and Plague Riot in Their Blood"

The Germination of a Thesis, 1906

We do not propose to have a Hindu town or bazaar rather, with its vicious evils and attendant undesirable element ... We shall have the plague, cholera and other deadly fevers and diseases here among us, if such is not stopped in time.

– Mary Wilson, Vancouver, December 14, 1906

The Hindu is not of us and can never be ... He brings nothing to our country but disease and filth and a little labor, in return for which he subtracts some of our capital.

– Bellingham Herald, *September 10, 1907*

SHORTLY BEFORE CANADIAN CONFEDERATION in 1867, future prime minister John A. Macdonald privately warned a friend that the new nation would have "a brilliant future ... were it not for those wretched Yankees who hunger & thirst for Naboth's field." He predicted with certainty another American invasion of Canada, in which, he wryly remarked, "India can do us Yeoman's service by sending an army of Sikhs – Ghoorkas, Beloches, etc. – across the Pacific to San Francisco, and holding that beautiful and immoral City with the surrounding California – as security for Montreal & Canada."[1] This remarkable statement escaped the attention of the contemporary press, much as the opening trickle of South Asian immigration into western North America four decades later has eluded the notice of most modern-day historians.[2] This chapter fills a critical gap in the literature by exploring the initial arrival of significant numbers of first wave South Asian immigrants in 1906, who entered at BC first and later at Washington State. The following pages explore the germination and growth of popular anti-Indian protests, along with official responses that were largely based on biological arguments that South

Asians were disease carriers, as well as the environmental and eugenic arguments that they were unsuited to the climate and to the rigorous labour demands of the Pacific Northwest.

The first phase of South Asian immigration to North America lasted just five years.[3] This short wave, which began in earnest in 1906 and had largely ended by the close of 1910, brought more than 12,000 South Asians to British Columbia, Washington, Oregon, and California. Most of these migrants were sojourners – single, male economic migrants of working age who, like the majority of the Chinese and Japanese who had preceded them to the continent, lacked the "cultural toeholds" of the sort that had facilitated the permanent settlement of European immigrants. Most of the new arrivals established temporary residence in Pacific coast communities while maintaining strong social, political, and economic ties to their home communities.[4] Their outsider status as the newest "Orientals" on the coast ensured that, almost immediately after their arrival, the seeds of popular protest against South Asian immigration and workforce participation took root among provincial and municipal politicians, the press, and the general public.

In Canada in 1906, Prime Minister Wilfrid Laurier was initially hesitant to bar South Asians. The Dominion's imperial connection with the British Raj, the government that had ruled India since 1858, placed Laurier in the difficult position of trying to appease BC residents while knowing that his government's actions could have serious repercussions in the Punjab. The Raj had long relied on Punjabi soldiers to enforce domestic stability and engage in military campaigns outside of India. The recent movement of Punjabi Sikhs to the Empire's other territories had therefore compelled Indian officials to attempt to manage the dual public relations problem of the discontent that resulted when migrants reported home about the political and economic disparities between India and these territories, and the reaction in Northern India to the poor treatment of Sikh labourers overseas.[5] Since the Empire's other white territories had already halted South Asian immigration – New Zealand in 1881, South Africa in 1897, and Australia in 1901 – Laurier was mindful that a Canadian exclusionary measure could exacerbate the growing tensions in the Punjab and in India generally.[6]

Vancouver, a growing municipality with a population of 26,000 in 1901, was the Dominion's main gateway for Asian immigrants. The Dominion's Immigration Branch office in Vancouver had opened in 1904 to manage the increase in incoming arrivals of Asians and others.[7] Only forty-five

South Asians arrived in 1904, but this number still triggered serious concern among municipal officials. In September, Thomas Guigan, Vancouver's city clerk, petitioned Richard William Scott, the Dominion's secretary of state in Ottawa, for federal intervention. Guigan argued that the first South Asians who had been brought to Canada could not perform manual labour because they were "naturally unfitted to stand the climate," which was "so different from their own."[8] Guigan was perhaps the first to espouse what I call the "climate theory" in BC's opposition to South Asians. The climate theory soon became a standard justification for municipal, provincial, and federal attempts to prevent South Asians from entering Canada in 1908. Linda Nash explains that nineteenth-century colonial theory held that "race" was both a consequence of geography and "the principal determinant of one's fitness for any particular land." Colonial discourse maintained that Europeans could not thrive in hot environments; typically this was attributed to the assumption that whites were uniquely vulnerable to dangerous "miasmas" (atmospheric contaminants) in warmer territories. Similarly, races from semi-tropical and tropical climates like India were viewed as unsuited for temperate regions like Canada because they could be sickened by fatal miasmas there. Although the Miasmatic theory of disease causation was falling out of favour "in most quarters" by 1900, as it had been largely supplanted by the germ theory that infectious diseases were caused by bacteria, various races were still "deemed more likely to 'carry' disease into otherwise healthy locations and to be more susceptible to certain kinds of illness" once they migrated.[9]

Initially, federal officials dismissed Guigan's concerns. W.G. Parmalee, Canada's deputy trade minister, informed the secretary of state that only ten South Asians had arrived in BC in 1903, that there were no records for earlier immigration, and that there was no cause for alarm about the number arriving in the current year. The deputy minister conceded that "they no doubt have their peculiarities," but he believed they had shown themselves to be reliable labourers in Trinidad and British Guiana. In his view, the work done by South Asians in those territories accounted for the commercial superiority of those colonies over others in the West Indies. He concluded that he was "not greatly impressed with the complaint" of the Vancouver authorities.[10]

Unlike Parmalee, officials in BC viewed the new arrivals – indeed, all Asian immigrants – with growing apprehension. This concern was rooted in the well-established belief that Asians were racially and culturally unable to integrate into white culture.[11] But in addition to that, the economic argument that Asians stole "white" jobs appealed to the large percentage of citizens who did not personally benefit from Asian labour.[12] After the Canadian Pacific Railway was completed in 1887, many Chinese had accepted work in domestic service, gardening, and laundering, which encouraged the stereotype of the subservient Chinese sojourner who worked in fields formerly dominated by white women. After their arrival in significant numbers beginning in 1900, Japanese immigrants came to be seen as the greater threat to white labour, as they became associated with the traditionally white male–dominated fields of resource extraction and fishing. Japan's 1905 victory in the Russo-Japanese War strengthened the popular stereotype that the "militaristic" blood of Japanese workers made them ruthless labour competitors whose unwavering loyalty to Japan could endanger BC's domestic security. Furthermore, unlike most Chinese, Japanese immigrants could bring their families with them to Canada, which made their presence seem especially threatening to the nation's long-term economic interests.[13]

Another important anti-Asian argument pertained to medical inspection procedures at BC ports. The initial arrival of significant numbers of South Asians roughly coincided with the emergence of Dominion medical inspectors as front-line guardians of the public health. Nineteenth-century cholera outbreaks had prompted provincial public health controls, including immigrant detention and fumigation at quarantine stations. These miasmatic and contagionist apparatuses for disease control had been established with the wide observation that "crowd" or group diseases had traditionally followed immigrants during the early European settlement of Canada.[14] When Confederation transferred quarantine powers to the federal government, the nation's infection control strategies became, as Mark Osborne Humphries reminds us, "as much about protecting the social body from unwanted groups as they were intended to protect Canadians from real diseases." This explains why the US border was never considered a significant threat to population health. Conversely, the quarantine apparatus in effect at the nation's seaports was designed to protect against sick immigrants, with infectious disease "acting as both a symptom of a larger socio-economic problem as well as a convenient excuse to deny undesirables entry to the country."[15]

The South Asians arriving at BC ports in 1906 came on the heels of a shift from regional to federal policies of disease prevention at Canada's borders. The appearance of cholera from Europe in 1831, which was followed by two major epidemics within two decades, led to the colony's first medical inspections at Grosse-Île station in Quebec. Given that both sick and healthy passengers underwent quarantine together at this facility, it is not surprising that this measure failed to halt the progression of both cholera and typhus along the St. Lawrence to Montreal and Kingston. In 1842, a decade after Lower Canada made Grosse-Île a permanent quarantine station, the neighbouring colony of New Brunswick buttressed its own immigrant inspection procedures with a head tax to protect against ill or impoverished arrivals. Most of Canada's other colonies adopted similar head tax and inspection measures in response to the arrival of hundreds of thousands of Irish immigrants fleeing the 1840s potato famine.[16] After the arrival of a British vessel prompted a cholera scare in 1866, the Province of Canada increased the scope of inspections at Grosse-Île. The introduction of the first federal Immigration Act in 1869 empowered Dominion inspectors at all ports and border points to reject "infirm" immigrants if they suspected they would become a public charge. Legislation passed three years later mandated quarantine at Grosse-Île for all vessels arriving from infected ports and for ships reporting a passenger death from illness. In 1887, mandatory quarantine for cholera and other contagious diseases was expanded to include all ships passing through the St. Lawrence.[17]

The rise of germ theory in the late nineteenth century had confirmed previous contagionist views of the body and its wastes as sites of disease. It also brought the belief that sickness always came from a human carrier. The establishment of the nation's permanent public health systems following the 1866 cholera scare resulted in an approach to disease control in which immigrants, as a recent source of cholera, were the chief causes of infection.[18] More broadly, the transition from regional to federal inspection and quarantine occurred under the umbrella of what Alan Sears calls the Dominion's post-1900 interventionism to control "social reproduction." In Canada as in the United States, Galtonian theories of race categorization, which positioned Anglo-Saxons at the top of the racial pyramid in the late nineteenth century, endured through the turn of the century and did much to transform immigration policy. This pyramid was the product of what David Goldberg describes as a state's typical two-step reaction to threats to the racial or social status quo. The state would first "conceptualize order anew" and then "reproduce spatial confinement and separation in renewed terms."[19] This hierarchy held broad appeal across Canada, where cholera epidemics in the 1830s, 1840s, and 1850s had been tied to Irish immigration, and where, despite the broad acceptance of bacteriology by the century's end, some (although not all) theorists maintained that infections and physical disorders were wholly attributable to, and explainable by, the separate evolution of distinct races.[20]

Appointed in 1902 as the first head of the Medical Division of the Immigration Branch, Dr. Peter H. Bryce emphasized the need for medical inspection to determine an immigrant's health and suitability for Canada. Bryce's early adoption of germ theory and his views on the importance of laboratory science to medical knowledge reflected the strong connection between Canadian and British medicine at this time.[21] Humphries points out that, far from being objective, this inspection was at its outset a "racialized process" designed to root out "foreign" disease by those tasked with protecting "the public purse, the public health, and the public morals."[22] Since race could "double as [an] indicator of disease," the medical inspection of immigrants generally "medicalized racial and nativist biases" by using medical terminology and descriptions of physical fitness to screen out those deemed undesirable. Overall, the contagionist view of disease transmission offered white Canadians "a guilt-free means of expressing latent fears and anxieties about a rapidly changing world."[23]

However, setting aside the controls on Chinese immigration first put in place in 1885, nineteenth-century medical inspections were targeted at protecting the public from fatal contagious diseases, not screening for non-fatal infections or chronic conditions that might impede an immigrant's labour productivity. Yet when the high industrial demand for unskilled workers brought an increase in "new" immigrants from eastern and southern Europe and Asia by 1900, threatening to supplant the "old" immigrants from Britain and northwestern Europe, the Immigration Branch began to selectively screen for various non-fatal infections. For example, medical inspectors at BC ports inspected Asians (but not Britons or other first-class passengers) for trachoma, a contagious bacterial eye infection that can cause blindness.[24] Despite these procedures, provincial and municipal officials warned that BC was becoming the "dumping grounds" for trachomatous Asians in the early years of the new century.[25] The revisions to the federal Immigration Act in 1906, introduced close to the beginning of significant first wave South Asian immigration to Canada, broadly addressed these concerns by standardizing new health screening requirements and by barring those who were mute, blind, epileptic, insane, or "infirm," as well as those with a "loathsome" contagious ailment. The destitute, including beggars, were also barred, as were those with a criminal record in prostitution or other crimes of "moral turpitude." The same act mandated that all immigrants be vetted by a Board of Inquiry, comprising a medical inspector and at least one immigration agent, appointed by the interior minister. That minister would also judge all appeals of board decisions. Finally, the act introduced a provision allowing for the deportation of any immigrant who, within two years of entering Canada, was found to be reliant on charitable or government assistance.[26]

While the 1906 Act tightened immigration controls at BC ports and border points, the Dominion government initially did little to directly discourage Indian immigration. Since 1898, the Laurier government, always cautious in diplomacy, and especially reluctant to inflame tensions with Japan, had repeatedly disallowed a series of anti-Asian immigrant literacy tests (called "Natal Acts") passed by BC's provincial government. But in 1906, Laurier understood that his Liberal Party's re-election two years later would depend on the votes of the working class and the trade unionists, who were the most passionate opponents of Asian immigration. Ironically, a significant slump in Chinese and Japanese immigration in the summer, paired with a growing demand for unskilled work, led to a severe scarcity of cheap labour in the province.[27] This labour shortage coincided almost exactly with a sharp rise in South Asian arrivals at BC ports in the summer.

In the second half of 1906, South Asians were aboard most of the CPR vessels arriving from Asia, sometimes in dramatically high numbers. Table 1 shows that, while fewer than 400 had landed by June, 2,242 entered at Vancouver and Victoria between July and December.[28] On their arrival, some joined other Asian workers in railway maintenance work, but soon most were employed as unskilled workers in lumber mills in the Fraser Valley and the BC interior and on Vancouver Island. The rapid increase in South Asians in these months catalyzed the massive public outcry against the new immigrant group. Vancouver newspapers abounded with stories of the dangers associated with the "Hindoo invasion." Beginning in 1906, the city's two major dailies – the Liberal *Daily World* and the Conservative *Daily Province* – offered more news coverage on this group than on almost any other ethnicity.[29] Both papers and the smaller *Daily News Advertiser* characterized the new arrivals using Orientalist concepts of India, especially in the arena of public health.

Peter Ward reminds us that the "public conceptions of India" as "a land of teeming millions, of filth and squalor, of exotic, peculiar customs" preceded South Asians to BC, just as similar ideas about the Orient as a

TABLE 1
Asians Immigrating to Canada, 1904–21

Year	South Asian	Chinese	Japanese
1904	45	4,847	0
1905	367	77	354
1906	2,124	168	1,923
1907	2,623	291	2,043
1909	6	2,234	7,801
1910	10	2,106	495
1911	5	5,320	271
1912	3	6,581	437
1913	6	7,445	765
1914	88	5,512	724
1915	0	1,258	856
1916	1	89	593
1917	0	393	401
1918	0	769	648
1919	0	4,333	883
1920	0	544	1,178
1921	10	2,435	711
Total	5,282	44,402	20,083

Source: "Movement to Canada of Indians," F.C. Blair to Pope, July 25, 1922, RG 25, G1, vol. 1300, File 1011, FPI, LAC; and "Record of Oriental Immigrants, 1901–1920," *Canada Year Book* 1930, 174.

place of "virulent, disgusting diseases" pre-dated nineteenth-century Chinese arrivals to the province and remained pinned to them well into the new century.[30] While some medical officials asserted that the Chinese, though "diseased" as a race, did not threaten public health by virtue of their spatial segregation in Chinatowns,[31] the "unclean Chinese" stereotype persisted in the popular press, not solely for health reasons, but also because many, as single males, could save money by living in cheap accommodations, which gave them a "competitive advantage" over other residents of the city. Press reports on living conditions were often embellished, even after health ordinances were strictly enforced in the Chinatowns of Vancouver, Victoria, and other cities. Yet since, unlike South Asians, most Chinese worked in domestic service and other fields not served by white male labour, the "unclean" stereotype had little impact on Chinese employment status in the province.[32]

Orientalist associations seem to have influenced early medical opinion on South Asians as the latest Asian arrivals to the province. After Superintendent of Immigration W.D. Scott ordered his two chief medical inspectors in BC to investigate the "Hindoo influx," both physicians included generalizations about life in colonial India in their assessments of the group's health. It is surprising that Drs. G.L. Milne and A.S. Munro have been largely overlooked in the literature on South Asians in Canada, for these Dominion Immigration Branch medical inspectors played key roles in the evolution of Canada's official response to Indian immigration. Milne at Victoria opined that South Asians in India were "not a strong race, being in many cases weak and lazy" and "not robust or hardy." Furthermore, he contended that their "peculiar" eating habits (vegetarianism in the case of Sikhs)and their caste system prevented the easy absorption of South Asians into the workforce. Writing his own first impressions from his office at the Port of Vancouver, Munro similarly averred that while Indians in BC were benefiting from the local "dearth of labor" precipitated by the increased Chinese head tax, they were clearly "inferior" workers. Munro added that

> although tall in stature and presenting as a rule a fine appearance, they are not nearly so strong or so well fitted to perform arduous work as the other classes. They are dirty and unsanitary in their personal habits and we have endless trouble with those held in the Detention hospital in this respect. In character they are in many aspects like children, very ignorant, never satisfied. They are the most cringing and servile people I ever met with and for lying they have no equals.[33]

Surprisingly, Munro soon changed his position on the undesirability of the new arrivals and actually began to help them. Since many South Asians arrived in Vancouver with little money, Munro often detained some of the men until work could be found for them, which prevented them from becoming public charges. For example, in October he reported to Ottawa that he had housed, presumably at the CPR's expense, one hundred South Asians at that company's detention shed in Vancouver to see if employers would offer them work. This aspect of Munro's response to the immigrants is interesting, first because it represented a clear departure from his previous approach to them, and second because it indicated that some flexibility still existed in the branch's enforcement of the newly introduced 1906 Immigration Act.[34] Central Canadian press coverage from this month indicated that, unlike most Westerners, many in the east supported Munro's desire to assist the new arrivals. R.G. Macpherson, the MP for Vancouver and an Asian exclusionist, complained in the same month that the "conservative press in the east" had been "filled lately" with sympathy for the immigrants and criticisms of BC's reaction to them. While Macpherson exaggerated the amount of coverage that central Canadian papers devoted to the topic, the *Ottawa Citizen*'s editor LAC dryly remarked that there was "really nothing against [South Asians] but their colour."[35]

In early August, the Vancouver branch of the Trades and Labour Congress (TLC), part of the BC Federation of Labour, called for a provincial investigation of this "most undesirable class" now on mainland BC and Vancouver Island. The Victoria TLC went a step further by publishing an "emphatic protest" to Indian immigration in an open letter to the province's workers.[36] Similar terminology appeared in the *Victoria Daily Times*. After Victoria residents complained when fifteen South Asians set up camp in that city while looking for work, a *Times* reporter opined that "it would be amusing, were it not so pathetic, to see the brightly robed sons of the tropics wandering aimlessly around the streets." He concluded that they appeared "a most wretched group." Press reports throughout the summer continued to register alarm at South Asian arrivals. On an August morning when almost 250 South Asians were let out of quarantine in Vancouver, a *Vancouver Province* journalist reported that Westminster Avenue (now Main Street) had been turned into an "Eastern Bazaar," where "the jabbering of the motley gang of bronzed warriors from the East" made "a tumult like the roar of the sea in a tempest when they were all going at once, which was very often." The scene attracted the attention of white labourers, whose remarks about the group would "make good pointers for any politician who wished to play a winning game with the labor vote." The journalist reminded readers that these men came from India, a nation "reeking with the foul emanations" of plague, "the most deadly of all diseases."[37] Chapter 2 will show that the latter point soon became an important thread woven throughout the fabric of exclusionist discourse on the coast.

Brief though it was, the Westminster Avenue incident was the first time that a large number of Vancouver residents encountered the visual spectacle of hundreds of South Asians arriving in their city. It is likely no coincidence that on the day of the incident, a Vancouver carpentry union declared by petition that South Asians "do not assimilate with the White Race."[38] The incident also attracted the attention of Dr. Frederick T. Underhill, Vancouver's Medical Officer of Health, who complained in a strongly worded letter later forwarded to Ottawa that his health inspectors had found Indians "breaking every City by-law and every ordinary rule of health." He accordingly requested that council take steps to "guard this

City" against the men. At a board meeting in September, Underhill again urged "instant action" to overcome what was already "an evil calling for remedy."[39] Others in Vancouver shared Underhill's view that Indians were dirty and unimproved by Edwardian standards of hygiene and disease prevention that had been established with germ's theory's acceptance in Canada. For example, in September the *Vancouver World* declared that a "Horde of Hungry Hindoos," recently arrived from the SS *Tartar* were "almost pitiable to look at," and that most were "badly in need of a bath." Yet despite his previous statement to the contrary, Munro disagreed that the group was dirty by nature. He recognized that local environmental factors, specifically the limited "facilities for their system of bathing" in the housing where most of the men lived in BC, were responsible for any lack of cleanliness. Munro offered this candid assessment to a *World* journalist just as his supervisor left Ottawa to assess the nature of the "Hindu" crisis.[40]

William Duncan Scott, a former land agent from Manitoba, was the newly appointed Dominion Superintendent of Immigration. From the time of his appointment in 1906 until his retirement in 1923, Scott devised and introduced various immigration policies under the supervision of the elected interior minister. In his September visit to BC, Scott investigated the new arrivals by meeting with his Immigration Branch inspectors, along with various city officials and employers. Scott, although not a medical official, later used these interviews to argue the idea, already challenged by bacteriology, that since South Asians came from a warm climate, their transfer to a northern climate "must of necessity result in much physical suffering and danger to health." He thus asserted, just as Munro and Vancouver's city clerk had before him, that they were not "physically fitted" for work in BC, and he therefore advised that Canada exclude immigrants from India.[41]

Despite Scott's recommendation, the Dominion government took no immediate steps towards exclusion. In September, Laurier privately informed a friend that Canada would not enact an exclusion policy "except after very serious consideration." The stalling frustrated Vancouver's mayor, Frederick Buscombe, who telegrammed Frank Oliver, the interior minister, requesting "immediate action" on the Indian issue. *World* editor Louis D. Taylor declared that "it was all very well" to talk about South Asians being ex-soldiers and subjects of Britain, but this did not change the fact that they were "crowding like rabbits in unsanitary shacks or camping out." A Vancouver resident agreed in an editorial that "every wage earner" in BC wished "to prevent BC becoming a dumping ground for the refuse of filthy and plague-ridden India." Local labour leaders quickly adopted the "Hindu disease" theory and employed it with gusto. At a national TLC meeting in Victoria, members resolved that "the vast majority of the Hindus now arriving in Canada are, by reason of venereal and other diseases, absolutely unfitted to be allowed into this country." A TLC affiliate later petitioned Imperial officials with the fantastic claim that a recent Pacific coast inspection of 260 South Asians had "proved every 'man' to have gonorrhea, [and] over two hundred have practiced sodomy!"[42]

There is no evidence to support Taylor's or the TLC's assertions about infections or venereal disease. Moreover, of the one hundred South Asians rejected among the close to 2,000 arrivals at BC ports from January to November 1906, all were diagnosed with either an eye condition or a physical deformity, or had been barred because they were deemed likely to become a public charge. Since gonorrhea was also grounds for deportation as a "loathsome and contagious" disease under the wording of the revised Immigration Act of 1906, it can be assumed that none of the Indians who had arrived in Canada had been diagnosed with the gonorrhea bacillus. The TLC's assertions about Indian venereal diseases and sexuality were also false. Although the Act did not explicitly define acts of homosexuality as deportable offences, the 1892 version of Canada's Criminal Code criminalized sexual acts between males under the broad category of "gross indecency." It is unlikely that one Asian immigrant suspected of sodomy would have been admitted into Canada; the idea that more than two hundred homosexual South Asians could be admitted en masse is unbelievable; yet the wildly erroneous claims made in this piece of trade union propaganda are important, because they help demonstrate the level of anxiety caused by the entrance of South Asians into the Canadian labour market.[43]

The TLC and other western labour organizations openly opposed the immigration of South Asians and other Asian groups for economic reasons; however, much of this opposition was ideologically rooted in the anxieties and beliefs associated with social morality and what Mariana Valverde calls the "social-purity ideas about vice and sexuality" linking Asian males with sexual deviance.[44] Susan Koshy avers that during the early twentieth century, white Americans saw Asians as "moral and public health danger[s]" and "carriers of unusually virulent strains of venereal disease." Both venereal disease and sexual deviance were widely understood as products of an "imagined Oriental licentiousness" rampant in "island paradises in the Pacific, treaty ports, and colonial possessions." Ian Mackay adds that these stereotypes typified the broader racist discourse of the Canadian Dominion, which "resonated with the idea and practice of race" in this era.[45] Overall, there appears to be no evidence to support the idea that South Asians in Canada were disproportionately afflicted with venereal disease.

TLC members were correct, however, that some South Asians were arriving with other conditions or infections. In September, the *Province* reported that an immigrant named Nara died in the Vancouver CPR detention sheds from "an attack of tropical fever, combined with lack of proper nourishment and care while crossing the ocean"; the victim's death certificate shows that he died of typhoid. An informant who was consulted in the 1984–87 Indo-Canadian Oral History Collection, a two-part series of university-led interviews with South Asian immigrants and their descendants in the Vancouver area, reported that her husband and many of his fellow passengers arriving in BC around this time had become sick on board ship and had sore eyes from the strong wind conditions during the voyage.[46] One South Asian was later admitted to hospital for tuberculosis, while others who may have been susceptible to it implemented safety measures to avoid it on their arrival. At Butchart Cement Works on Vancouver Island in 1907, several South Asian workers camped off-site, an arrangement that may have saved their lives, since a number of Chinese workers living in the company's on-site bunkhouses reportedly died of tuberculosis that fall. The tubercular symptoms of the Chinese workers had been exacerbated by the fact that they did not use dust masks, while the South Asians at Butchart carefully protected their lungs by applying the Indian method of using turbans and cloths.[47] This account reveals that, contrary to BC popular opinion about South Asians, at least some were invested in safeguarding their health.

BC newspapers continued to criticize South Asian health and hygiene throughout the fall. The *Victoria Colonist* reported that Dr. Milne at Victoria had rejected ten of a group of "unwholesome looking," "half-starved and decrepit" South Asians; the journalist argued that "only by ocular demonstration at Dr. Milne's office" could one grasp the importance of his screening work. The *Province* later reported that Indian arrivals in Vancouver were "trying to deceive" Dr. Munro's staff that "their diseases are mere trifles." The article quoted one South Asian "of long standing" in BC, who called these new arrivals "dirty" and recommended they "learn to take a bath." The journalist agreed, adding that "a thick, heavy odor floating shoreward from the afterdeck of the Empress" would remain "until the steerage is swabbed out with chloride of lime."[48] Given that they had spent six to eight weeks at sea with no showers, we can assume that these men were indeed dirty and appeared unkempt. But by magnifying the initial state of the passengers on their arrival, and relating their condition directly to their race, the reporter portrayed South Asians as naturally dirty people who, even when free of the ship, would have difficulty maintaining good hygiene. Certainly, it was helpful to find an Indian who shared this opinion.

It would be impossible to deny that South Asians were a dirty group if one was describing their condition on arrival; from this, it could be inferred that they were also immoral, for at this time, cleanliness was one mark of respectability, while to be unwashed "was to be a physical and moral menace." Church home missions and other Canadian community organizations emphasized the need for personal hygiene and home sanitation, because, as Mariana Valverde explains, "in the minds of social reformers soap and water were spiritual as well as physical cleansers." Debates arose over the personal and moral hygiene of various immigrant groups, and many observers believed that the dirt and unsanitary living conditions of some Asian dwellings broadly demonstrated a racial tendency towards spiritual and moral failings. More broadly, the Edwardian obsession with cleanliness reflected a sanitary protocol in which "cleanliness and morality" were firmly connected in a "hygienic code that linked transgressions – real and imagined – to physical sickness."[49]

Reporting on South Asians peaked during a crisis on Vancouver's waterfront on October 14, when Mayor Buscombe ordered police to detain one hundred South Asians recently landed from the SS *Empress of Japan* at the immigration shed. The *Province* reported that Buscombe had ordered that "not a Hindu will be allowed out of the building" until Council was assured that the Indians could support themselves. This illegal order was precipitated by the pressure caused by the sharp increase in South Asian arrivals during the summer months, which sparked both racial intolerance and genuine concerns over the ability of Indians to find work. Instead of taking steps to end the situation, Laurier in Ottawa decided that, while Buscombe had acted "illegally," it was better "to go cautiously" on the matter as feeling in BC was "very strong against having these people in our country."[50]

As the South Asian group sat imprisoned in the detention shed in Vancouver, Victoria's TLC petitioned Scott that "however strict the medical examination at our ports" had become since the introduction of the 1906 Immigration Act in June, there was "a constant danger of these people being the means of transmission of diseases to our people." Union members reminded the superintendent that India had "long been recognized as a hotbed of the most virulent and loathsome" infections such as "bubonic plague, smallpox, Asiatic Cholera and the worst forms of venereal diseases."[51] Shortly thereafter, a Vancouver resident informed the editor of the *Vancouver News-Advertiser* that "we do not propose to have a Hindu town or bazaar rather, with its vicious evils and attendant undesirable element," because "we shall have the plague, cholera and other deadly fevers and diseases here among us, if such is not stopped in time."[52] *World* editor Louis D. Taylor similarly stated that Vancouver's Chinese were "bad enough," but "these Hindoos," he argued, menaced society with their "leprosy and that most awful and deadly of all diseases, the bubonic plague, rioting in their blood and infecting their garments." He later warned that without federal intervention, Vancouver could become "a vast outhouse" of "dark-skinned Indians" and their "disgusting diseases."[53]

Retired Anglo-Indian army officer Colonel Falk Warren, who now lived in Vancouver, took issue with these statements in an October letter to editor Taylor.[54] "As to their being diseased," he argued, "I can testify to the national cleanliness of the race, though a long journey and difficulties in carrying out ablutions go against their outward appearance." He added that, despite recent accusations about the group's "sicked practices," none of the new immigrants had been convicted of any crime, and he did "not believe anyone can suggest what sin is alluded to."[55] However, Warren was in the minority on the issue. Hundreds of his Vancouver neighbours flooded City Hall on October 15 to hear Mayor Buscombe pontificate on the "Hindu crisis." A *Province* journalist observed that, although almost all in the crowd were white, some "Hindus managed to secure standing positions near the doors" as they waited to hear the meeting's outcome. While discussions were in progress, police at the nearby CPR wharf rounded up the first *Empress* passengers who had been released from federal quarantine. The mayor eventually agreed to allow some of the men to stay for one night before leaving for the interior; others among the group, however, remained illegally imprisoned in the shed. Buscombe ended the meeting at City Hall with a resolution to Ottawa requesting Indian exclusion.[56]

Nearly 1,850 South Asians had arrived in British Columbia by mid-autumn. While almost 1,000 more Japanese than South Asians arrived over the year, joining at least 20,000 other Japanese and Chinese immigrants in the province, coverage of the South Asian situation dominated Vancouver and Victoria press reports and held the attention of municipal and provincial politicians. In early November, R.G. MacPherson, MP for Vancouver City, warned the interior minister that there was "absolutely no work" for the 850 more Indians who were expected shortly. Numerous newspaper articles about the BC labour shortage at this time indicate that his statement about the lack of work was entirely false,[57] yet MacPherson recommended that Ottawa immediately pass legislation requiring that each Indian show $100 on arrival. Oliver responded merely by contacting CPR steamship officials, who denied that they were advertising Canada in India. But the minister's modest effort did nothing to resolve the immigration issue in the short term.[58]

By October, South Asians had begun to avoid Canadian ports, in part because of the strong public reaction against their presence in BC. Those who chose to stay in the province and found temporary shelter in Vancouver had difficulty meeting their basic needs; the city was already overcrowded, and even immigrants with money struggled to secure lodging from landlords unwilling to rent to them. The Vancouver Health Department continued to monitor the sanitary condition of South Asian camps, particularly those in Cedar Cove and along the Fraser River, where South Asians resided while searching for work.[59] Some camp residents who could not find employment were forced to beg for food in the West End and the suburb of Burnaby. One Indo-Canadian Oral History interviewee recalled that his father, who had likely arrived that fall on the *Tartar*, walked with a group of fourteen other passengers to seek work. When they eventually came across a house on the outskirts of the city, the homeowner understood their sign language asking for food and kindly provided them with a meal, which tided them over until they could find work with the CPR or a local mill shortly thereafter.[60]

Other local residents were less sympathetic to the camp residents in their time of need. The *World* reprinted a letter to the editor from "Housewife," who wrote that, like "hundreds of other housewives," she was suffering from "an invasion of Hindoo beggars." Two days later, journalists reported that a woman on Bridge Street had been forced to defend her home against similar beggars, while two South Asians had attempted unsuccessfully to steal food from the wife of a prominent banker on Nicola Street.[61] These stories were precursors to a dramatic allegation in November that South Asians had gang-raped a white woman in the suburbs, which further cemented popular opposition to the South Asian presence.

On the evening of November 14, Vancouver resident Alfred Laviolette returned to his house on Homer Street to find his wife Harriett unconscious in an upstairs bedroom. When she awoke, she claimed that she had been robbed and sexually assaulted by several South Asians. The men had hit her, and, after she fainted, dragged her into the bedroom and raped her. Later that evening, city police began combing the city for the perpetrators. The *World*'s coverage, beginning with the cover story "Masked Hindoo Sandbags Vancouver Woman," employed language clearly calculated to incite panic; the journalist covering the story reasoned that the crime was the natural outcome of the arrival of so many South Asians in the city. Indeed, a sexual assault was the inevitable result of allowing South Asians to walk the streets in only the "scantiest of raiment" and "filthy towels about their heads." The writer concluded that immediate action was required to stop the South Asian "carnival of crime."[62]

The press coverage reflected an almost carnivalesque environment. On the 16th the *Colonist* printed Mrs. Laviolette's updated account that only two South Asians had been involved, one of whom had worn both a mask and "a tall hat." The victim could not recollect the assault, but did remember previously reporting to police an encounter with South Asian beggars. The *News-Advertiser* reported more cautiously that the police had denied receiving any previous complaints from Mrs. Laviolette about Indians. The journalist continued that although "the air is full of rumors of Hindus begging and frightening women and children, no definite complaints have been made to the Police." The writer added that a "prominent citizen who understands the Hindus thoroughly" – probably Colonel Warren – had told him that it was unlikely that South Asians would attack a white woman, as they feared authority and regarded contact with whites "with superstitious dread, as if it were pollution."[63] However, the other papers reporting on the incident continued to sensationalize the case while overlooking the emerging cracks in Mrs. Laviolette's story.

The alleged rape of Mrs. Laviolette had a dramatic effect on Vancouver's populace. At a meeting of the Vancouver TLC, several members noted that the incident had led them to purchase revolvers for their wives for protection against South Asians. Delegates made a "veritable storm of threats," and the *Province* reported that a vigilante posse might soon form "to close out the heathen population" if another South Asian assaulted "defenceless white women." Delegates spoke out against "those degraded natives of India" who could become "thieves and outragers of womanly virtue." The reporter concluded that the city's Indians had "about reached the end of their tether with many of the working men."[64]

In an abrupt reversal the next day, the *Province* partly retracted the story under the headline "White Man May Have Assaulted Mrs. Laviolette." According to this report, Vancouver police now doubted the veracity of Mrs. Laviolette's allegations; if the incident actually occurred, only one South Asian had been involved, along with one white man. No arrests had been made thus far, and none were expected, as police detectives now suspected that the woman had, in fact, imagined the attack, given that the details she provided had changed remarkably since the initial investigation. For the police, the most incredible thing about her latest story was that, if a white man had actually been involved, "what was he doing traveling with a Hindu?" The police reasoned that, in such a scenario, the white man would have seen Mrs. Laviolette through her Homer Street window, entered the alley behind her house and then, by complete coincidence, been "joined by a Hindu there." The journalist concluded, however, that detectives were already in consensus that the entire incident likely never happened.[65] None of the other papers printed this retraction, although perhaps it would not have mattered if they had. The original allegation alone had already further damaged the South Asians' reputation in Vancouver.

Unfortunately, press accounts offer the only evidence of Mrs. Laviolette's allegations, as a police record of her claim no longer exists.[66] This news story broke during what was, thus far, the apex of mass hysteria and public outcry against Indians in Vancouver. Sociologist Stanley Cohen's classic definition of "moral panic" describes it as a social phenomenon that ensues when a group or community perceives an individual or group as a major threat to societal norms and values. This phenomenon encapsulates the vociferous public opposition to South Asians in Vancouver. The story that South Asians had raped a white, middle-class woman appeared to confirm TLC allegations that South Asians represented a fundamental danger to Canadian society – a danger specifically linked to a supposedly inherent Indian predilection for deviant sexuality.[67]

A similar incident occurred in 1914, when Jack Kong, a juvenile Chinese servant, murdered his employer, C.J. Millard, the wife of a Vancouver steamship official. It was not clear whether Kong hit Millard or if she fainted, but when the servant believed she was dead, he cut up her body and burned her in the furnace. The public's initial response was, as with

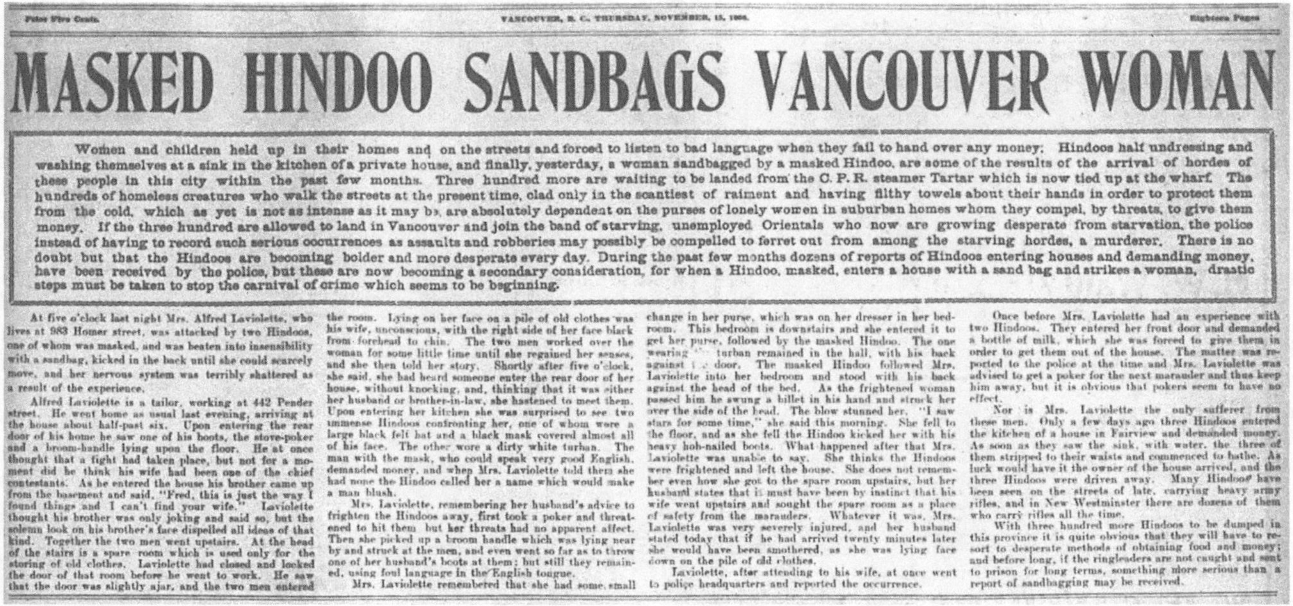

Police First Column

Nineteen Pages

MASKED HINDOO SANDBAGS VANCOUVER WOMAN

VANCOUVER, B.C., THURSDAY, NOVEMBER 15, 1906.

Women and children held up in their homes and on the streets and forced to listen to bad language and finally, yesterday, a woman sandbagged by a masked Hindoo, are some of the results of the arrival of hordes of these people in this city within the past few months. Three hundred more are waiting to be landed from the C. P. R. steamer Tartar which is now tied up at the wharf. The hundreds of homeless creatures who walk the streets at the present time, clad only in the scantiest of raiment and having filthy towels about their hands in order to protect them from the cold, which as yet is not as intense as it may be, are absolutely dependent on the purses of lonely women in suburban homes whom they compel, by threats, to give them money. If the three hundred are allowed to land in Vancouver and join the band of starving, unemployed Orientals who now are growing desperate from starvation, the police instead of having to record such serious occurrences as assaults and robberies may possibly be compelled to ferret out from among the starving hordes, a murderer. There is no doubt but that the Hindoos are becoming bolder and more desperate every day. During the past few months dozens of reports of Hindoos entering houses and demanding money, have been received by the police, but these are now becoming a secondary consideration, for when a Hindoo, masked, enters a house with a sand bag and strikes a woman, drastic steps must be taken to stop the carnival of crime which seems to be beginning.

At five o'clock last night Mrs. Alfred Laviolette, who lives at 862 Homer street, was attacked by two Hindoos, one of whom was masked, and was beaten into insensibility with a sandbag, kicked in the back until she could scarcely move, and her nervous system was terribly shattered as a result of the experience.

Alfred Laviolette is a tailor working at 442 Powder street. He went home as usual last evening, arriving at the house about half-past six. Upon entering the rear door of his home he saw one of his boots, the shoe-maker and a broom-handle lying upon the floor. He at once thought that a fight had taken place, but not for a moment did he think his wife had been one of the chief contestants. As he entered the house his brother came in from the basement and said, "Fred, this is just the way I found things and I can't find your wife." Laviolette thought the brother was only joking and said so, but the look on his brother's face dispelled all ideas of that kind. Together the two men went upstairs. At the top of the stairs is a spare room which is used only for the storing of old clothes. Laviolette had closed and locked the door of that room before he went to work. He saw that the door was slightly ajar, and the two men entered the room. Lying on her face on a pile of old clothes was his wife, unconscious, with the right side of her face black from forehead to chin. The two men worked over the woman for some little time until she regained her senses, and she then told her story. Shortly after five o'clock, she said, she had heard someone enter the rear door of her house, without knocking, and, thinking that it was either her husband or brother-in-law, she hastened to meet them. Upon entering her kitchen she was surprised to see two immense Hindoos confronting her, one of whom wore a large black felt hat and a black mask covered almost all of his face. The other wore a dirty white turban. The man with the mask would speak very good English, demanded money, and when Mrs. Laviolette told them she had none the Hindoo called her a name which would make a man blush.

Mrs. Laviolette, remembering her husband's advice to frighten the Hindoos away, first took a poker and threatened to hit them but her threat had no apparent effect. Then she picked up a broom handle which was lying near by and struck at the men, and even went so far as to throw one of her husband's boots at them; but still they remained, using foul language in the English tongue. Mrs. Laviolette remembered that she had some small change in her purse, which was on her dresser in her bedroom. This bedroom is downstairs and she entered it to get her purse, followed by the masked Hindoo. The one wearing turban remained in the hall, with his back against the door. The masked Hindoo followed Mrs. Laviolette into her bedroom and stood with his back against the head of the bed. As the frightened woman passed a bullet in his hand and struck her over the side of the head. The blow stunned her. "I saw stars for some time," she said this morning. She fell to the floor, and as she fell the Hindoo kicked her with his heavy hob-nailed boots. What happened after that Mrs. Laviolette was unable to say. She thinks the Hindoos were frightened and left the house. She does not remember now how she got to the spare room upstairs, but her husband states that it must have been by instinct that his wife went upstairs and sought the spare room as a place of safety from the marauders. Whatever it was, Mrs. Laviolette was very severely injured, and her husband stated today that if he had arrived twenty minutes later she would have been smothered, as she was lying face down on the pile of old clothes.

Laviolette, after attending to his wife, at once went to police headquarters and reported the occurrence.

Once before Mrs. Laviolette had an experience with two Hindoos. They entered her front door and demanded a bottle of milk, which she was forced to give them in order to get them out of the house. The matter was reported to the police at the time and Mrs. Laviolette was advised to get a poker for the next marauder and thus keep him away, but it is obvious that pokers seem to have no effect.

Nor is Mrs. Laviolette the only sufferer from these men. Only a few days ago three Hindoos entered the kitchen of a house in Fairview and demanded money. As soon as they saw the teakettle, with water, they stripped to their waists and announced their intention of taking a bath. At least it is obvious that if this was their intention the luck would have the corner of the house arrived, and the three Hindoos were driven away. Many Hindoos have been seen on the streets of late, carrying heavy army rifles, and in New Westminster there are dozens of them who carry rifles all the time.

With three hundred more Hindoos to be dumped in this province it is quite obvious that they will have to resort to desperate methods of obtaining food and money; and before long, if the ringleaders are not caught and sent to prison for long terms, something more serious than a report of sandbagging may be received.

FIGURE 1 "Masked Hindoo Sandbags Vancouver Woman." | *Vancouver World*, November 15, 1906.

its reaction to the "rape" of Mrs. Laviolette, to attribute Kong's actions to the inherent immorality and violence of his race. Millard's murder "revived the idea that the thoughts of the Chinese run in morbid, unhealthy channels" and that "'the Oriental is more of a brute than a man.'" Yet, since many middle-class households employed Chinese servants because they were reliable and accepted low wages, the press asserted that "it would be unjust to 'hold a whole race responsible for even the most brutal crime of one of its members.'"[68] This final point offers a stark contrast to the press reporting on the "rape" of Mrs. Laviolette, which occurred less than a decade earlier. Only one newspaper ultimately retracted its allegations that the "Hindu" crime had occurred, and every editorial on the topic asserted that the incident was merely the next logical step in the Indian "carnival of crime," even though this contradicted statements made by city's police. Overall, the differences in public reception between these two cases demonstrate the unique extent to which Vancouver popular discourse vilified South Asians, even in the first year of their arrival in large numbers.

Extensive reporting on the activities of South Asians continued in the incident's aftermath, particularly in Vancouver, where the housing shortage was now acute. On the evening of the Homer Street incident, the SS *Tartar* had anchored off William Head Quarantine Station, Victoria, with more than eight hundred South Asians on board. The men were carefully screened by quarantine staff Dr. A.J. Watt and Dr. Anderson, and almost all of them were found to be healthy. Only thirty were refused admission for being either old, infirm, addicted to opium, or lacking sufficient funds.[69] Many of those admitted proceeded to Vancouver, where the lack of rental accommodations forced them into temporary shelters. On November 17 the *World* reported that seventy South Asians had spent the night in a condemned three-room shack, which the journalist dubbed the city's "Black Hole of Calcutta." The report was in reference to an event associated with Robert Clive and the 1756 Battle of Plassey; Bengali leader Saraj ud-Daulah locked 146 Englishmen into a tiny cell, where most of them died. This tale, which may have been fabricated, persisted in popular culture; sociologist Harold Isaacs found in 1958 that the "dungeon-like pit" from the story was the image most Americans thought of when picturing India and "things Indian." The term "Black Hole" has since fallen out of favour in the humanities, but it has been resurrected in physics. Physicist Jean-Pierre Luminet avers that Edwardian era feelings about the incident parallel the fear many feel today about stellar black holes. This useful comparison helps contextualize the *World* reporter's use of the term to describe South Asian housing – the black hole image would have titillated and horrified Vancouver's readers.[70]

The sensationalist press description of the state of the "Hindu quarter" reflected wider societal concerns over the problems associated with increased urbanization. Public health campaigners believed that overcrowded and unsanitary slums were, like infectious microbes, foreign imports. As such, politicians, labour leaders, temperance organizations, and other community groups promoted increased immigration screening as a "panacea that would solve a host of moral and social ills," including the emergence of unsanitary immigrant ghettos.[71] As Sylvia Reitmanova explains, the goal was to "protect the purity and healthiness of Saxondom" from the "'racial poisons'" of the slums: sexually transmitted infections, substance addiction, and tuberculosis were all viewed as imported problems, especially after British physician Caleb Williams Saleeby, a proponent of Francis Galton's eugenic theory, asserted that immigrants who lived in these neighbourhoods were racially "predisposed" to various diseases. This theory gained popularity among those concerned over the province's recent population explosion. BC's 1901 population of 178,657 was almost twice what it had been in 1891, and the trend's continuation in the new century led some to believe that the province was growing too quickly compared to the rest of Canada, especially since much of the increase was attributable to "new" immigrants from eastern Europe and Asia settling in BC cities.[72]

The housing shortage caused by Vancouver's rapid population growth made it difficult for Munro, the federal medical inspector who had secured work for a group of South Asians who would otherwise have been rejected on landing, to find accommodations for the new arrivals. Even so, interior minister Frank Oliver declined doctor's request for federal funds for temporary housing. Vancouver municipal officials similarly did little to relieve the desperate housing situation, and one alderman actually made the problem worse. At a council meeting, Health Committee chairman Francis Williams called for the immediate eviction of any men living in unsanitary housing. He stated that "no mercy should be shown" to South Asians, so that they would see that "the City was not in sympathy with them." This statement generated significant political fallout, in part because Williams also criticized acting mayor George Halse for supporting Munro's position, but also because the city was experiencing a serious cold snap. The *Vancouver World* reported that Munro had collected $6 from each homeless South Asian to supply him with boots and clothing, without which "many would have been dead" in November. To resolve the issue, an assembly was called, to which was invited Munro, who was now fixing up an old cannery in Eburne for Indians to rent. According to the *News-Advertiser,* this turned out to be "the most sensational committee meeting ever held in the City Hall."[73]

The *News-Advertiser* reported that during the meeting, Munro "reached over and SEIZED A MASSIVE GLASS INK-WELL and drew his arm as if to hurl the object" at one alderman who criticized his work with the Indians. The *Province*'s recounting of the melodramatic scene recalled Dr. Munro rising from his seat and grasping the inkwell, which "properly directed with sufficient force, would have crushed a man's head like an egg shell." After "a silence deep as death," Munro lowered the inkwell and apologized, saying he had been insulted. Order was restored only after all parties involved apologized, and Munro was personally thanked for his ongoing humanitarian efforts. Overall, despite the drama and ensuing press reportage, the meeting had accomplished very little. Munro defended the new arrivals, stating that many had come to Canada with the same amount of money as the average European immigrant landing on the Atlantic coast. City Medical Officer of Health Underhill remarked, and Alderman T.W. Joffe, also a medical doctor, concurred, that the "greatest danger was the spread of tuberculosis," for some South Asians with the disease were "spitting all over the place." Although Munro vehemently denied letting any tubercular immigrants into Vancouver, he conceded that Dr. Milne at Victoria had admitted many of the Indians now in BC.[74]

After an Eburne cannery owner had finished retrofitting his property for human habitation, Munro enlisted Underhill to transport South Asians who were camping in the city to their new rented accommodations. With health inspector Robert Marrion and two constables, Underhill evicted men living in shelters unfit for habitation, including a morbidly ill man found in a cupboard in New Westminster. From the timing of this finding and the description of the man's condition, it is almost certain that this man was one Easer Singh, who died in Westminster three days later. Although the *Province* speculated that he was consumptive – and indeed, he may have been – Singh actually died of pneumonia, a serious inflammatory lung condition that, compared to tuberculosis, carries a relatively low risk of cross-infection in healthy populations and can develop without human transmission. City health officials differentiated between the two diseases at this time: all physicians were required to report cases of tuberculosis as an infectious disease, but not pneumonia. The press's presumption that Singh had tuberculosis – which was unsurprising, given medico-racial discourse – may have prompted Alderman Williams to declare, two days later, that South Asians presented a serious health menace to the city by having that wasting sickness, the "scourge that was to be greatly feared." Council members responded by petitioning Laurier to enact Indian exclusion, warning that "several" South Asians had died of the disease.[75]

Prior to Robert Koch's discovery of the bacterial causes of the disease in 1882, etiology held that tuberculosis, a leading killer among communicable diseases in nineteenth century, was brought about by genetic predisposition, unhealthy habits, and poor living conditions. Popular attitudes about the disease were slow to change in Canada, where eugenicists asserted that susceptibility to tuberculosis was a consequence of weak genetic inheritance. While infections were declining as the new century dawned, a spike in deaths from tuberculosis and other pulmonary diseases had influenced Frank Oliver to tighten health requirements for immigrants in the 1906 Immigration Act. By that year, the disease had become widely associated with immigrants, especially Asians and poor Europeans. This association was largely influenced by what Sylvia Reitmanova calls the emerging eugenic "ideology of racial ordering" in Canada's public health discourse. Canadian responses to the threat of infectious disease generally, and tuberculosis in particular, became rooted in a "pseudoscientific" racial framework that conflated Koch's germ theory of tubercular transmission with race-based theories of biological determinism.[76] This helps explain why civic officials so readily associated South Asians with tuberculosis, the most significant of a growing list of diseases now linked to that group.[77]

Williams had wildly exaggerated the South Asian connection with this illness. Before antibiotics, medical treatment for the disease was not always effective; it follows that if many South Asians actually contracted it, there would have been a significant number of South Asian fatalities. A low mortality rate did not necessarily indicate a low infection rate from the disease, since many people likely carried it without knowing it; at the same time, the living conditions of many of the South Asians in Vancouver (particularly their exposure to the elements) would have exacerbated tubercular symptoms and accelerated death in extreme cases of the disease. Yet the death certificates of the seven South Asians who died in the province in 1906 indicate that only two of the men actually died from tuberculosis; the remaining five succumbed to industrial and domestic accidents or other causes. Furthermore, during a December trip to Vancouver to deport indigent and ill South Asians, W.D. Scott's Assistant Superintendent of Immigration, E. Blake Robertson, found just one tubercular South Asian.[78]

Robertson, who arrived in December from Ottawa three months to the day after his supervisor Scott had come to investigate the "Hindu" problem, was initially optimistic that he would find sick and indigent South Asians on the streets of Vancouver; once found, he would deport them and "the problem [would] thus adjust itself." But after meeting with the mayor, the police chief, Underhill, and other city officials, Robertson discovered there had been no convictions of South Asians for any offence and that no South Asians were public charges. Robertson could only deport immigrants who, within two years of landing in Canada, had committed a crime "involving moral turpitude" or who had become institutionalized in a jail, mental asylum, hospital or charitable housing. Since he found only one person in this situation – the above-mentioned tubercular patient who was too sick to be deported – there was nothing he could do to remove the city's South Asians, who were neither unemployed nor diseased. Although he had not found sufficient evidence to support the climate theory that South Asians were especially prone to Western hemispheric diseases like tuberculosis, he left the coast with special orders for federal inspectors Drs. Munro and Milne:

> I instructed the agents of the Department at Vancouver and Vancouver to pay particular attention to the general physique of Hindus in future and examine carefully all those who were anemic, narrow chested or showed other symptoms which would appear to place them in a class likely to contract or develop tubercular trouble as such diseases seem to be the ones to which Hindus in B.C. are most likely to fall victims.[79]

Robertson's assertion that South Asians were especially at risk for tuberculosis was the first admission of its kind from a federal official, and it seems possible that the assistant superintendent came to this conclusion after his meetings with the mayor, Underhill, and other city officials just two weeks after city council petitioned Ottawa on the issue.

Like Robertson, Vancouver journalists and city councilors alike affirmed Williams's view by quoting the assertions of unnamed "medical men" that "many" South Asians, especially the close to 10 percent who had shallow chests or other predictors of "incipient tubercular trouble," would die from tuberculosis "if they remain long in this climate."[80] Yet this argument was not universal. In December, the writers of the Toronto-based *Canadian Annual Review of Public Affairs* pointed out that the South Asian immigration crisis in BC was "exaggerated and misrepresented as a matter of course" and that the "chief real argument against them" – "their alleged inability to withstand the climate" – had yet to be proven. The writers also noted that allegations that South Asians had "loathsome habits and diseases and obnoxious modes of living," were "of a character hardly borne out by other evidence and the actual facts."[81] Furthermore, a report by Dr. Robert McKechnie, Munro's assistant physician in charge of the Vancouver Detention Hospital on the wharf, challenged the argument that South Asians were especially prone to tuberculosis. McKechnie reported to Ottawa that while "the Hindoos are dirty, live [*sic*: lice] being their chief pest," they were otherwise healthy, and he underlined the point that *"Genuine cases of Trachoma are not so frequent as among the Chinese or Japs."*[82] Although the doctor did not discuss tuberculosis, logic dictates that he would have made some mention of it if the disease was actually a serious problem among the South Asian population of Vancouver during this time.[83]

In December, after several months of popular and official protest in BC against South Asians, officials in London and Ottawa alike conceded that some action was necessary to discourage Indian immigration to Canada. Opposition party members in the British House of Commons asked the ruling British Liberal government to help His Majesty's "two thousand" unemployed South Asian subjects in BC, who, being "constitutionally unfit to stand the severity of the Canadian winter," might require mass deportation back to India.[84] Canada's governor general, Albert Grey, Britain's 4th Earl Grey, who served as the liaison between the Canadian government and the Colonial Office in London, also got involved. Grey's position was in many ways a ceremonial one, but he often met with Laurier and his cabinet on domestic policy matters. In December, using Scott's recent report that the South Asians were not "physically fitted" for work in BC, Grey asked the Indian and Hong Kong governments to warn South Asians not to immigrate to Canada.[85]

A total of 2,350 South Asians had landed in BC by year's end, representing an increase of over 1,000 percent from 1905.[86] By then, many were already leaving, drawn by the promise of better wages in the United States. Along with the three hundred who arrived directly at Pacific coast ports in 1906, another three hundred entered Washington via the US

Immigration Service (IS) station in Vancouver. Although Indian immigrants had been periodically entering the United States since 1899, their numbers had been "hardly noticeable" for the IS. Officials took notice, however, when a significant number began to enter in 1906. In November, L. Edwin Dudley, the US Consul at Vancouver, warned the State Department that almost four hundred Indians from the *Tartar* had immediately left for Seattle after landing in Victoria. He included an informant's assertion that the group was "dangerous to the American people, as their ways of living and characters are quite like wiled [*sic*] men."[87] Dudley personally believed that the group were "a strong race of men, who might render most excellent service in lumber camps and other places where manual labor is needed," but he was concerned that India's population of more than 350 million could overwhelm North America with immigrants and that many in BC could easily cross the loosely controlled border with Washington.[88]

At the time Dudley penned his report, anti-Asian ideology was well established in the US Pacific coast states. The large majority of Washington, Oregon, and California residents who were not directly invested in Asian labour had long opposed what Joan Jensen calls the "very characteristics which made Asian workers attractive to employers" – their tendency, at least in the minds of white observers, to work and live separately and maintain separate subcultures.[89] This opposition was also based on the established American racial dichotomy of "white" and "other" and on worker frustrations over the financial and aspirational limits of wage labour. California's economic recession in the 1870s, which coincided with the rapid growth of the Chinese community in that state, had sparked the initial anti-Chinese movement, which was then politicized by the class politics of Jacksonian democracy.[90] A second prominent argument against the Chinese arose from concerns that they could not assimilate because their "moral code" supposedly threatened domesticity (by raising the spectre of opium and prostitution).[91] These same stereotypes had initially been pinned to Japanese arrivals, until the emergence of a specific anti-Japanese movement in the 1890s that identified a "greater" Japanese threat. Exclusionists pointed to Japanese successes in agriculture, fishing, and other industries and especially to the fact that, unlike the Chinese who had preceded them, many were making permanent homes and establishing families. The Japanese were also seen as more deceitful, immoral, and violent than the Chinese, especially after the 1905 Japanese victory in the Russo-Japanese War.[92]

Despite these concerns, for many Pacific coast politicians, labour leaders, and reporters, and for the public servants and politicians who shaped immigration policy, the arrival of the "Hindu" represented a greater menace to society than either of these groups. Indeed, even before their first arrival in significant numbers in 1906, South Asians were popularly portrayed as less desirable than other "Orientals" because of their associations with disease and immorality. Important groundwork for the Indian disease thesis was laid in 1906, and the Immigration Service (IS) played a critical role in its germination. Given the fluidity of immigration across the 49th Parallel in the early twentieth century and the porous nature of the "world's longest undefended border," it is perhaps not surprising that the story of the IS response to South Asian immigration began in Canada.

In the fall of 1906, agent John H. Clark, the IS's foremost source on Canadian immigration, reported to Washington, DC that a large number of South Asians were applying to enter the United States at the IS outpost station in Vancouver, where US Boards of Special Inquiry (BSIs) had examined more than one hundred between July and September. Two weeks later, Clark left his office in Montreal to travel to BC to investigate the "Hindoo" firsthand. There he met with officials at the IS branch offices in Vancouver and Victoria, where an official drew his attention to the fact that Canada had rejected, for medical reasons, 100 of the 2,500 South Asians who arrived in 1906. This number was "most suggestive," Clark argued, given that immigrants could avoid deportation if they could pay for treatment. Overall, Clark believed that BC's general public disliked South Asians because of their "peculiar habits" and "their unclean and unsanitary method of living." He believed that some Vancouver residents had set fire to South Asian shacks during his visit, not from racist feeling, but because they were fed up with the immigrants' living conditions. Most importantly, he also detailed his visit with Dr. W.C. Billings, the US Public Health Service's (PHS) medical gatekeeper at Vancouver. Clark recalled that

> having been present at the Bureau's office at Vancouver while Medical Examiner Billings was inspecting a number of these Hindoos who applied for admission to the US, Dr. Billings took occasion to point out the inferior physique of these people, and stated that while in some instances they were able-bodied persons, that as a rule they were men of poor physique and in all likelihood would be unable to stand the hard work usually expected of aliens from other countries.[93]

It is worth noting that five years later, Billings, then chief medical officer at Angel Island, no longer believed that this type of simple external inspection could actually reveal the health or labour potential of an Asian immigrant. He believed that "at least when dealing with oriental races," a glance or even a standard physical examination was insufficient to "penetrate" the inscrutable Asian body. Instead, bacteriological testing was required to detect internal problems and disease. But in 1906, satisfied with Billings's initial belief that "poor physiques" made poor workers – a charge that would soon become key to South Asian exclusion – Clark ended his report by stating that his personal observation of the new immigrants and the animosity they faced in BC, where they were members of the same Empire, indicated that South Asians would have "great difficulty" succeeding in the United States.[94] C.W. Bennett, San Francisco's British Consul General, echoed Dudley's concerns. In a letter to H.M. Durand, Britain's Ambassador to the United States, Bennett doubted that the South Asians could succeed where "all is so strange with them." He recommended that America extend Chinese exclusion "so as to operate against Brit East Inds [*sic*]."[95]

The sharp spike in South Asian immigration in 1906 – largely detailed in Table 2, along with other Asian immigrant statistics for the US in the years 1899–1921 – placed Billings and other federal medical inspectors in an important but challenging position as guardians of the public health. Unlike the Chinese, South Asians and Japanese immigrants could enter the United States if they arrived healthy and paid the general immigrant entry tax of $2. It thus fell to PHS officials to filter the initial inflow of arrivals from India. Alan Kraut explains that, since the debates over Chinese exclusion emphasized the need for better immigrant screening, "unhealthy ... became a convenient metaphor for excludable, legislation for remedy, and public health bureaucrats – first state, later federal – the instruments of cure."[96] This line of reasoning influenced the introduction of the 1891 Immigration Act, which in effect conflated nativism, bacteriology, and eugenics. Although 1882 legislation barred "lunatics" and those "likely to become a public charge" (LPC), the new Act, which created the Bureau of Immigration, dramatically increased screening procedures, which would include mandatory inspections by the Public Health Service. For the first time, incoming immigrants were to be issued medical certificates stipulating whether they had a "loathsome or contagious disease." A 1907 amendment would bar those with tuberculosis and/or physical defects and make the LPC charge a "Class A" (exclusion mandatory) condition.[97]

TABLE 2
Asians Immigrating to the United States, 1899–1921

Year ending June 30	South Asians	Japanese	Chinese
1899	15	3,395	3,925
1900	9	12,626	3,802
1901	20	4,908	1,784
1902	84	5,325	1,273
1903	83	6,990	1,523
1904	258	7,771	1,284
1905	145	4,319	1,348
1906	271	5,178	714
1907	1,072	9,948	788
1908	1,710	7,250	1,298
1909	337	1,593	1,818
1910	1782	1,552	1,777
1911	517	4,520	1,400
1912	165	6,114	1,765
1913	188	8,281	1,303
1914	231	8,929	1,481
1915	161	8,613	2,660
1916	112	8,680	2,460
1917	109	8,991	2,237
1918	130	10,213	1,795
1919	171	10,064	1,964
1920	300	9,432	2,330
1921	511	7,878	4,009
Total	8,381	162,570	44,738

Source: Report of the Immigration Commission, 1911, vol. 25, 5; *Annual Report of Commissioner General of Immigration* 1912, 89; ... 1913, 40–41; ... 1914, 36–37; ... 1915, 60; ... 1916, 14; ... 1917, 14; ... 1918, 57; ... 1919, 85; ... 1920, 90; 1921, 28; Erika Lee, *At America's Gates*, Table: "Chinese Admitted, By Class, 1894–1940," 101–2.

Note: Numbers do not include South Asian admissions from US Pacific territories and Canada, and do not include Japanese arrivals from Hawaii.

The 1907 amendment was to have important consequences for South Asian immigration. Clark had indicated in his 1906 report that Billings "simply gave [South Asians] a stringent medical examination before permitting them to enter the United States." This was an imperfect means of restriction: a large majority of the 235 examined that year at Vancouver passed inspection, as did 247 of the 271 South Asians who landed directly at American ports in 1906.[98] Just as Clark had reported from BC that many in this group were of "poor physique," other stereotypes preceded South Asians to some parts of the coastal states. The editor of the *Blaine Journal* reported that, while he had never seen a South Asian in the flesh, those living in nearby Bellingham were "said to live like so many dogs, are

charged with being chicken thieves and very undesirable citizens generally." He added ominously that Bellingham was thus "having trouble" with
its growing community of South Asian mill workers – a conflict that would
have important ramifications in the fall of 1907.[99]

 This chapter has shown that racially based discourse on the "Hindu"
problem in 1906 had many roots and was deployed in multiple ways. In
BC, where the arrival of significant numbers of South Asians coincided
with a severe labour shortage, Vancouver civic officials nevertheless sought
Dominion intervention to halt the increase in South Asian immigration,
a request echoed by the province's federal MPs, Immigration Branch
agents stationed at Pacific ports, and the Superintendent of Immigration
himself. In Vancouver, popular associations of South Asians with bubonic
plague, and the highly publicized claim of city officials that South Asians
were especially susceptible to tuberculosis, together appeared to validate
the widespread biological argument that South Asians endangered public
health, as well as the environmental argument that these immigrants could
not cope with cold conditions. Although one Dominion physician was not
convinced that these views were legitimate, immigration agents shared
them, as did many BC reporters, union leaders, and members of the
general public. The disease and environmental issues were compounded
by the allegations of sexual violence in the Homer Street incident, which
for many observers proved that the new arrivals were sexual deviants. As
South Asians started to enter Washington State late in the year, American
immigration officials, like their counterparts in Canada, began to associate
the new arrivals with disease and physical weakness. The next chapter will
show how these ideas continued to inform official and popular anti-Indian
protest over the following year and strongly influenced the subsequent
introduction of controls on South Asian immigration in both countries.

2

Riots, Plague, and the Advent of Executive Exclusion

They swarm down through Washington and are entering California ...
bringing with them that common aftermath of every famine-induced
pestilence, the bubonic plague, the presence of which the San Francisco
authorities are so eager to conceal."

– International Woodworker, *October 1907*

IN EARLY 1907, CANADIAN prime minister Wilfrid Laurier publicly declared
that South Asian exclusion was unnecessary and that the argument that
the new immigrants were diseased "was not borne out" by facts.[1] However,
he and his Immigration Branch soon abandoned this view after the increasing numbers of Asian arrivals precipitated race riots in Bellingham
and Vancouver. This chapter will show that 1907 was a pivotal year for
South Asian settlement in North America. In the days following the riots,
Immigration Branch officials in BC would rely heavily on public health
arguments to justify the executive restriction of South Asians at BC ports.
Reports of the unsanitary living conditions of South Asians, and their
purported unsuitability for Canada's climate, cemented public opinion
against the newcomers. Meanwhile, in the United States, the appearance
in 1907 of meningitis in Washington and bubonic plague in San Francisco
reinforced the popular association between South Asians and disease.
This chapter will also show that, since political considerations prevented
US president Theodore Roosevelt from restricting the inflow of arrivals
from India, IS officials at US Pacific ports and border points would echo
their Canadian counterparts by using similar health-based arguments to
reject South Asians.

The rapid rise in Asian arrivals to BC in the early months of 1907 indicated to white observers that the recently increased Chinese head tax had
not stopped the inflow of workers from other parts of Asia. Chinese

immigration may have temporarily ceased, but almost 1,000 Japanese arrived in the first three months of the year. Provincial premier Richard McBride responded by calling for the BC legislature to pass yet another "Natal" (Asian exclusion) Act. Provincial legislators voted in favour of the bill; however, BC Lieutenant-Governor James Dunsmuir – who personally employed many Asians – used his right of "reservation" to effectively cancel it before it became necessary for Laurier's government to disallow it at the federal level. McBride responded by increasing pressure on Ottawa for Asian exclusion. Most MPs from the province shared McBride's sentiments, as did virtually every municipal politician and editor. Consequently, while comparatively few South Asians landed at BC ports between January and March – less than one-tenth the number of Japanese – the timing of their arrival ensured their negative reception.[2]

The South Asian issue was brought further into focus in February, when officials at Vancouver General Hospital complained to the Immigration Branch that Ameela Singh, a South Asian patient with a chronic case of bronchitis, was unable to pay his bill. City Council unanimously agreed that the man should be deported. This unfortunate man's situation was by no means exceptional, as the city was forced to help many whites in similar predicaments. For example, Dr. Frederick T. Underhill, the city's Medical Officer of Health, complained in January that "helpless and indigent persons" from across the continent were routinely "dumped on the city" because BC was known to have a climate conducive for recovery. Several Vancouver patients who had died from tuberculosis in January hailed from other provinces, including one Cape Breton man who passed away shortly after his arrival from Nova Scotia.[3]

While the Ameela Singh case easily fell within the Immigration Act's deportation parameters, Dr. G.L. Milne, the Immigration Branch's medical inspector in Victoria, reported to the immigration superintendent in Ottawa, W.D. Scott, that he had been mostly unsuccessful in his attempts to deport other South Asians. It was difficult to prove that they were likely to become public charges, even though many could not find lodging. When Milne personally intervened in the case of some who had been caught begging (normally a deportable offence) and found them work, interior minister Frank Oliver quickly condemned Milne's actions. Although Milne explained that the men were not vagrants but had simply been unable to obtain work, Oliver informed Scott, Milne's supervisor, that "if Dr. Milne can't or won't deport vagrant Hindus we will engage another medical officer who will. Make that restfully clear to both Milne and Munro."[4] For Oliver, Milne's failure to enforce the Immigration Act amounted to a serious departure from Immigration Branch policy. Before legislative exclusion, Dr. Milne in Victoria and Dr. A.S. Munro, the medical inspector in Vancouver, had been the Immigration Branch's main line of defence against the perceived onslaught of South Asian immigrants. Although the particular group Milne helped had passed medical inspection, their failure to find work offered the opportunity to rid Canada of at least some of them.

Scott's general policy at ports of entry was that "there are certain nationalities who are required to pass more stringent regulations than other[s]." For example, in the pre–First World War period, the Canadian government offered medical examiners a cash bonus for each prospective black immigrant they rejected at the border, where they turned away immigrants on the "wildest of pretenses," including a range of diseases not ordinarily associated with infection, such as hernia. This process essentially followed Erika Lee's description of American "gatekeeping," whereby state protection against "'alien invasions'" was "instrumental to articulating a definition of American national identity and belonging at the turn of the twentieth century." Defining and controlling "foreign-ness" through immigrant medical inspection and deportation helped foster a construct of "American-ness," on which Americans built their national identity.[5]

If, as Lee asserts, immigration regulation drove American nation-building at the turn of the twentieth century, so too did restrictive controls inform (and reflect) notions of statehood and citizenship during this period in Canada. In their frequently cited social theory of racialization, Michael Omi and Howard Winant contend that racial subjugation occurs when the dominant group sees racial classifications as a type of "common sense" explained by "an amateur biology" in which "temperament, sexuality, intelligence, athletic abilities etc. are presumed to be fixed and discernible from the palpable mark of race." The authors explain that although stereotypes can change over time, "the presence of a *system* of racial meanings and stereotypes, of racial ideology," appears to be inexorably anchored in culture.[6] By early 1907, Oliver's Immigration Branch staff had become decisively opposed to Indian settlement for racial reasons. For example, Scott privately revealed that "the Department does not regard these people as desirable immigrants." J.B. Williams, one of Scott's immigration officers, also expressed this opinion, in a 1907 *Canadian Magazine* article in which he evoked a caricature of the South Asian on the Pacific coast. Williams declared pityingly that "it is a daily sight to see them wandering here, there, and everywhere, half starved, half naked, hording in wretched hovels, ordered here, excluded there, and despised everywhere."[7]

Punjabi scholar Saint Nihal Singh presented an opposing position in the same article, arguing that many South Asian shacks in Vancouver were very unsanitary, but that this was not the fault of the men themselves, as they could not find better housing. Moreover, their exposure to the cold presented no special risk to either themselves or to community health, as they were accustomed to Punjab's annual rainy season and many had been soldiers in the colder climates of China, Tibet, and Afghanistan. Singh's opinions represented the minority viewpoint in popular and academic literature. In May, Fred Lockley, editor of *Pacific Monthly* magazine, penned a contradictory diatribe against South Asian immigration. Although he argued that Indians "had not the faintest idea of sanitation," he also favourably presented the views of British politician William Gladstone's nephew, who held that "the Sikhs are scrupulously clean and I regard them as a very fine race of men." Yet Lockley reminded readers that India was a land cursed by "poison-breathing plague," with air "filled with infected dust." India's famines were followed by cholera, fever, smallpox, and plague, which "originate in the overcrowded and foul slums of India."[8]

The contradiction in Lockley's assertions about South Asian hygiene and health demonstrates the paradox inherent in early-twentieth-century concepts of disease causation. In the late nineteenth and early twentieth centuries, British officials in colonial Bengal struggled to reconcile emerging medical knowledge about malaria with established hereditarian ideas about racial taxonomies. For 1902 Nobel Prize–winning British physician Ronald Ross, Bengal's enduring malaria problem explained the poor appearance of many Bengalis and had, over several centuries, transformed a strong and healthy populace into "an ancient race outworn." The association of malaria with racial typologies was at its height in India's scientific community between 1890 and 1920, when India's physicians gave "scientific specificity" to European understandings of the perils of tropical climates – perils that previously had been explained as "fatal miasmas" and as caused by the impact of hot weather on Western dispositions. There is no question that India underwent a series of disease outbreaks in the years preceding Lockley's article; indeed, between 1890 and 1910, malaria, plague, cholera, and leishmaniasis devastated many parts of the colony.[9] Yet by characterizing entire peoples as weak in the shadow of India's great past, and by framing race as an inherent element of the epidemiology of malaria, Ross and others perpetuated the link between the Indian "races" and disease – a link that endured despite recent advances in the germ theory of disease transmission.

With Lockley contending in his article that South Asians were bringing cholera, smallpox, and bubonic plague to North America, it should have followed that some of them were dying of these fatal diseases. Yet no Indian died of those diseases in the province in 1907; ten of the thirteen death records that list a cause of death identify such commonplace causes as old age, exposure to the elements, pneumonia, anemia, tuberculosis, or, in one well-reported instance, murder. Furthermore, immigration statistics reveal that only about 50 of the 2,200 South Asians in BC were unemployed in early 1907 and that none had sought public relief or been deported after landing. Between January 1906 and February 1907, just 125 were refused landing for medical reasons. Put another way, only 5 percent of Indians attempting to enter Canada were rejected for medical reasons.[10]

In late June, Vancouver's acting mayor George Halse telegraphed Ottawa requesting controls on Indian immigration, even though only 500 South Asians had arrived since December. This number was small compared to the 1,200 Japanese who landed from a single vessel just a few weeks later. Oliver later addressed the Asian immigration issue publicly during a trip to Vancouver that summer, announcing that he stood for "a white Canada"[11] – a statement that reflected his broad approach to immigration policy. Clifford Sifton, Oliver's predecessor as elected interior minister from 1896 to 1905, had emphasized immigration based not on race but on occupation and working ability. After taking the helm in 1905, Oliver favoured a much more selective admissions process designed to ensure the assimilability of immigrants into Canadian society; this was clear from the unprecedented controls enshrined in his 1906 Immigration Act. The interior minister, however, was forced to delay legislation on Japanese and South Asian exclusion for fear of generating hostility with Japan, an important British ally, and of inflaming public opinion in India.[12]

The rise of Japan to "imperial status" after its triumph in wars with China (1894–95) and Russia (1904–5) strongly influenced Britain's response to Japan's lobbying for better treatment for Japanese immigrants in Canada. The Meiji government's serious lobbying for a redrafting of Japan's unequal treaties (in place since 1858) led to the Anglo-Japanese Treaty of Commerce and Navigation in 1894, which according to John Price was a "major step" towards the termination of the unequal trade relationship between the two nations. An important element of the treaty was that subjects of Japan and Britain were given "full liberty to enter, travel or reside in any part of the dominions and possessions of the other contracting party" after 1899. The Anglo-Japanese Alliance of 1902 further crystallized diplomatic relations between the two empires. Japan's subsequent victory in the above-mentioned war with Russia in 1904–5 enhanced Japanese imperial prestige, but this status became a "double-edged sword" in North America, as it "resuscitated fears of the 'yellow peril,' which Price defines as "an imagined Asian expansion through military might and mass migration that threatened white supremacy."[13]

Japan's widening sphere of influence in the Pacific marked its emergence as a force to be reckoned with on the world stage; India could make no such claim. Since the founding of the British Raj in 1858, India's native population had remained firmly under the rule of the British minority, which controlled the colony's treasury, domestic governance, military, and foreign affairs. Since the realities of living under British rule in the colony significantly "deviated from these principles upheld by the metropole," Indian nationalists began to criticize the flaws in colonialism and to confront British imperialism. This marked the birth of Indian nationalism, which led to the founding of the Indian National Congress (INC) in Bengal in 1885 and, as importantly, to rioting in the Punjab, which was the main source of the colony's army.[14] All of this suggests why the Indian government watched events in North America with growing concern, especially in September 1907, when increasing racial tensions in Bellingham, Washington, erupted into a massive "Anti-Hindu" riot that drove several hundred Punjabis out of that city and into Canada.

On the night of September 4, close to four hundred white residents of Bellingham, seventeen miles from the Canadian border, roused several hundred South Asian mill workers from their beds and drove them out of town. The police did nothing to help the workers, except to lock some of them in the county jail for "their protection." The mob's work caused the exodus of the entire group of South Asians by the following day; most of them crossed the border into BC. The riot was both racially and economically motivated. Contemporary accounts indicate that the South Asians had not been hired to replace white workers or to break strikes; rather, in the words of a US immigration inspector, there was "a scarcity of men to do the rougher and heavier work" in the region. But this distinction was not widely known.[15]

The British response to the attack on the South Asians, who were British subjects, was wholly inadequate. After a consular official in Washington State investigated the incident and its aftermath, Britain's Ambassador to the United States reassured his Secretary of State in London that it seemed unlikely that another riot would occur and expressed hope that press reports of the violence of the incident were "exaggerated."[16] Meanwhile, the local people overwhelmingly supported the mob's actions. The *Bellingham Herald* asserted that while the rioters' methods had been extreme, there was no question that "the Hindu is not a good citizen" and that "it would require centuries to assimilate him, and this country need not take the trouble." *Herald* editor Werter D. Dodd observed that "our cloak of brotherly love is not large enough to include him as a member of the body politic."[17] The local City Council resolved on September 9 that local mill owners, not the rioters themselves, were at fault for the violence because they had hired the immigrant workers. One council member also condemned the landlords of the city's South Asian shacks as well as the city's health board, arguing that "if the board had done its duty ... every Hindu would have been driven from the city" for violating civic health ordinances. The *Herald* quickly picked up the story, opining that "the Hindu is not of us and can never be," for "he brings nothing to our country but disease and filth and a little labor, in return for which he subtracts some of our capital." Similarly, Bellingham resident A.W. Magnum, a soil scientist in the Puget Sound area, informed his mother that the riot had occurred because "these Hindos (sic) are very undesirable citizens." Demonstrating that perceived labour competition was a key factor driving anti-Indian racism, he explained that "they are dirty and mean and will work for wages that a white man can't live on." Magnum concluded that "they are worse than the Japs and *Chinamen*."[18]

Magnum and Dodd's perception that South Asians were inherently inferior to other races was emblematic of nineteenth- and early-twentieth-century discourse on racial ordering. As early as the 1860s, Pacific coast doctors had argued that significant genetic disparities existed between Asians and whites. California physician Arthur B. Stout first made this argument in his 1862 paper "Chinese Immigration and the Physiological Causes of the Decay of a Nation," which employed, according to Alan Kraut, "a collection of dubious data, much of it merely the common wisdom of racial nativism."[19] These ideas continued to prevail in American academic discourse well after Congress excluded Chinese immigrants in

1882. In 1901, famous sociologist Edward A. Ross affirmed and expanded on the biological theory of racial ordering by contending that the Chinese immigrant was "mediocre and intellectually sterile," whereas the Anglo-Saxon was the "Superior Race" of "born pioneer[s]." His theory of "Race Suicide" included a future America where whites, although a "superior caste," would be "hopelessly beaten" by resident Asians.[20]

The reaction to the riot among the broader Pacific coast press demonstrated that, like Ross, many coast residents opposed immigration from Asia, and especially India. Much of the popular resistance to Indian immigration stemmed from concerns over the impact of cheap Indian labour on Pacific coast wages, yet some local residents genuinely feared the South Asian newcomers. Indeed, a Washington newspaper later reported that an Olympia woman, who had become "crazed by spiritualism" as a result of too much study, had a recurring hallucination that she was being "pursued by Hindus." The journalist elaborated that "she believes that the Hindu section hands on the Northern Pacific [railway line] are coming to her window in the evenings and making faces at her," which caused her to become so violent that she had to be restrained.[21]

After news of the Bellingham riot reached California, the *San Francisco Call* called the mob's efforts "vital to the preservation of their own status as Americans," and the editor of the traditionally pro-Asian *Los Angeles Times* declared that "at home, the orthodox Hindu is scrupulously clean about his person, but filthy as regards his surroundings, a defect which the US will not tolerate for one moment." While Joan Jensen argues that the Bellingham Riot ultimately "led to opposition to Indian workers in other parts of Washington," early 1907 editorializing by the *Blaine Review* shows that this had in fact already existed elsewhere in the state since at least May, including in areas where South Asians had never been.[22]

In the wake of the riot, the editor of the *Blaine Review* printed a returned missionary's anonymous assertion that the South Asians living along the coast were diseased. This missionary was Methodist bishop James Mills Thoburn, who had spent twenty-seven years in India. He believed that South Asians had caused the recent appearance in Washington of cerebro-spinal meningitis. Meningitis, which had taken the lives of several Washington residents that spring, was "exactly like one form the plague takes in India"; for this reason, he blamed the South Asians for the outbreak, explaining that "the filth in which the natives live" heightened cross-infection between South Asians and whites. The *Bellingham Herald* picked up the story the following day, declaring that although "it has frequently been argued that the natives of India would bring disease into this country," the missionary's statements would "do more than anything else to prejudice the people of the Northwest against the Hindus." The *Herald*'s editor also remarked that "it is true that the coming of the Hindus and the dread disease was simultaneous."[23]

Other observers connected South Asians with the recent resurgence of bubonic plague in San Francisco. That city's first plague outbreak, which occurred between 1900 and early 1904, was reportedly linked to an Asian carrier in Chinatown. However, a European appeared to have reintroduced the disease a year after the city's catastrophic 1906 earthquake; this second outbreak lasted more than eighteen months and led to 78 fatalities, none of whom were South Asian.[24] After 1900, many residents believed that plague was a uniquely "Asian" disease that was encouraged or even caused by filthy living conditions in Chinatown. The city's decision to quarantine the entire Chinese quarter and remove whites from that area further strengthened the already popular case for racial separation. Nayan Shah argues that while the wide scope of the quarantine along racial lines was in itself "extraordinary," it was "consistent with the logic of public health measures that routinely conflated deadly disease with Chinese race and residence."[25]

Although in 1902 Robert Koch had first theorized that healthy carriers could infect others with the typhoid bacillus, most epidemiologists and members of the public were not aware of that possibility until a few years later. But by that time, California authorities already maintained that Asians were likely to carry certain diseases, especially plague. Alan Kraut points out that the 1906 discovery in New York City that Typhoid Mary (Mary Mallon), a seemingly healthy Irish woman, had spread typhoid, "brought no harm to the Irish" in the long term in that city, as Irish nationals did not face an enduring public perception that they were diseased. Yet when San Francisco officials traced a plague outbreak to Chinatown resident Chic Gin in 1900, this discovery affirmed Orientalist stereotypes and exacerbated existing racial tensions in the region. Chinese "visibility," largely caused by "racial distinctiveness," heightened the group's susceptibility to "stigma and smear." The "racial hysteria" resulting from the first outbreak unquestionably "distort[ed] public health policy" as city physicians "[failed] to progress beyond the racial prejudices and stereotypes pervasive in American society."[26]

The timing of the second plague outbreak and the Bellingham Riot was crucial. South Asians were in BC, Washington, and even Oregon by late

1906, but they only began arriving in significant numbers in northern California in mid-1907, just as plague reappeared in San Francisco. Furthermore, the Bellingham Riot occurred only days after a rash of new plague cases were reported in August. Both incidents, which were widely reported in the Pacific states,[27] put considerable focus on the new arrivals in California and raised suspicions about their culpability in the outbreak, even after it was established that the second epidemic originated with (and chiefly afflicted) whites, not Asians. For example, shortly after the riot, the Chicago-based Amalgamated Wood-Worker's Union of America, which represented Washington's unionized sawmill workers, linked the two phenomena in an article accusing South Asians of coming to the country to escape India's plague. Because of "their weakened condition from famine and pestilence," most Indians had chosen to enter the country from BC, where "inspection is weak or absent entirely" at border points, as opposed to inspections at American ports, where Indians were "physic-ally unable to pass our immigration stations." After crossing the border and "swarm[ing] down through Washington," where they had acted as strikebreakers in Puget Sound, South Asians were now arriving in Califor-nia to work on the railways, "bringing with them that common aftermath of every famine-induced pestilence, the bubonic plague, the presence of which the San Francisco authorities are so eager to conceal."[28]

Bellingham Herald editor Werter Dodd combined the findings of a recent British medical study with the statements of an American tropical disease specialist to argue that South Asians carried a mysterious "oriental disease" similar to plague. The British study, a doctor's investigation of skin disease in India, looked solely at conditions in India and not the health of mi-grants, yet Dodd declared that the study "gives some good advice to the US regarding Hindu immigration." Dodd asserted that the plague-like "'oriental sore' which Hindus are likely to bring with them" was "far more virulent when contracted by people other than Hindus." Dodd added that Dr. Charles W. Stiles, hookworm expert with the Roosevelt Country Life Commission, had told a Spokane paper that the "real yellow peril to be feared on the Pacific coast" was the "invasion of oriental diseases." Al-though Stiles had not mentioned India or Indians, Dodd predicted "ter-rible results if these diseases should be transmitted by Hindu immigrants to the people of our own farming communities."[29]

Well-publicized plague outbreaks in China and India in the 1890s had influenced the North American view that Asians were racially susceptible to plague, and this opinion was especially prevalent on the Pacific coast.[30]

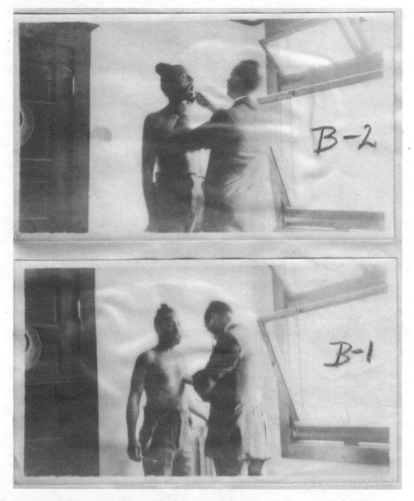

FIGURE 2   A South Asian being medically inspected at Seattle? 1907. | "Exhibit B, Public Health Service Medical Inspection at Seattle or Portland, 1907," for *Report of Inspector Braun, September 1907*, E9 51630 44C Exhibits, NARA, Washington, DC.

Since 1893, Marine Hospital Service inspectors stationed in overseas ports had checked both passengers and cargo before vessels arrived in the United States, and a "Disease Early Warning System" in Japan, the Philippines, and Hawaii regularly updated US mainland ports on disease outbreaks in those territories. In the event of an epidemic abroad, either US mainland ports were closed temporarily to ships from Asian countries, or passengers were detained for extended quarantine before being admitted. American inspectors stationed in Japan would often reinspect ships from

China after Japanese officials had passed them. Robert Barbe points out that before its annexation, Hawaii, which shared the American "obsession with trans-Pacific hygiene," also rescreened Asian passengers en route to Honolulu. Screening became more stringent during a global plague outbreak that began in China in 1894 and spread to India, parts of Africa, and finally Europe in 1896. This pandemic occurred at a time when scientific and popular knowledge about the etiology of plague and all communicable disease was "in a state of flux," even after Alexandre Yersin and Shibasuburo Kitasato theorized in 1894 that plague was spread through the rat flea. By the time plague erupted in San Francisco in 1900, the advent of bacteriology had altered only "the language of the scapegoating, not the target." Many physicians conflated anti-Chinese racism with the emerging germ theory by arguing that the plague bacillus originated or thrived in Asian homes or uniquely affected Asians.[31]

The connection between South Asian immigrants and plague is not surprising, given that the disease took one million lives in India in 1907.[32] Pacific coast newspapers often reported on plague on the Indian Subcontinent, and many Americans genuinely believed rumours that South Asians carried the invisible seeds of plague – that they were what Alan Kraut would call the "silent travelers" of disease.[33] Yet it is important to note that exclusionists eagerly capitalized on these fears, using them to inflame popular opinion against South Asians, whose initial arrival in California coincided with San Francisco's second plague outbreak. The *Blaine Review* resorted to hearsay testimony to argue that South Asians had spread meningitis in Washington State; other nativist newspapers used questionable evidence to support similar assertions. For example, the front pages of two coast newspapers carried the sensationalist warning of Pacific coast visitor R. Aylmer Winearis that "India Reeks With Dread Bubonic." Winearis, a South African war veteran from a Canadian regiment, spoke with coast reporters shortly after the return of plague in San Francisco. After the war he had worked as a health inspector in Durban, the Transvaal, where he investigated two plague outbreaks around 1903. In this capacity he had realized "the serious menace that lurked in the Hindoo immigration." One outbreak "was traced directly to the Hindoos," while the second was attributed to blankets from India. Winearis cautioned that since "India from end to end is reeking with disease," "for your own good they should not be allowed here." He continued that Indians could also gain control of a nation's economy, if given the opportunity; this sentiment appears to have influenced Winearis's diatribe against South

Asians, as he added that "the Indians at that time [1903] practically owned the whole of Durban and their hoarded wealth could only be guessed."[34]

Kornel Chang explains that "labor circuits" between British Imperial territories and North America in the early twentieth century became "conduits for racial knowledge, which facilitated the transmission of racial ideas and identities, spawning anti-Asian racism that reached across national and imperial boundaries." Chang offers the example of Edward Terry, a miner who worked in South Africa and California before settling in BC. Terry was called before the 1902 Royal Commission on Chinese and Japanese Immigration "precisely because of his knowledge of the 'Oriental question' in different colonial settings."[35] While Winearis delivered his remarks in a less official capacity, his experience with South Asians in Durban offered *Vancouver World* and *Bellingham Herald* readers an invaluable window onto the "Hindoo" problem in other regions of the Empire. Like Winearis, famous Anglo-Indian novelist Rudyard Kipling connected the group with plague during his own trip to the coast in the fall of 1907. Kipling told local reporters that he had "come six thousand miles" to study the continent's South Asian problem. Speaking extemporaneously, he argued that the Pacific northwestern climate likely made South Asians "more timid and weak than is their wont"; more importantly, he attributed the South Asian arrival to "restlessness occasioned in India on account of the plague," which had entered the Punjab "by every road."[36]

The assumption that the push factor of plague had brought South Asians to the continent ignored the major pull factor of North American wages. Punjabi labourers could earn up to $2 a day in Pacific coast lumber mills, ten to fifteen times what they could earn at home. Interviews with descendants of some of these migrants showed that they immigrated to make money, not to flee disease. One interviewee stated that "opportunity" was the reason his grandfather left India in 1906; the relative of a current MP also came for "economic opportunity." News reports at the time widely publicized this as the reason for Indian immigration.[37] Why, then, did Kipling and others assume that South Asians came to the continent to escape plague? According to medical historian Morton Beiser's "Sick Immigrant Paradigm," the notion that immigrants were diseased was a prevailing assumption in North American public health discourse before the mid-twentieth century. The theory further held that immigrants were the "least well-integrated" of their home societies and that Asians and southern Europeans were the primary culprits of disease importation and transmission. The disease thesis was based on the fact that Europeans had brought smallpox, cholera, measles, and other diseases to the continent after the fifteenth century. Sylvia Reitmanova adds that "it was assumed that diseases are often the reason which forces immigrants to leave their homelands."[38] This context offers a useful lens for interpreting Pacific coast American perceptions of South Asian disease.

The Americans' association of South Asians with the return of plague also resonated in Canada, where nativists already connected the newcomers with that disease. In 1906, *Vancouver World* editor Louis D. Taylor, a future mayor of Vancouver, had launched a week-long editorial "battle royale with '"Gwen," the anonymous female colonist of the *Vancouver News-Advertiser*, over Taylor's assertion that South Asians were importing plague into the city.[39] The fact that no South Asians in North America had developed plague symptoms disproved this assertion, yet when the disease resurfaced in San Francisco, BC residents quickly propagated the plague connection. In October 1907, the Province of British Columbia legislated that "all sick Chinese, Japanese, Sikhs or other Orientals must send or give notice of their illness" to their district's "Health Officer or Police Constable." This reactive measure followed the pattern established in the province in 1892, when an outbreak of plague in Hong Kong caused the province to introduce a bill to create the first BC Health Act; later outbreaks in Japan and Hawaii impelled the passage of the Act and the creation of a board of health. Shortly thereafter, the BC legislature resolved that the Health Act be strictly implemented in the province's Chinese neighbourhoods because "the dirtiest, filthiest, and most repulsive people in the province" were "prejudicial to the general health." When plague reappeared in China in 1900, Health Board secretary C.J. Fagan recommended that the bodies and homes of all Asians in the province be subjected to annual physical examinations. The epidemics generated serious anxiety among those concerned with the hygiene of the province's Chinese districts, but no plague cases and no deadly disease outbreaks of any kind were linked to these neighbourhoods.[40]

Despite ongoing concerns about hygiene in BC's Chinese residences, it is telling that Vancouver's broad enforcement of the October 1907 Act began not in Chinatown but in the city's "Hindoo Quarter." City Medical Officer of Health Underhill's team, in a search for plague at city wharves and in Asian residences, found no trace among the city's South Asians; nevertheless, the *Saturday Sunset* reported that "the Hindus, by methods more forcible than polite, were given to understand that the premises occupied by them must be kept in a sanitary condition."[41] The reports of

Underhill's health inspectors indicate that many of the city's Indians did live in unhygienic conditions. One inspector's summary of these 1907 visits offers valuable insight into the city's extensive surveillance of Indian-occupied properties along Water, Main, Cordova, and Hastings Streets. Underhill and his team of seven assistants found that many of the Indian-occupied dwellings had outdoor commodes, shoddy plumbing, and inadequate sites for food preparation – all infractions that were "a serious menace to Health." The worst locations were near the Carnegie Library on Hastings, where forty men resided in "indescribable" conditions, and on Main Street, where thirty more lived near City Hall. The inspectors evicted the latter group, forcing them to move to South Vancouver and Cambie Street, "where a goodly number" still lived at the time of the report.[42]

The *World* publicized the results of the inspections in its front page article "Hindoo Houses Were Unsanitary," which praised the city's health authorities for their "vigilance in connection with the bubonic plague scare." Two South Asians had been fined $10 plus expenses for violating health ordinances at a Fairview house and at the overpopulated "Maple Leaf" boarding house, where a health inspector reported that the men there "live[d] more as beasts than as human beings." Earlier in the fall a *Province* reporter had called the Maple Leaf house "dirty beyond imagination," in part because it had only one basin, and also because "the steam from the over-worked cook stove floats heavily through the door to a high smelling mist that renders darkly indistinct the nut-brown bodies of the lithe Hindus." Nevertheless, inspectors found no trace of bubonic plague in these or any South Asian residences in the city.[43]

The search for plague in "Oriental" residences in Vancouver followed a major anti-Asian riot in that city on September 7, three days after the events at Bellingham, following a demonstration by the newly formed Vancouver chapter of the San Francisco-based Asiatic Exclusion League (AEL). Chinese and Japanese immigrants, not South Asians, were the primary targets of the Vancouver riot, which damaged Chinatown and destroyed significant property in the city's Japanese section, but rumours about the arrival of the Bellingham refugees swelled the number of participants in the protest that preceded the riot and thus may have amplified the evening's violence. Indeed, within hours of the riot in Bellingham on the September 4, Vancouver newspapers had issued alarmist reports that hundreds of South Asian refugees were walking towards the Dominion's border.[44]

Not surprisingly, local newspapers largely downplayed the damage in-
flicted that night. The *World* editorialized that while there had been a
regrettable destruction of property in Vancouver's Chinatown, no Asian
had been physically hurt, as "tall Sikhs and little Japs passed among the
crowd without molestation, even when the excitement was at its greatest."
This observation failed to capture the intense racial hatred expressed that
night, which later influenced a shift in Laurier's approach to the Asian
issue. The riots demonstrated to Ottawa the degree of racial tension on
the Pacific coast and further reminded the Dominion government that
BC was "virulently anti-Indian." Jensen argues that this "helped sway Canadian public policy" against South Asian immigration and that the riots
marked the turning point when the Canadian, British, and Indian governments began efforts to bar Indians from Canada.[45] However, this explanation only partly accounts for the Liberal policy shift towards Indian
exclusion, which was also rooted in the political fallout from the arrival
of nearly 1,000 South Asians just four days after the riot.[46]

The SS *Monteagle* landed at Vancouver on September 11 with 914 South
Asians, 149 Chinese, and 114 Japanese aboard. The vessel's arrival drew
further public focus to the South Asian immigration issue and exacerbated
tensions between city officials and the Laurier government. As Lord Grey
secretly wrote to Lord Elgin (born Victor Bruce), Britain's Secretary of
State for the Colonies, "the recent arrival of 900 Hindus in one vessel
(September) when the lumber mills, the principal outlet for Hindu labour,
were commencing to shut down, has revived the old alarm, and has caused
my Ministers to be apprehensive" about riots in the city. When Dr. A.S.
Munro cleared almost eight hundred of the South Asians for entry, the
new mayor, Alexander Bethune, immediately asked Laurier for permission
to house them at federal expense in the city's Dominion Drill Hall. When
Laurier denied the request and stated that the group could be deported
as paupers, the mayor was forced to admit to Laurier that the men were
not paupers but simply needed housing. The idea to request use of the
Drill Hall probably came from Indian expatriate Taraknath Das, secretary
of the Vancouver Hindustani Association and a political activist, who
complained that many of the *Monteagle* immigrants were being forced to
camp in unhygienic conditions. Despite Bethune's telegrams and Lord
Grey's personal request for aid, Laurier merely dispatched Frank Oliver
to BC to assess the situation. In the meantime, Bethune created a private
fund to send the immigrants to Ottawa by rail, and the *World* solicited
reader donations for the fund. A *World* journalist compared the Indians

waiting for housing to "sheep" awaiting a pasture, and developed the analogy by recalling that two hundred *Monteagle* South Asians had run "like hungry cattle after a load of hay" behind an employer's wagon after receiving a job offer. He concluded that, like an animal, "the Hindoo's individualism is a negligible quantity."[47]

The Orientalism expressed in this assessment exemplifies Edward Said's well-known work on Western understandings of Asian-ness and the Asian mind.[48] For the *World* journalist, the South Asians were not individuals but were all of the same mold. There is no question that Vancouver's Asian exclusionists consistently perpetuated a view of South Asians as "other." In the wake of the arrival of the *Monteagle*, a contingent of South Asians approached Dr. Frederick T. Underhill, Vancouver's Medical Officer of Health, for help to improve living conditions and sanitation in their Vancouver housing. Picking up the story, a *World* editorial dryly advised that Underhill should speak to the group in "their own language" to motivate them to clean up their camps; the editor suggested that, for this purpose, "an opinion that these unworthy ones deserve that wild asses shall walk on their ancestors' graves or words to that effect, will probably help some." This depiction of South Asians as superstitious and illogical illustrates how, in the *Province* and *World* from 1905 to 1914, South Asians ranked second to last, ahead of only the Italians, of sixteen national groups when it came to denigrating news stories about their status and social, moral, and religious customs. Said's assertion that Orientalism "has less to do with the Orient than it does with 'our' world" explains how the Vancouver press continually associated immigrants from India with "immorality, dirt, disease and abhorrent cultural practices" that "clearly validated the social, cultural and ideological privileges" of Anglo Canadians.[49]

The arrival of the *Monteagle* was especially significant because Dr. Munro's stringent medical examination of its Indian passengers signalled the start of Canadian executive restriction against South Asians. Years before the US Congress legislated South Asian exclusion in 1917, American immigration officials were rejecting Indians for bogus reasons – medical or otherwise – to limit the entry of Indian arrivals.[50] Although Jensen defined this process of executive restriction solely in an American context, the term also describes what happened in Canada when the *Monteagle* docked at Vancouver. At this time, Munro informed Oliver that "Hindus ex Monteagle subjected rigid physical examination all old men and those physically unfit rejected and ordered deported." Meanwhile in Victoria, Milne acknowledged receipt of the minister's instructions on South Asian immigration. While the record of Oliver's instructions no longer exists, Munro's telegram appears to indicate that Oliver had ordered the doctors of both ports to zealously search for physical faults in all South Asian arrivals.[51]

The *Province*, which described the *Monteagle* passengers as the "Hindu Eclipse of the Brownie Moon," recalled that Dr. Munro, unaccountably assisted by the city's Dr. Underhill, was able to reject only 103 of the 921 South Asian passengers for old age and various medical complaints, including "narrow chests with a possible predisposition to tuberculosis." Although the journalist stated that the men presented a "physically fit and handsome" appearance, the *Saturday Sunset* warned that Munro, as the only federal representative on the pier, was unable to properly screen and assist the large number of immigrant arrivals entering his port, especially since

> Vancouver ... is ever subject to the inroads of infection as brought in through the liners from the Orient and coasting steamers from Southern Pacific ports. If [an immigrant] passes [his] inspection he is turned loose at the lower end of the city and, a stranger in a strange land, is compelled to make the best he can of his conditions. Take, for instance, the large number of Hindus who arrived at this port last year and, even nearer, the hundreds of that race who came over on the Monteagle last week. Under what deplorable conditions did they make their entrance into the Dominion and what a veritable menace were they to themselves and the public in general?[52]

Shortly after the *Monteagle's* arrival captured city headlines, Laurier in Ottawa confided to Governor General Earl Grey that the South Asian situation was "far more serious" than that of the Japanese. Although the ongoing negotiations with Japan would limit immigration from that nation, "to speak frankly," the prime minister wrote, "I see no solution ... except quietly checking the exodus from India." He later added that the ongoing "rushing in of Hindoos" was preventing Vancouverites from forgetting the causes of the Vancouver Riot, as the South Asians were "an element to which the people of BC have a still greater aversion than to the Japs." On September 19, immigration superintendent W.D. Scott returned to the city, one year after his first trip to Vancouver. W.L.M. King, the deputy labour minister, confided to his diary that Scott was officially investigating the riot but that the superintendent had also been sent to find a way to end Indian immigration. King wrote that although Laurier hoped to further restrict (not entirely end) migration from Japan and China, the prime minister privately told King that "we would have to stop the Hindu immigration altogether."[53]

Like Laurier, Governor General Earl Grey observed that Indians were "still more unpopular than the Japs" in Vancouver; he later asserted that the arrival of the *Monteagle* and the Bellingham refugees was reigniting the tensions in Vancouver that had caused the riot. Writing on behalf of himself and Laurier, Earl Grey confided to John Morley, India's secretary of state, that "the Hindu difficulty alarms us more" than Japanese immigration. If the "Hindu inflow" was caused not by vigorous campaigning by steamship companies but by the "startling contrast" in wages between India and BC, the flood of South Asians would continue "until the people in their fear as to the results of this invasion raise the dykes against all Asiatics." Earl Grey asserted that Laurier, who was concerned about American agitators, feared that any new arrivals from India would put "a lighted match to a lot of explosive material – mainly of American manufacture, knocking about Vancouver." He later warned Secretary of State for the Colonies Elgin that the arrival of another shipload of Indians would only heighten tensions in the city. He concluded that "the only way out of the difficulty that I can see" was for India to prohibit emigration without a passport.[54]

Laurier continued to stall on the issue, hoping that India would restrict its own emigration. In October, reverting to the well-established argument that South Asians were unsuited to Canada's climate, he ordered the Immigration Branch to prepare a request that India limit passports for labourers. Thomas R. McInnes, a secret agent for the Immigration Branch, echoed the climate argument in a confidential report to Oliver, which detailed the testimony McInnes had recently collected from immigration officials, the AEL, and six resident South Asians. McInnes's findings reflected anti-Asian anxieties in the province. While employers wanted more cheap labour, the American exclusionists currently in BC increased McInnes's (and Laurier's) concern that hostility towards South Asians could soon extend to the Japanese, who would fight back in the event of another riot. Like Scott, McInnes believed that the South Asians were "physically unfit" for BC's climate; he added that despite press reports of Indian criminality, city records indicated that Indians were "remarkably inoffensive and peaceable, getting into trouble far more frequently with health officers than with the police."[55]

McInnes also reported Dr. Munro's concern that many South Asians would die of tuberculosis over the winter, due to exposure to the cold and the lack of adequate food and clothing. According to Munro, Filipino sawmill workers had brought the disease to Seattle four years earlier, and more than two hundred from that group had died from it; although he did not assert that South Asians had actually imported the disease, he forecast a similar fate for them. McInnes thus recommended that Canada adopt an examination similar to that of the US Vancouver office, which "subject[ed] all Hindus and Japanese to a very stringent medical inspection." This would "prevent the steamship companies dumping the more squalid misery of India in increasing proportions upon our Coast."[56] The suggestion was predicated on the idea that the Indian arrivals were either ill or weak. However, McInnes admitted that US officials passed 118 of 133 Indians who had applied to enter from Vancouver in the past three months. If these men were in fact unfit to work, how could most have passed two inspections, one to first enter Canada, and another particularly "stringent" test to enter the United States? Nevertheless, McInnes's findings increased Laurier's apprehension about the situation and persuaded the Governor General that exclusion was needed. Earl Grey accordingly informed Laurier that he hoped that McInnes's "apparently accurate diagnosis of the whole situation" would convince India to halt emigration to Canada.[57]

The SS *Tartar*, one of the last vessels to bring South Asians to Canada in large numbers, arrived at Vancouver shortly after McInnes submitted his report. Before the ship anchored, Munro cabled Ottawa for instructions on how to examine the passengers. While there was no official financial requirement for any immigrant arrivals, Laurier personally instructed Superintendent of Immigration Scott, who was still in Vancouver, to assist Munro in rejecting Indians who might become public charges. Accordingly, on Scott's last day in the city, the pair rejected 75 of the 518 *Tartar* Indians for disease or physical unfitness and another 106 for being Likely to Become a Public Charge (LPC). It is very possible that many of the *Tartar* passengers rejected for physical reasons were not ill but were merely recovering from the effects of a remarkably difficult ocean crossing. The *World* reported that a strong wind during the voyage had delayed the vessel's arrival in Vancouver by five days. Furthermore, the men suffered from both from the cold and from seasickness, which likely explained their "worn and haggard appearance when they landed."[58]

Pahan Singh, one of the *Tartar* passengers rejected because he was deemed LPC for having insufficient funds and was assessed as having a "defective physique," launched a legal appeal against Munro's decision to deport him. The above-mentioned Taraknath Das, a translator for the American IS stationed in Vancouver who had been seconded as the interpreter in Singh's trial, later recalled that the appellant and many of his fellow passengers had been physically disqualified after being examined "at a rate of six a minute." Singh, who had arrived with $10, argued that Munro and Scott had not given him the chance to explain how he would avoid destitution. Using the precedent of a 1906 ruling that immigrants had the right to defend themselves, a federal judge surprised the Immigration Branch by ruling that Singh had not been given a fair examination, and he was released into Canada on a writ of habeas corpus three months later.[59] The father of Kartar Singh Ghag, a participant in the Indo-Canadian Oral History Project, likely arrived on this voyage of the *Tartar*. In a 1984 interview, Ghag recalled that his father had told him that the men in his group had felt particularly "harassed" by immigration officials when they arrived in Vancouver. Immigration officials scrutinized the men carefully for trachoma and later deported several for having the disease.[60]

Some South Asians escaped deportation through medical treatment. One Indian migrant who arrived in the fall of 1906, likely on the *Tartar* in September, was initially rejected at Hong Kong for cataracts or redness in the eyes, which he attributed to the summer in India. According to my 2010 interview with his nephew, this individual was able to obtain a medical clearance card from another passenger who decided not to go to Canada, and used the card to buy passage to Victoria. On board ship, the same doctor who had previously examined him told him "I rejected you," but cured his medical condition, and he travelled to Victoria, where friends at the Butchart cement mill helped him secure employment there.[61]

Kartar Singh Nawanchand's autobiographical account offers a similar example of sympathetic treatment by medical officials. Nawanchand likely arrived with Ghag on the *Tartar* in 1907. In Hong Kong he bought a ticket to Vancouver because he had heard that BC medical inspections were less strict than those at San Francisco. Passengers were twice examined by the ship's doctors, although some who failed still came aboard after bribing the vessel's commanders. On reaching Vancouver, passengers wore their best clothing to the Immigration office at the pier, where a physician, most likely Munro, checked their eyes and in some cases their clothing. After his inspection, Nawanchand was locked in a room, and since the interpreter had not arrived, he was enlisted to translate questions about diseases and Indian customs, including polygamy. The stenographer put medicine in his eyes [likely for trachoma] and told him to get follow-up treatment in Vancouver. She told him that if he could not find a doctor, he was to return to the port for a free treatment. She asked him to keep in touch, and told him he should come back to the pier if he needed her help.[62]

In October, a physician visiting Vancouver appeared to validate Dr. Munro's medical rejection of an unprecedented number of Indians from the *Tartar*. Wilfred G. Fralick, a Queen's University–educated doctor whom the *World* called "one of the most noted New York physicians," declared to a *World* reporter that poor health was the "greatest menace" of Asian immigration because of the Asian susceptibility to disease. Fralick warned that Canada should bar Asians or, at the very least, strengthen inspections at BC ports. The *World* neglected to mention Fralick's highly unorthodox ideas about germ theory. In 1901, Fralick had demonstrated a "new cure" for tuberculosis that "remov[ed] every trace of bacteria" from a person's system. A culmination of seven years of research, the cure called for injecting a "clear and colorless liquid" into a patient to flush out bacteria. This method failed to produce significant results, despite Fralick's declaration that it "must succeed, or the whole germ theory is false." Yet the *World* championed Fralick's 1907 assertions, adding that Asians were "impervious to modern ideas of sanitation" and carried "the oriental pestilence" of bubonic plague.[63]

After stalling on the issue for over a year, Minister of the Interior Oliver finally moved to restrict South Asian immigration in October. With McInnes's report in hand, he asked Governor General Grey to approve a proposal for a revision to the Immigration Act that would curb Indian immigration. Oliver argued that the past fourteen months of South Asian immigration was causing "considerable alarm" for both the community's health and its labour force. In particular, he cited the following evidence from Scott's first-hand report on the *Tartar*: "The first obstacle in the way of these people is our climate. Last year some twenty-five of them died from exposure and this is likely to be repeated this year ... Then their habits of living are such that they cannot be considered as desirable immigrants ... People say to me that 'as for the poor Hindoo it would be a mercy to keep him out.'"[64]

As noted in Chapter 1, BC death records for 1906 indicate a total of seven South Asian deaths, not twenty-five, no more than three of which could have resulted from exposure to the elements. Despite Scott's glaring miscalculation, Oliver used this report to recommend that all South Asians be required to show $500 on entry.[65] This order was scrapped when Earl Grey, whose opinion held some influence among the Laurier cabinet, withheld approving it until he had more information; as Grey secretly revealed by letter to Elgin in London, he believed the provision was problematic because it explicitly discriminated against a class of British subjects. Although he felt that the men were "not suited physically" for Canada, he still hoped that India would pre-empt the need for Canadian legislation.[66] W.L.M. King's arrival in BC in October further delayed this decision.

While the deputy labour minister was in Vancouver investigating the city's riot, Laurier ordered him to also begin a Royal Commission inquiry into the causes of Asian migration to Canada. King interviewed six South Asians who had been rejected and were awaiting deportation, and several others, during the Commission's regular sittings, which began shortly after two South Asians escaped from the Vancouver immigrant detention hospital, embarrassing Dr. Munro and probably reaffirming for King the urgency of the situation.[67] For the Laurier government, King's most useful observation was that every South Asian who came to Canada changed ship at either Hong Kong or Yokohama because no steamship company offered direct passage from India. The consultations also confirmed Laurier's suspicion that steamship companies were at least partly responsible for the recent increase in South Asian arrivals – a point later confirmed in testimony recorded in the Indo-Canadian Oral History Project. One individual recalled that his father sailed for Vancouver in 1907 because a man, presumably representing a steamship company, had come to his village in India, disseminating "propaganda" about BC. This convinced more than two hundred men from the man's village to go to Canada that year.[68]

Laurier, like Earl Grey, had remained hopeful throughout 1907 that Canada and India could find a diplomatic alternative to exclusion. Such an arrangement would likely be better received in India than an outright exclusion measure; it would also resolve the problem Grey had mentioned to Elgin: unlike other Asians, South Asians were British subjects, which meant that barring them solely on the basis of citizenship was nearly impossible. After the British colony of Natal in South Africa in 1897 barred Indian workers, Australia's 1901 Immigration Restriction Act had circumvented this imperial issue by compelling all prospective Asian immigrants, including South Asians, to pass a highly difficult dictation test. Since 1898, Laurier had vetoed a series of above-mentioned acts with literacy clauses passed by BC's legislature. According to Jensen, Laurier's initial reluctance to explore non-diplomatic options – evidenced by the fact that he did not ask Oliver for a draft exclusion bill until October 1907 – stemmed from his leadership style, which emphasized party consensus and a prudent approach to reform. W.L.M. King, and others who were "full of nervous reform energy" in Laurier's cabinet, objected to his careful approach, although Laurier was slowly changing his position, given that his party had to appeal to the nation's workers and trade unionists to stay in power.[69]

Earl Grey's prediction that the arrival of more South Asians would generate protest bore out in December, when the *World* decried the arrival of more than one hundred South Asians aboard the SS *Monteagle*. That number would not have received front-page press coverage earlier in the year. Enforcing his recent policy of executive restriction, Dr. Munro rejected forty of the men for reasons of disease or insufficient funds. However, not all were sent away. As Peter H. Bryce, the interior department's Chief Medical Officer, reminded Munro at the end of November, the Immigration Branch's policy at this time was to allow prospective immigrants, including Asians, to pay for the medical treatment of curable diseases in the Vancouver Detention Hospital. Since some individuals left Asia healthy but were "accidentally affected on board ship during their long voyage," Bryce felt that it would be unfair to deport those who were willing to pay for treatment. This policy presumably allowed some South Asians to be landed after treatment, as several landed on December 16; however, the *Monteagle* was the last ship to bring South Asians to Canada in large numbers before legislative exclusion.[70]

This chapter has shown how the coincidence of the initial South Asian arrival in the Pacific coast states with the appearance of meningitis and bubonic plague cemented the Americans' association between the new arrivals and disease, especially after a major riot erupted at Bellingham in September 1907. A chaotic week in BC, which saw the arrival of the Bellingham refugees, a major race riot at Vancouver, and the landing of eight hundred South Asians, marked the beginning of executive restriction at BC ports. Laurier, Oliver, Grey, and especially King used aspects of the now-popular health and climate arguments to justify the need for exclusion. That position was echoed and reinforced by BC federal representatives, editors, and others who argued that South Asians could not assimilate into Canadian society. Statements made by Rudyard Kipling and other high-profile international visitors to Vancouver, who purported to have first-hand knowledge of the racially or culturally inherent characteristics of the group, appeared to affirm the legitimacy of the argument. The next chapter will show that the resulting introduction of legislative exclusion in 1908 virtually halted South Asian immigration to Canada. Meanwhile, in the Pacific coast states, a sustained campaign of executive restriction at ports and border points brought about a similar result for Indian immigration to the United States. When these policies were challenged several times over subsequent years, Canadian and American officials continued to employ climatic and especially health-based arguments to maintain exclusion.

3

"The Public Health Must Prevail"
Enforcing Exclusion

The only solution I can see of the Hindu difficulty is to prohibit your Hindus from coming into our icebox without a passport ... I know it is difficult, but the law of common humanity like that of the public health must prevail!

– Governor General Earl Grey to John Morley, March 23, 1908

IN JANUARY 1908, WILFRID Laurier's government finally excluded South Asian immigrants from Canada with PC 920, an order-in-council prohibiting the admission of any immigrant who had not arrived by continuous journey (on one ticket) from their land of birth or citizenship, along with a second order, PC 926, that significantly increased the money qualification for Asian immigrants.[1] The continuous journey stipulation, which was impossible for Indian residents to meet, virtually ended South Asian immigration to Canada. Although some South Asians circumvented exclusion in 1908 and 1913 by finding technical flaws in the order, continuing anti-Indian activism in British Columbia ensured that this legislation essentially remained in effect even after religious and community organizations began petitioning for a relaxation of PC 920. This chapter will show that the popularly theorized link between South Asians and disease offered a convenient answer to challenges to Canadian exclusion in the prewar period and, in the Pacific coast states, strongly influenced efforts to bring about executive and legislative exclusion.

Previous chapters have shown that South Asian immigration, and the resulting theory of South Asian "otherness," came at a critical juncture in the history of immigration to BC. The September 1907 riots in Bellingham and Vancouver had proven two things. First, Britain's muted reaction to the violent treatment of hundreds of Indians in Bellingham indicated that the British and Indian governments would not protect the interests of South Asians in North America generally. Second, official correspondence between Earl Grey and others after the Vancouver anti-Asian riot revealed that British and Canadian federal authorities were seriously concerned that further immigration from India would increase agitation in BC against the thousands of Japanese residents of that province; the Japanese, who had chased rioters out of their neighbourhoods during the Vancouver Riot, might respond with even greater force in the event of a second anti-Asian riot. Since the result could "bring on trouble between Canada and Japan," Grey and Laurier agreed that South Asian exclusion was necessary to preserve good relations with Tokyo.[2]

Herein lay the need for PC 920, which carefully excluded South Asians and also Japanese migration via Hawaii but did not affect the token Japanese immigrant quota that Laurier's government also put in place in 1908 to appease Japan's government. At the same time, Chinese immigrants could still pay the $500 head tax that had been in place since 1903. The near-absence of documentation on the evolution of PC 920 makes it difficult to prove that it was specifically introduced to bar Indians. However, retrospective statements made by interior minister Frank Oliver and others offer compelling evidence that South Asians were the legislation's intended target. In April 1908, Oliver informed a British official that because popular opinion in BC regarding Asian immigration was "aggravated and had to be dealt with," both PC 920 and PC 926 had been drafted in late 1907 "to keep out as many of those we do not want as possible." Moreover, Henry Herbert Stevens, MP for Vancouver, candidly revealed in 1923 that "this Order-in-Council was passed some years ago to prevent Hindus coming to Canada from Hong Kong and other Asiatic points." Having first been elected in 1911, Stevens was not involved in the 1908 order's passage, but his deep involvement in immigration issues would have made him privy to the rationale behind it.[3]

Erika Lee describes Chinese exclusion in the United States as an "institution" that legally affirmed racial categories. As a general account of state gatekeeping against foreign nationals, this depiction offers a useful framework for understanding exclusion ideologies and practices. The institution's principles and operational systems variously branded immigrants as "undesirable" and "diseased." The same process occurred in BC, where by 1908 popular discourse had helped solidify these definitions and firmly anchor them to South Asians. The first such "undesirable" South Asians rejected under the continuous journey regulation arrived from Fiji in mid-February. Oliver, anticipating the arrival of more on other

vessels destined for BC, wired Drs. Milne and Munro requiring Indians
to have "through tickets" from India; he also ordered that provisions for
exclusion for "health or character are to be rigidly enforced" on all South
Asians. Matters were complicated when BC passed its most recent "Natal
Act" requiring Asians admitted to Canada to pass a language test. The
first to face this test were 160 South Asians who had arrived on the SS
Monteagle in late February. Although Munro released those who could
show through tickets from Calcutta, under the provincial Natal Act these
men were immediately held without bail in the provincial courthouse.
The Immigration Branch ordered the other Indians deported. Earl Grey
informed Secretary of State for the Colonies Elgin that while Laurier
regretted this development, he "realizes the consequences of an attack
on Hindu arrivals by Van rioters would be still more serious."[4]

The practical application of the continuous journey provision was initially tricky, as officials struggled to interpret it correctly and apply it to
all ethnic groups. Some Indians could show through tickets indicating
that they had paid for their entire journey in Calcutta, although most had
been forced to buy a second ticket after transshipping at Hong Kong or
Japan. Furthermore, after Munro rejected a German immigrant travelling
from Australia in January, Laurier admitted in Parliament that this rejection was "carrying a good principle a little too far." Secret agent Thomas
R. McInnes, who advised Laurier that Europeans arriving from Japan had
also been denied entry, similarly opined that the order "was never intended
to be enforced in this absurd manner." Britain's parliamentary opposition
thrice forced Elgin's Under Secretary of State for the Colonies Winston
Churchill, and Secretary of State for India John Morley, to admit the order's failings, which included its general application to all nationalities.[5]
Writing from Ottawa, Earl Grey thus privately asked Morley to keep Indians
out of "our icebox" by withholding Indian passports. He argued that exclusion was necessary because "the law of common humanity like that of
the public health must prevail!"[6]

Shortly after a BC Supreme Court Justice declared BC's Natal Act invalid
in March and freed eighteen South Asian provincial prisoners, the Court
ruled that the continuous journey order was worded imprecisely and was
thus technically inoperative in its current form. The Immigration Branch
was forced to liberate more than 150 South Asians from the Dominion
detention shed. Oliver immediately introduced a revised version of the
order in the House of Commons. The Vancouver press was largely skeptical
of the new bill, which was very similar to the first version. A *Province*

editorial cartoon depicted a turbaned head coming through a wall into the province, pushing out the broken planks of the "Order in Council." After Ontario Conservative John Graham Haggart, the only MP to oppose the bill, warned against drawing "a colour line," Vancouver's R.G. Mac-Pherson ended the debate by stating that "I would rather draw the colour line now than draw it fifty years later." American history had shown that it could take "years of fighting" and millions of dollars to resolve a race issue.[7]

That the Indian issue had become Canada's own race problem shows the pervasiveness of BC's anti-Indian racism by 1908. Ideologies like racism "can and do" become organized into "social practices and material arrangements," which Timothy Stanley contends "make the logics of these ideas appear all the more convincing and self-evident." Michel Foucault and others define this process as a "discursive formation," yet Stanley expands the term to include "material consequences and arrangements" and also "symbolic processes of representation and the circulation of meanings," which allowed anti-Asian racism in BC to become "a texture of life."[8] By expanding Stanley's ideas on racism to South Asians, it can be shown that Canada's legislative South Asian exclusion was the direct outcome of a sustained and highly vocal two-year campaign built upon the principle of South Asian racial "otherness."[9]

A majority consensus of the ruling Liberal and opposition Conservative parties resulted in the codification of the second continuous journey order-in-council in April 1908, which required immigrants to come directly (on one ticket) from the land of their "nativity and citizenship." The new act widened the government's exclusionary power to bar, for example, a prospective immigrant of Indian ancestry born in Hong Kong.[10] Laurier could not have anticipated the astounding success of the continuous journey legislation – only about one hundred Indians entered Canada between 1908 and 1915 – yet he continued to hope for a diplomatic answer to the issue. In January he sent deputy labour minister W.L.M. King on a secret mission to Washington, DC. US president Theodore Roosevelt had made the highly unusual request that King act as Roosevelt's emissary in London, to ask Britain to convince its Japanese ally to restrict immigration to America. Roosevelt, fearing diplomatic and even military conflict with Japan over the issue, further suggested that King advocate a shared Anglo-American policy of excluding Japanese labourers from the United States and Canada. Laurier agreed to the plan, despite his reservations about its diplomatic impropriety. Since, according to R. MacGregor Dawson,

Canada "could not possibly announce that King was going to England at Roosevelt's request," Laurier sent King to London under the guise of conducting a Royal Commission into the causes of Indian immigration.[11]

Even before King left Ottawa, at least one senior cabinet member believed that the trip was pointless. In his diary, King recalled that agriculture minister Sydney A. Fisher had told him that "as to the India question and Canada, it was doubtful what could be accomplished."[12] Fisher rightly predicted that King would be unable to convince India to restrict the emigration of its subjects, and thus King's subsequent report on his mission merely affirmed the need for Canada's continuous journey order. The report described his interviews with Elgin, Morley, and other British and Indian representatives, as well as India's assurances that Canada, as a self-governing British colony, was justified in controlling its own immigration. Indeed, the Indian government had suggested ways for Canada to indirectly bar Indians, including a more stringent "physical fitness" standard for immigrants. King's meetings also affirmed the popular Canadian belief that immigrants of Indian extraction were unsuited to Canada's climate and had "manners and customs" that would prevent their assimilation.[13]

In the BC press, coverage of King's spring trip to London was mixed. *Saturday Sunset* editor J.P. MacDonnell panned King's attempt to warn Indians that BC's "climate is damp and that wet feet start consumption in the lungs"; he reasoned that the "starving, plague-ridden, dissatisfied and restless natives of India" would likely be more successful in Canada than in their home country. Possibly for the first time in a Vancouver editorial, *World* editor L.D. Taylor admitted that King's use of the climate argument would not work "for the very good reason" that it was "not altogether true." Although Bengalis "suffer[ed] terribly" in cold weather, "stories of the evil effects of the climate" would not discourage immigration to Canada since virtually all of BC's Indians were the "hardier races from the hill country" of the Punjab, and appeared to survive "under conditions of clothing and shelter which would put the average white man in hospital."[14] Similarly, Lionel Curtis, an Oxford-educated lawyer based in Johannesburg, informed a friend that "there is a certain amount of hypocrisy" in Canada's use of the climate argument. "On the whole," he added, "I suspect that the Asiatics from the tropics can acclimatize themselves to colder regions better than Europeans to tropical regions." However, he supported exclusion, arguing that "if the British Empire means handing over the balance of the habitable globe to Asiatics, it is a vast mistake."[15]

Despite exclusion, small numbers of South Asians – mainly return visitors – arrived after King's return to Canada. In May, Peter H. Bryce, the interior department's Chief Medical Officer, informed Scott that ten South Asians had been detained for observation in Vancouver along with other Asians. Although by June the Vancouver detention hospital no longer treated any immigrants, those with minor illnesses could still pay for private treatment. During Bryce's visit to the hospital that month, the only patient was one South Asian who had been reported sick by municipal authorities. After two weeks in hospital, the patient was found to be dying, not from infectious disease, but "probably from some internal cancerous growth, or general blood condition." Dr. A.S. Munro at Vancouver later reported to Scott that, despite the closure of the hospital, Indians continued to cause "considerable trouble" by "constantly coming to the office" for information and help "of every kind." Munro may have exaggerated the frequency of these visits, as he used them to justify requesting a pay raise to Dr. Milne's level.[16]

In late August, the *Province* reported that Munro had begun "a campaign to rid Vancouver and New Westminster of sick and indigent Hindus before the advent of winter." Fifteen had already been deported, and ten more were waiting to leave. Many of them were consumptives whose exposure to the cold of the previous winter had made them "easy victims to tuberculosis." In reality, only thirteen were deported in 1908; some of these left voluntarily, while others were expelled as public charges or for entering Canada illegally. Unfortunately, Immigration Branch records offer no clue about whether some, or indeed any, of these men had tuberculosis or other diseases.[17]

By fall, BC's continuing anti-Indian sentiment impelled the Dominion to consider expelling the South Asians who had entered before exclusion. Canada had investigated transplanting the group to Hawaiian sugar plantations in 1907, but this idea fell through after a sugar company employee met with Indians on the Pacific coast. While a coast newspaper reported that the Hawaiian Planters Association had canned the proposal because the Indians' "low standard of living and uncleanly habits do not appeal to us," Jensen posits that company officials likely abandoned the plan because they realized that Indians would not be happy with Hawaii's lower wages.[18] The same issue caused a similar plan to fail the following year, when Brigadier General Eric Swayne, the Governor of British Honduras, a colony that is now Belize, suggested to British officials that BC's Indians could solve Honduras's labour shortage.

When he arrived on the Pacific coast, Swayne found only around three thousand of the approximately five South Asians who had originally entered at BC, as many had left for the United States. Swayne became concerned, however, that the men who remained were earning much more than they could in India and had also been exposed to the west coast labour movement's socialist and anarchist doctrines. These factors, and their possible impact on India's political situation, affirmed Swayne's decision to pursue the plan. Swayne also fatefully recommended that Canada hire William Charles Hopkinson.[19]

While employed by the Dominion's Immigration Branch from early 1909 until his murder in Vancouver in 1914, Anglo-Indian Hopkinson, formerly a police inspector for the British Raj in Calcutta, was responsible for monitoring the activities of Pacific coast Indians. After his arrival in Canada, his fluency in Punjabi and Hindi quickly propelled him into a key role as Canadian immigration inspector in BC.[20] In October 1908, Hopkinson, along with Frank Oliver's private secretary J.B. Harkin and two "Hindu" representatives, travelled to Honduras to investigate Swayne's proposal for a voluntary mass relocation. Even before the scouting team arrived in Honduras, some members of BC's South Asian community opposed the move, likely because provincial labour conditions were improving. For example, a large sawmill on mainland BC announced that it would soon be hiring a thousand men. Even so, after the Honduras scouting company landed in November, Earl Grey strongly advised Laurier that Canada go ahead with the plan because it would "postpone for another generation the conflict between the White and Asiatic races."[21]

It was clear by December that J.B. Harkin's mission to Honduras had failed. When he travelled to Vancouver to present his findings that month, he found that the community was unwilling to move, in part because of the arrival of Indian independence activist Teja Singh. Singh, who had purchased a $40,000 industrial property for a "Hindoo Colony" in North Vancouver, offered work to all of the city's unemployed South Asians who were considering leaving Canada.[22] These efforts ensured the failure of the Honduras plan and frustrated the efforts of J.H. MacGill and other Immigration Branch officials in Vancouver who were attempting to deport indigent South Asians. In November, MacGill reported to Scott that he had made "no progress" in this regard, as Teja Singh's hiring of jobless Indians had resulted in 100 percent South Asian employment in the city. Furthermore, no Indians had visited the office to request help in finding work, evidently because community leaders had instructed the group to stay away from the authorities. Nevertheless, Scott instructed MacGill that all new Indian arrivals were to be excluded if they had not come on a through ticket from India; Scott added that "it is particularly desired that the Law should be strictly enforced with respect to immigrants of this class."[23]

The collapse of the Honduras plan forced officials to reconsider the climate argument that Indians were more comfortable in a tropical setting. As Earl Grey privately observed to Elgin, "[although] we have used the climate of Canada as a reason for prohibiting Hindu emigration," this "will not apply to the Sikhs, who have slept in the snows of the Himalayas." For this reason, he doubted that Canada could continue to bar Sikhs "without tasting trouble." The Governor General's opinion points to the difficulty Canada faced in finding and maintaining a non-racial rationale for keeping South Asians out of the Dominion. Grey suggested that Canada might be able to justify continuing Indian exclusion by arguing that it would maintain "the Purity of Race" by keeping "each colour to its own zone."[24] James Shaver Woodsworth, missionary, writer, and future founder of the social democratic Co-operative Commonwealth Federation – the forerunner of today's New Democratic Party – maintained that the Sikh physique and diet made the group constitutionally unfit for Canada's "rigorous climate," but he also agreed with Grey that the races should remain separate. In his important 1909 book *Strangers within Our Gates*, which called for increased government resources for immigrant welfare in Canada, Woodsworth explained that Indians could not compete industrially because they were slow and incapable of "hard, continuous exertion." Although "opinions differ as to the cleanliness of these Sikhs" in that they seemed "punctilious" in their "ablutions while in India," after arriving in BC "they have lived herded together in the most wretched fashion." Their refusal to give up their turbans gave the men a "grotesque" appearance. Overall, while Woodsworth sympathized with the group, he believed that their struggles were attributable to the fact that "however estimable they may be in India, they are sadly out of place in Canada."[25]

Woodsworth's emphasis on South Asian unassimilability embodied what Richard Day terms the popular "design theory of identity," which dominated early-twentieth-century Canadian nation-building, wherein the Dominion generally strove to exclude or deport non-white immigrant "classes" while encouraging immigration from Europe.[26] Most Canadians, including academics, continued to champion the preservation of ethnic and cultural homogeneity through assimilation. Woodsworth and others prescribed the use of socialization (by whites) to "convert Foreign Others into Anglo-Saxon selves."[27] Many in Ottawa shared Lord Grey's and Woodsworth's desire to maintain the spatial separation between Europeans and Asians. Some espoused this view more publicly than others; after Oliver openly called for total South Asian exclusion in a speech at Nelson, BC, in November, Laurier expressed dismay that his interior minister had forgotten Canada's imperial ties by "commit[ing] himself to this policy of blind exclusion." Yet King complained in his diary that Laurier privately shared Oliver's "narrow view" on Asian exclusion, as the prime minister often did on "matters of foreign policy and relations." This was partly because he was "surrounded by narrow men," but King also believed that Laurier "fears little from the Orient, and recognizes little or nothing in the way of Imperial obligation."[28] King further confided to his diary that the prime minister, and all Canadians, should understand that "if we are to have the protection of the British flag, we must share in the obligations its protection affords," including some concession on the immigration issue.[29] Unsurprisingly, King reversed his support for limited Indian immigration when he became prime minister thirteen years later, even when Opposition leader Arthur Meighen would have likely supported such a policy.

The South Asian immigration issue was already slipping out of public focus by the time King left for what Jensen has called his December "goodwill tour" in India.[30] On Earl Grey's advice, King followed a diplomatic trip to China with a visit to India, where he met with officials, publicized his 1908 Royal Commission report, and promoted good relations between Canada and India. In Calcutta he found that any government resentment of Canada's PC 920 had already ended: the Colony's Anglo-Indian officials told John Morley that they "raised no objection" to exclusion and did not plan to in the future. Overall, although King had failed in London that spring to compel India to restrict its own emigration, the continuous journey provision precluded the need for further discussion of the matter.[31]

BC's small South Asian community repeatedly protested the continuous journey provision in 1908 and 1909, but it was far too successful for Laurier to abandon. In May 1910, Oliver renewed PC 920 and PC 926. After the Immigration Branch learned that the Canadian Pacific Railway (CPR) might reintroduce South Asian immigration through direct ticketing from Calcutta, Scott privately suggested to Oliver that "as the question of subsidies for the CPR Pacific" would soon come up, "I think this would be a good time" to confer with the company on the issue. This supports Donald Avery's contention that the Dominion government's "strong pressure" discouraged the company from establishing a direct passenger service between Calcutta and Vancouver.[32]

With the important exception of Hopkinson's ongoing community surveillance in the province, federal involvement with BC's South Asians briefly subsided after 1908. The *Canadian Review of Public Affairs* eruditely recalled that compared to that year's dramatic exclusion of South Asians and failed Honduras scheme, "Canada's touch upon India was but slight" in 1909.[33] This trend continued in 1910, although the year saw important community organization, especially in Vancouver. The vast majority of the settlers from India were Sikh, but some were Muslim or Hindu, and members of these religions treated the newly established Vancouver Sikh temple as a "secular rallying point" where they engaged in regular religious meetings and social events. Others met at the Swadesh Sewak Home on Fairview Street, a hostel and Gurumukhi-language newspaper office established in 1908 by writer and activist Guran Ditt Kumar. In April 1910, Kumar collected signatures for a petition to the India Office protesting against legislative exclusion, although this brought no result.[34]

An average of only twenty-two immigrants from India arrived annually over the next five years, most of whom were previous residents. In contrast, an average of 610 Japanese and 4,464 Chinese immigrants entered each year over the same period. BC's South Asian population continued to shrink as its members left for the United States or returned to India. Virtually all left voluntarily, although one South Asian was ejected in June 1910 for having tuberculosis. With the exception of an immigrant sent back to India at his own request in 1908, this patient was the only South Asian to be deported for having that disease, although Hopkinson reported to Ottawa in 1910 that G.D. Kumar was also hospitalized for it. While Hopkinson predicted that the Indian political activist would soon pass away, in early 1911 Kumar surprised Hopkinson by fully recovering from what the inspector now realized was appendicitis.[35] The same year, the Immigration Branch made Hopkinson a permanent inspector in order to continue monitoring settlers from India, a full three years after exclusion had ended Indian immigration. This demonstrates the extent to which Immigration Branch officials prioritized the surveillance of the province's small number of South Asians.[36]

While Laurier had stemmed the flow of Indian immigration to Canada in 1908, political considerations prevented US president Theodore

Roosevelt from following suit. Roosevelt, whose term in office coincided with the height of first wave South Asian immigration to the Pacific coast states, refused to introduce an Indian exclusion measure because western congressional requests for South Asian exclusion almost always included a call for Japanese exclusion – something Roosevelt hoped to avoid. The president, who had moderated the Treaty of Portsmouth following Japan's naval victory in the Russo-Japanese war, realized that America's expanding presence in the Pacific depended on cordial relations with Japan. When San Francisco authorities disrupted these relations by segregating Japanese students in 1906, Roosevelt contained the situation first by ordering the city to desegregate its schools, and second by forging the informal 1907 Taft–Katsura "Gentlemen's Agreement" with Japan, a diplomatic solution to the Japanese immigration issue under which Japan agreed to restrict immigration to the continental United States. To satisfy nation-wide demands for tighter immigration controls on all racial groups, Roosevelt also expanded the moral and physical qualification for entry and doubled the general immigrant head tax from $2 to $4. These concessions appeased exclusionists to an extent sufficient to secure the Republican Party's nomination for Roosevelt's hand-picked successor, William Howard Taft, who would also oppose legislative South Asian exclusion.[37]

It thus fell to immigration officials to bar South Asians. While Joan Jensen asserts that executive restriction was initiated in 1908 at Pacific coast ports, especially San Francisco,[38] rejection statistics from Vancouver and Seattle in 1907 expand the parameters of this theory in both time and space. Just as Canadian officials introduced stringent screening measures to slow South Asian admissions at BC ports in the fall of 1907, Immigration Service (IS) and Public Health Service (PHS) officials used the same approach to decrease South Asian admissions at Vancouver and Seattle that year. Despite Dr. Billings's assertion in 1906 that the new immigrants were of "poor physique," this was a contestable grounds for exclusion, and officials thus rejected only 24 of 295 South Asian arrivals that year. However, a 1907 amendment to the US Immigration Act barred immigrants with physical defects and made the "Likely to Become a Public Charge" (LPC) designation a "Class A" (exclusion mandatory) ruling. Although "poor physique," a term generally associated with narrow-chestedness and susceptibility to tuberculosis, remained a "Class B" (appealable) designation, IS officials began to use a PHS "poor physique" label – which Howard Markel and Alexandra Stern call a "favorite 'wastebasket' label of nativist groups" – to assert that an immigrant was LPC.

The IS also deemed South Asians LPC for a major non-medical reason that will be discussed below. Together these efforts ensured the rejection rate of 417 in 1,072 arrivals at these ports in 1907, as shown in Table 3.[39]

In her discussion of the general enforcement of the US Immigration Act in this era, Amy Fairchild explains that, as major epidemics were generally in decline, and as passengers suspected of serious infection were generally quarantined before undergoing off-vessel inspection, PHS officials focused less on finding epidemic infections and more on identifying any physical and physiological factors that might impede an immigrant's working ability and social potential.[40] Anne-Emanuelle Birn adds that PHS inspectors used both "hereditarian theories of disease" and what Elizabeth Yew calls the "more democratic germ theory" to diagnose physical defects. Officials blamed "faulty genes" for mental and physiological deficiencies and poor constitutions, and blamed germs for contagious infections, including trachoma and tuberculosis.[41] Although bacteriology indicated that germs spread indiscriminately among every ethnic group, by the turn of the century PHS physicians had subscribed to the idea that certain races were inferior to others and therefore more likely to have certain

TABLE 3

South Asian Immigrant Admissions, Rejections, and Exits in the United States, 1900–14

Year	Admitted	Debarred	Returned
1899	15	0	0
1900	9	0	0
1901	20	1	0
1902	84	0	0
1903	83	0	1
1904	258	7	2
1905	145	13	0
1906	271	24	2
1907	1,072	417	0
1908	1,710	438	9
1909	337	331	1
1910	1,782	411	4
1911	517	862	36
1912	165	104	11
1913	188	236	32
Total	6,656	2,844	98

Source: "Memorandum regarding Hindu Migration to the United States," January 23, 1914, 1, E9, 52903, 110C, Records of the Immigration and Naturalization Service, Record Group 85, NARA.

Note: These figures do not include arrivals from US Pacific territories and Canada.

diseases and moral vices. Thus, PHS officers on the east coast carefully inspected Russians, Greeks, Armenians, and Syrians for trachoma, Jews from eastern Europe for both trachoma and favus, and Italians and Russians for mental deficiency. Overall, however, inspection at East coast ports facilitated inclusion much more than it did exclusion, which explains why less than 3 percent of Europeans were rejected for medical reasons at New York's Ellis Island in this period.[42]

While science on the east coast was employed to meet national industrial demands for a steady stream of healthy workers, along the Pacific it was instead used to "manage cultural and biological anxieties" by rigorously screening Asians. This approach was at least partly rooted in a tradition of racial stereotyping against Chinese peoples that had resulted in the initial inclusion of the LPC provision in the 1882 Immigration Act. Most medical rejections of Asians were for skin infections and especially trachoma, and the group was also checked for the easily diagnosable conditions of favus and head lice.[43] Yet since only a small fraction of the South Asian arrivals at Pacific Northwest PHS stations had these infections or any other "loathsome and contagious" disease, the LPC designation was a far more effective means of exclusion. At its highest rate of application at US ports and border points in 1908, the certification was applied to 25 per 100,000 immigrants of all nationalities, and usually reserved for chronic, non-contagious conditions such as deformities or heart and vision problems that could impair labour productivity.[44] Japanese immigrants were more likely to be designated LPC at Pacific ports, but the certification in these cases, "while annoying," was "not crucial." Roger Daniels points out that the LPC charge was used in only 7 percent of Japanese rejections in this period; in stark contrast, most of the 417 South Asians rejected at Pacific Northwest ports in 1907 were certified as LPC. Table 4 includes these rejections, along with US Pacific coast rejections of South Asians for other causes in the years 1900–13.[45]

Since the PHS labelled only some South Asian arrivals as having "poor physique," the majority of rejections were based on the assumption that the arrivals were likely to become public charges for another reason. IS agent J.H. Clark, the agent who first warned Washington officials in 1906 about the "Hindu menace," suggested that the IS brief its agents at northern Pacific ports on current "industrial conditions in Pacific Coast states," so that inspectors could use this information to assess South Asians hoping to reside in those areas.[46] In 1908, IS officers at Vancouver, Seattle, and Portland adopted this recommendation with gusto. Clark observed in

TABLE 4

Numbers of South Asians Rejected at US Pacific Ports, by Cause, 1900–13

Year ending June 30	Tuberculosis	Trachoma	Loathsome or contagious diseases	Surgeon's certificate*	Likely to become a public charge	Contract labourers	"Idiots"	Criminals	Polygamists	Other	Total	Deported
1900											0	0
1901					1						1	0
1902											0	0
1903											0	1
1904			3		4						7	2
1905					12	1					13	2
1906			6		10	5	2			1	24	2
1907			102		286	29					417	1
1908	1	192		107	118	20					438	9
1909		94	2	54	146	17		2	16		331	1
1910		161	7	18	200	7			18		411	4
1911	1	105	150	34	536	8	1		27		862	9
1912	1	7	21	5	58	4		2	3	3	104	3
1913	3	18	20	8	159	23		1	3	1	236	23

Source: "Number of East Indians Debarred during the Years 1900 to 1910, by Cause," *Reports of the Immigration Commission*, vol. 25, 61 Cong., 2 Sess., *Sen. Doc.* 633 (1911), 326. 1911 data from Table 17, "Aliens Debarred from Entering the United States, Fiscal Year Ended June 30, 1911, by Races or Peoples and Causes," *Report of the Commissioner General of Immigration* (Washington, 1911), 76–77. 1912 data from Table 17, "Aliens Debarred ... [to] 30 June 1912" *Report ...* (..., 1912), 130–31, and Table 18. "Aliens Deported to Countries Whence They Came, 1912," 134–35. 1913 data from Table 17, "Aliens Debarred ... [to] June 30, 1913" *Report ...* (..., 1913), 106–7, and Table 18, "Aliens Deported ... [to] June 1913," 110–11.

December that "our officers at Vancouver are exercising great care" in examining South Asians applying to enter Washington via that office. Many whites in Puget Sound were currently out of work, and thus the state's labour prospects were "decidedly unfavorable to the admission of Hindus"; this was a factor in the minds of the examining officers. In Portland, F.H. Larned, who had become Commissioner-General of Immigration after Sargent's death in the fall, dismissed the Board of Special Inquiry (BSI) appeal of two healthy South Asians, reasoning that Bhagwan, one of the men, probably would not be able to secure "employment of any kind" because "at this time racial prejudice and adverse labor conditions in the North-West will doubtless mitigate against him."[47]

Executive South Asian exclusion at these ports was attributable mainly to the consistent application of the LPC designation. The second justification for exclusion stemmed from an observation made by A.S. Hollis, an American Consul in South Africa in 1907. After the Bellingham Riot, he warned the State Department that most South Asians in the United States were polygamists. He asserted that since "every Mohamedan [*sic*] in the world is a polygamist," and since "a great proportion of the natives of Hindustan" were Muslim, America could easily exclude them as "alien polygamists" under the 1891 Immigration Act. However, since he doubted that most IS officials could "tell a polygamist when they see one," he declared that "whenever you find a circumcised colored man who is not a Christian, you can be absolutely sure that, at heart, he is a polygamist, no matter how much he may deny it."[48]

Immigration officials began to use the polygamy charge in combination with the LPC certification, especially at Seattle, where Commissioner P.L. Prentis declared that his Boards of Special Inquiry (BSIs) had turned away "every Hindu laborer" in 1910 for believing in polygamy or for being LPC, or for health reasons. Prentis elaborated that the polygamy charge qualified some, if not most, for blanket rejection; this finding exemplifies what Nayan Shah described as the IS's use of "racial taxonomies to predict male predisposition to polygamy."[49] Shah adds that "just as individual charges of polygamy were laid at the door of the entire ethnic group," another sexual issue also became an important barrier to South Asian admissibility. Since 1906, some western labour groups had maintained that South Asians were especially disposed to homosexual behaviour. Immigration officials agreed and expanded the LPC classification to include individuals likely to engage in "moral" offences; even a suspicion of sodomy could bar an otherwise ideal South Asian labourer from entry.[50] For this reason and the others discussed above, no new South Asian immigrants were admitted at Vancouver, Seattle, or Portland by 1909, although some circumvented executive restriction by entering illegally from Canada.

Illegal border crossings had long concerned IS agents in Washington, but the Bellingham and Vancouver Riots of 1907, and the entry at BC ports of 4,000 Japanese from Hawaii that year, exacerbated concerns that Asians were circumventing border controls. Puget Sound's many islands had long made it a "paradise" for human smugglers transporting Chinese immigrants from Canada, especially after the CPR mandated in 1903 that Chinese passengers proceeding directly from Vancouver to the United States had to cross a designated entry point for Chinese arrivals. Like the US border with Mexico, the border with Canada was becoming "part of the visible apparatus by which states attempt to effect state power." However, Patrick Ettinger explains that the "gradual elaboration" of the border occurred "in the midst of consistently successful efforts to undermine it," as the era saw both "the simultaneous 'drawing' and 'erasing'" of the international boundary by officials and human smugglers.[51]

Oral history accounts do suggest that surreptitious border crossings occurred during this period. First wave arrival Imanat Ali Khan, a participant in the Indo-Canadian Oral History Collection, recalled walking across the international border during his seasonal migrations in this period. After working until the fall at an Astoria mill earning $2 a day, Khan and several friends avoided unemployment in the winter by securing lower-paying mill work in Fraser Mills, BC. The group accomplished border crossings into the United States by bribing IS officials or by crossing the borderlands on foot early in the morning and hiding at a "white saloon" until nightfall, when they walked up to ten miles to reach a rendezvous point in Washington.[52]

In late 1907, immigrant inspector Marcus Braun arrived in Washington to report on surreptitious border crossings. Kornel Chang shows that Braun's investigation was the result of public outcry over "the popular image of a leaky US–Canadian boundary being deluged by sneaky Orientals." After recent investigative work in Europe and along the Mexican border, Braun had become a key IS advocate for better border patrol, as he believed a well-protected border to be, in Chang's words, "a vital operational feature of the modern state." Braun's report on conditions along the Washington–BC international boundary "confirmed public sentiments" by describing the border as a "porous line" easily susceptible to Asian human smuggling. To remedy this situation, Braun recommended that the IS station sixty additional agents along the border, which was the same number of agents responsible for patrolling the 1,900-mile-long US–Mexico border in 1907.[53] This request for increased border supervision might have been overlooked if not for September's anti-Asian riots. "Indeed," Chang argues, "perhaps no single event or development did more for the cause of border security than the anti-Asian upheavals in Vancouver and Bellingham," as the racial tension precipitated by the riot "helped to spawn a new system of surveillance and control that would make a once invisible boundary in the Pacific Northwest visible."[54]

Although Commissioner-General of Immigration Frank Sargent warned his superiors that some of Braun's statements were "based upon erroneous premises and assumptions," he echoed Braun's opinion that "if the immigration of Hindus is not soon controlled there will arise on the Pacific coast a 'Hindu question' which will make the 'Japanese question' look like child's play." Braun had erroneously asserted that South Asians were being brought in as contract workers who were already illegally employed before their arrival; he was accurate, however, in stating that feeling against the group was "more bitter than against any other class of Asiatics." Sargent commented that these findings showed the "gravity of the situation" and would hopefully "make possible even a closer scrutiny and examination [of South Asians] than in the past" at Washington ports and border points.[55] Heeding Braun's warnings, Sargent ordered an increase in inspectors at the port of Seattle and watchmen to patrol the numerous roads that crossed the international boundary line in 1908.[56] This, however, had almost no effect on Indian immigration, as the legislative exclusion in place in BC, and the executive exclusion in place at IS stations in Vancouver, Seattle, and Portland, impelled most South Asian migrants to land directly at San Francisco.

The previous chapter showed that in 1907, the simultaneous appearance of South Asians in California and reappearance of plague in San Francisco caused significant anxiety. Many California residents connected the two phenomena before actually seeing a turbaned worker in their community; for example, the *Los Angeles Herald* warned in September 1907 that "scores" of South Asians would soon be arriving in the southern part of the state, "carrying with them the germs of the dread bubonic plague."[57] While this assertion was never proven, surviving IS San Francisco rejection certificates from 1908 indicate that, like immigrants from other nations, some South Asians were sick; for example, at least sixteen of those rejected in 1908 had trachoma, while at least six others had physical deformities or were addicted to narcotics. Yet the low rejection rate due to disease before 1910 indicates that most South Asian arrivals were healthy; of the 438 excluded in 1908, only 118 were certified as having a medical defect or illness, while the rest were presumably LPC for the factors discussed above.[58]

At San Francisco, the last Pacific coast port accepting South Asians, arrivals dropped dramatically from 1,710 in 1908 to only 337 in 1909. The efforts of US consular officials in India offer one explanation for the decline. With the approval of the State Department, US Consul General at Calcutta W.H. Michael refused to issue visas to some prospective migrants on the grounds that conditions in the United States were unfavourable for South Asian immigrant labour. However, diplomats like Michael could not bar South Asians outright because, while a visa often ensured a smoother entry at US entry points, the document was not officially required until 1917.[59] Therefore, the main explanation for the decline was the IS's self-appointed policy of executive restriction. In 1908, William R. Wheeler, the acting labour secretary and an Asian exclusionist from San Francisco, sustained this policy, ordering immigration officers there to exclude South Asians en masse using the LPC designation. However, when labor secretary Oscar Straus returned from his vacation shortly thereafter, he "ordered the officers to resume the old policies." Consequently, although immigration officers were broadly implementing executive restriction by mid-1909, South Asians continued to be admitted at San Francisco, albeit in diminished numbers.[60]

Although they were less influential on admission levels, two other groups played a key role in the social transactions governing the popular reception of South Asians by California's white communities. First, politicians in California galvanized public opinion against Asians generally. Even after the conclusion of the 1907 Gentlemen's Agreement with Japan, and after Roosevelt, ever unpopular in California for his "soft" Asian policies, left office in 1909, state legislators, reflecting the wishes of their constituents, advocated tighter controls on Asian settlement and landownership. State politicians, whose predecessors had played a vital role in the passage of the federal Chinese Exclusion Act of 1882, continually protested against what they perceived as federal inaction on Asian immigration.[61]

The San Francisco–based Asiatic Exclusion League (AEL) also mobilized public opinion against South Asians. Just as the Bellingham press had blamed that town's riot on South Asian living conditions, AEL President A.E. Yoell asserted that the "immodest and filthy habits of the Hindoos" made them "at fault" for the "trouble, beatings and otherwise" they experienced in California.[62] Yoell, whose organization had recently been renamed from the "Japanese and Korean Exclusion League" to include South Asians, was referring to the local reaction to the newcomers in the city and in the Sacramento and San Joaquin valleys. In 1908, local whites in the town of Stege threw rocks at Indian–occupied bunkhouses, and citizens of Live Oak drove seventy South Asian Southern Pacific Railroad workers out of town; similar disturbances occurred in West Berkeley, where Indians lived in "three Hindoo colonies." Yoell attributed this response to the newcomers' "utter disregard ... [for] the decencies of life" and to their choice to "herd together in miserable hovels which, if permitted to exist, will soon invite disease and epidemic."[63]

In response to similar treatment in Oregon, a South Asian living in Portland appealed for fair treatment from the local populace by denying, in a letter to the editor of a local newspaper, that Indian immigrants were "Dirty or Undesirable." He argued that his countrymen were "decent, law-abiding men," and added that he was learning English at night school "and the practical things that will make me a good American." Legal scholar Hon. A.G. Burnett, an Associate Justice of the District Court of Appeals of California in Sacramento, similarly argued in a 1909 paper that "England's half-starved, superstitious, caste-bound Hindus," had actually been "none too truthfully portrayed" by "the fascinating pen of Kipling." However, this represented a minority opinion on the coast.[64]

In 1910, despite a decline in South Asian admissions the previous year, Yoell censured US labor secretary Oscar Straus for not implementing blanket Indian exclusion at San Francisco and for allowing in "a great many of those afflicted with Oriental diseases, particularly trachoma," at San Francisco's newly opened quarantine station on Angel Island in San Francisco Bay. Between 1891 and 1910, the island's north cove was the site of a PHS quarantine facility for vessels from Asia, while passenger inspection and formal processing was carried out at the Pacific Mail docks on San Francisco harbour. After it opened in January 1910, the shared IS/PHS facility on Angel Island's Winslow cove served as America's chief point of entry for Asian immigrants for thirty years, processing close to 341,000 immigrants and returning residents between 1910 and its closure in 1940. The *San Francisco Call* reported that one of the station's first residents was a "lone and gloomy Hindu" aboard a boat transferring Chinese detainees from San Francisco; close to 8,000 more South Asians would land at the station over the next few years. Here, all arrivals were separated by race, quarantined for several days, medically inspected by

PHS physicians, and interviewed and processed by IS agents. Continuing a policy established years before at San Francisco, all Asian arrivals were carefully screened for trachoma, lice, and other non-fatal contagious conditions.[65]

David Hernandez explains that the island, which opened in an era "where there was no military threat or crisis in which to rationalize the scapegoating of non-white migrants," was designed mainly to process Chinese students, tourists, merchants, and their families travelling in steerage and second class. The facility also served to contain fears of disease and to "stunt the reception and growth of the Chinese community." The Asian inspection process contrasted significantly with the experience of Russians and other Europeans who arrived at the facility. Whites arriving at San Francisco in steerage were also required to stop at the island, but they were inspected, detained, and processed separately from Asians and generally spent less time at the station.[66]

In their recent work on the history of the station, Erika Lee and Judy Yung detail Hyatt Hart North's brief career as the first commissioner of Angel Island, including the controversy surrounding his administration of immigration legislation. Lee and Yung explain that North's policy of "treat[ing] South Asians like other immigrant groups," and his insistence on "process[ing] them under the general immigration laws," conflicted with the policies of Asian exclusionists and even with some members of North's own staff, who wanted the commissioner to continue the IS's general strategy of using the LPC designation to bar South Asians. Inspector Frank Ainsworth, North's subordinate, personally believed that South Asians could not assimilate into American society, and therefore he urged North to sanction their wholesale exclusion. After North admitted several hundred South Asians into the country by mid-1910 – easily surpassing the number allowed in during the whole of 1909 – the AEL took its case to officials in Washington, DC. After a well-publicized series of allegations of misconduct flew between North and Ainsworth, North was removed from duty in late 1910.[67]

While North remained in charge in 1910, the *San Francisco Bulletin* urged him to apply the executive restriction of South Asians already in place at IS stations at Seattle, Portland, and Vancouver. The *Bulletin*'s editor and others advised him to simply reject the group as polygamists, but he refused to use this as a uniform exclusion tactic, for he had learned that most Indian arrivals were Sikh and thus were unlikely to have multiple wives. San Francisco's press perpetuated the Indian polygamy charge throughout the summer, especially after North let in close to one hundred South Asians per month and told the city's press that he could not exclude all South Asians en masse. However, press allegations of South Asian disease and uncleanliness greatly eclipsed the polygamy issue. For example, the *Chronicle* called South Asians "by far the worst of the Orientals in their personal habits"; although the writer optimistically projected that medical officials would find many diseased Indians among the two hundred who arrived on the SS *Manchuria* in February, the PHS rejected only nine, for what records indicate was trachoma. The *San Francisco Call* thus anxiously reported that more South Asians had entered by March than had arrived in the whole of 1909.[68]

By mid-year, the IS was faced with a difficult problem. Some of the South Asians arriving at Angel Island were being rejected by the PHS for "physical unfitness" or "poor physique," but most were free of "loathsome or contagious diseases." South Asian immigration continued at Angel Island because, in the continuing absence of congressional "anti-Hindu" legislation, North was refusing to follow the IS policy in place at Seattle, Portland, and Vancouver of barring the whole group outright as polygamists or LPC. In April, Daniel J. Keefe, the new Commissioner-General of Immigration and a former labour leader, attempted to solve the issue after his supervisor, assistant labor secretary Benjamin S. Cable, advised him that most Indians arriving at Angel Island were, in fact, LPC. Keefe reprimanded North for allowing in so many South Asians, reminding him that while no law excluded "Hindus as a race," there was "considerable prejudice" against them in the Pacific coast states. He ordered that "prejudice" alone should be "an important fact in determining whether an alien shall be permitted to land," and added that "these instructions should also be observed with regard to the primary inspection" and at BSI hearings.[69]

Keefe, who viewed South Asians as inassimilable in American society, championed the methods recently used by white British colonies to halt immigration from India, including rejection of indigents and the "contagiously diseased." Indeed, Keefe's objective, Shah explains, was for "zero admissions from India, using health inspections to satisfy a political constituency of white working-class residents" who vehemently opposed the South Asian presence in their communities. Keefe justified his approach by reasoning that South Asians could not secure or maintain employment because of the strong discrimination against them, and their resulting vagrancy would exacerbate existing tensions. After rejecting criminals and paupers, Keefe recommended, in Shah's words, "eliminating the rest by focusing medical scrutiny" on those with physical deformities or "poor physiques."[70]

Just as the early years of the century saw a rise in PHS rejections for various chronic, non-fatal conditions that could render an immigrant LPC, PHS agents at Angel Island, like their counterparts in other ports, applied a "Class B" designation when they suspected, but could not prove, infection or even susceptibility to non-pulmonary tuberculosis. Despite the Surgeon General's concern in 1907 that "the term has been considered by the board of inquiry as a stronger term" than the PHS intended, PHS physicians at New York City's Ellis Island also used this diagnosis, especially on eastern European Jews with "weak posture" or deformed shoulders. However, three factors tempered its effect on Jewish admission levels at Ellis Island. First, at this station as at every immigration facility, the PHS served as "advisers" to IS agents, whose ultimate decision it was whether to accept or reject an immigrant. The fact that "Class B" conditions were excludable at the discretion of the IS meant that BSI examiners could be swayed by "the immigrant's negotiating skills and resources." The second factor, local community involvement in New York City, helped many Jewish immigrants appeal rulings against them. Third and finally, since Jews as Europeans were eligible to naturalize after their establishment in the United States, their "citizenship status" on arrival was "more secure than that of Asian Immigrants."[71]

In his discussion of the treatment of eastern European Jews at the port of Galveston, Texas, Alan Kraut has shown that many of the 10,000 Jewish immigrants who arrived at that port in 1910 faced executive exclusion that more closely mirrored the South Asian experience at Angel Island. Under the direction of one anti-Semitic medical examiner, the number of rejections for "poor physique" rose dramatically in that year. Even after the PHS replaced the medical team at Galveston, "marginal calls often went against Jewish immigrants." Kraut asserts that overall, it is "very likely" that "local pressures to exclude as many eastern European Jews as possible ... created an atmosphere in which some Galveston medical inspectors were willing to cooperate with local immigration opponents by misdiagnosing diseases certifiable for exclusion."[72] There are several similarities between the Jewish experience at Galveston and the South Asian experience at Angel Island, which was the only station still admitting immigrants from India. Jews and South Asians were both legally entitled to immigrate, provided that they were healthy and met the moral and financial requirements of entry; but both groups lacked a local support network. Moreover, bowing to California exclusionists, Keefe advocated a policy of extra-stringent "primary inspection" to bar as many South Asians as possible, while medical examiners at Galveston intentionally misdiagnosed Jewish arrivals to limit their numbers.

Keefe's instruction that South Asians be examined more strictly increased the number of Indian rejections at Angel Island. Even so, the AEL, ratcheting up its campaign against North's leadership at the station, maintained that North's staff were still allowing undesirable South Asian labourers to immigrate; these newcomers would soon "constitute a serious menace to the health, happiness and welfare of the community." O. Tveitmoe, the AEL's new president, claimed that South Asians recently arrived on the SS *Manchuria* and *Siberia* in April would, like their countrymen already in California, soon become public charges because they were "unspeakably filthy and in nearly every instance suffering from contagious and incurable diseases." Another AEL member called attention to "the dangers of infection being carried into the city by the East Indians," and warned that the immigrants would bring about a new plague epidemic in the city. The *Call* added that some of the steerage stewards of liners from Asia called South Asians' personal habits "filthy," and that the employers of Indian immigrants found them "dirty, lazy and shiftless and altogether lacking in initiative."[73]

Congressman Julius Kahn, who represented California's 4th District, made similar assertions two weeks later in a letter to Keefe. During a western train journey, Kahn noted that most of the section crews he could see during his two-hundred-mile trip along the Western Pacific line were South Asian, and predicted that the group would soon replace whites in all occupations "within a couple of generations." In a private letter, he asked Keefe to stem South Asian immigration, noting that California's Indian immigrants were unkempt and in "poor physical condition" and that he had heard that these tropical immigrants "can not stand the rigors of a northern climate."[74] Many Californians would have agreed with his assertion that South Asians were dirty. In August, Leon Ray Livingston, a famous American sojourner who later published a book detailing his cross-country travels with the writer Jack London, asked the labor secretary to implement Indian exclusion because South Asians were "the lowest, filthiest, disgusting people I ever saw"; he warned that thousands of them were "overrunning" California. Similarly, even though shower facilities were almost non-existent on transpacific steamships, San Francisco reporters strongly censured Indians for arriving unwashed at Angel Island.

Paradoxically, journalists also criticized those South Asians who managed to arrive clean. The *Call* reported in August that a newly arrived group of Indians were "rather cleaner than some of the earlier arrivals" because, according to some of the ship's workers, the group had "luxuriated in scant and filthy attire during the voyage" until the day before they arrived, when each put on a "comparatively clean suit" over his underclothes and turned his turban inside out.[75]

San Francisco reporters announced with relief that Dr. W.F. McNutt, the city's Health Officer, had a plan to address the South Asian "invasion" in the face of North's inaction on the issue. In his annual report to City Council, McNutt recapped his May 1910 suggestion that

> inasmuch as this city is located on the Western hemisphere, and the influx of Hindus and other Asiatics with the consequent danger of the importation of tropical diseases such as Amoeba, Uncinariasis [hookworm], Beri Beri, etc., presented a conditions of affairs that would require the attention of the Health Department to properly regulate, it was recommended that the scope of the work of the Bacteriological Laboratory be enlarged to the extent of adding an assistant whose duty it would be to engage in research Work.

McNutt added that "the results obtained would not alone benefit San Francisco and the Pacific Coast, but the entire United States as well."[76]

This proposal appeared to represent a scathing critique of Angel Island's medical inspectors, who supposedly were holding open California's door to masses of disease-ridden South Asians. The AEL's Yoell concurred, securing written statements of support for his "anti-Hindu" campaign from six California state senators in response to his claim that fifteen South Asians who had recently landed at San Francisco had trachoma.[77] It is highly unlikely that these assertions were true. Like other PHS examiners at Pacific coast ports, inspectors at San Francisco had long abandoned the "line inspection" used at Ellis Island, where inspectors superficially examined large numbers of Europeans by observing them as a group. Instead, medical officers at Angel Island subjected South Asians, along with all other Asian arrivals, to thorough, hands-on inspections. At Angel Island, physicians used their "medical gaze" to examine naked or nearly naked Asians for easily recognizable medical conditions, used stethoscopes to listen to the heart, inverted eyelids to look for trachoma, tested saliva for traces of beriberi, and, with increasing frequency by 1910, conducted bacteriological tests for parasitic infection. While Asians and Europeans travelling first class were not required to stop at the station, virtually all Asians travelling in steerage – the vast majority of Asian travellers – were brought to Angel Island and subjected to these tests, regardless of social position.[78] According to Amy Fairchild, "disease interacted with race to undercut class distinctions prevailing in most other regions," especially after 1912, when Asians arriving by second class passage were also detained at Angel Island.[79]

But the greatest difference between Ellis and Angel Islands was in the philosophy governing the duties of medical inspectors. Physicians tasked with inspecting Europeans at Ellis Island spent less time with each immigrant, used less technology, and overall had "few resources devoted to exclusion." Fairchild explains that this was the direct "consequence of a decision to admit a tremendous and relatively unimpeded flow of immigrant labor." According to Fairchild, this policy "necessitated a processing or disciplining rather than a screening regimen at the nation's borders," which was why, generally, "the laboratory was not necessary" at eastern ports. Government policy regarding Asian admissions at Angel Island, the nation's major gateway to the Pacific, was dramatically different. Here, medical officers routinely "racializ[ed] disease" by applying what Shah calls "special scrutiny" to Asian groups, whom PHS physicians believed were at special risk for "Oriental" diseases and physical disorders. Paradoxically, the island's detention facilities for Asians placed these individuals at significant risk for cross-infection. When the station first opened in 1910, officials complained that the facility was a fire hazard, already unsanitary, plagued with vermin, and cramped; one room with cubic air space sufficient for ten individuals contained fifty-four beds. For these reasons, Daniel J. Keefe, the Commissioner-General of Immigration, soon recommended that the facility be scrapped and rebuilt elsewhere, but it remained open until a fire forced its permanent closure in 1940.[80]

But for as long as he remained in charge, until October 1910, North refused to summarily reject South Asians. The low disease rate among the group – probably due to steamship companies in Hong Kong performing scrupulous medical inspections of all South Asians before allowing their passage to America – continued to complicate matters for his staff and the PHS inspectors stationed there. Dr. M.W. Glover, a PHS physician stationed at the Island's detention hospital, reported that since opening in January, the hospital had treated 137 South Asians, compared to 136 Chinese and 6 Japanese; however, the majority of these Indians had trachoma, which passengers with financial means could pay station doctors to treat. Although treatment for trachoma could cost up to $300, most of those with the disease chose this option, and indeed in June the PHS certified and deported only seventeen South Asians for trachoma among the "large crowds of East Indians" who arrived on passenger vessels that month.[81]

But what to do with the rest, whom Keefe and the IS had expressly discouraged the station's officials from admitting into the country? Angel Island staff increasingly turned to the ambiguous LPC certification. In June, North overturned IS agent Frank Ainsworth's decision to use this reason to bar several South Asian passengers from the SS *Siberia*; Ainsworth's resulting appeal to Washington, DC led to the reinstatement of the original order. Keefe also sent commissioner Fred Watts to Angel Island, where Watts personally rejected eighty of a vessel's 164 South Asians for being LPC, after submitting them to a "rigid examination, which they could not pass." Despite these efforts, San Francisco residents were alarmed by the continuing arrival of South Asians at Angel Island, where, the *Call* blithely opined in August, "Sahib Hart North" heartily welcomed them to America after only a cursory examination. A *Call* reporter remarked that local residents regarded Sikh turbans in particular with "a good deal of suspicion"; after living alongside South Asians, many whites with "an elementary knowledge of the germ theory" were now convinced that "the turban was not a pleasant thing to have around." South Asians used it as a "combined hat, handkerchief and towel," and while the outside was generally clean, the reporter reasoned that "it would take a bacteriologist to write the story of the inside."[82]

For opponents of South Asian labour, the Sikh turban was perhaps the greatest symbol of the inherent foreignness and "caste prejudices" of South Asian workers. Herman Scheffauer's popular article "The Tide of Turbans" declared that the "affrighted pale-face[d]" western populations were under siege by the "turbaned'" Hindu. Like Scheffauer, many others attributed the turban, long hair, and other male Sikh customs to Hinduism. When, in 1907, Los Angeles mayor Arthur Cyprian Harper warned that South Asians would soon "flood" his city, the *Los Angeles Herald* printed "bright upstate" twelve-year-old Ica Schulz's advice on how to get rid of the new arrivals. She wrote that "I know of a way which worked like a charm in Chico. That is to get them when they first come and cut three or four of the Hindus' hair short. Then they will leave right away." Other California residents assumed that the Sikhs in their state were not Hindu but Muslim.

US federal Senator Frank Putnam Flint of Los Angeles declared that California had no place for "[Muslim] fakirs and mendicants." San Francisco's police chief also assumed that all Indian immigrants were Muslim, even in 1910, after thousands of predominantly Sikh South Asians had arrived in his state. At this time he purchased a copy of the Koran for Indian prisoners to swear upon in court, which he believed prepared his jail for "the threatened inundation of Hindoo immigrants."[83] These mistaken assumptions broadly affirm Jennifer Snow's argument that "one of the most striking aspects of the race–religion equation was the collapse, in the popular mind, of all Asian religions into one racial 'civilization.'"[84]

While the "Hindoo religion" resurfaced in press and other reports on South Asians in 1910, disease remained the dominant theme in US Pacific coast discourse on the "Hindu" problem. A special "Hindu" edition of the AEL's monthly magazine *The White Man*, whose subscribers included the California and Washington branches of the Central Labor Council and Trades and Labor Assembly, described South Asians as bearers of "moral and social diseases" and the "virus of Asian degeneracy." Editor A.F. Fowler, who had risen to some prominence during Vancouver's 1907 riot, described South Asians as "the Filth of Asia" who spread "leprosy, bubonic plague, beri beri, trachoma and other terrible diseases of the body." Fowler also made the sensational claim that "weird orgies take place in the Hindu settlements throughout the state," and added that the Sikh burial custom of cremation contaminated California's countryside. He argued that "sanitary science should be applied sociologically" to halt Indian immigration and prevent the nation from becoming "a modern Babylonia, saturated with the physical and moral rottenness of the world."[85]

Fowler's contentions about South Asian health won him at least two major supporters in California. Governor Hiram Johnson backed Fowler's call for an end to Indian immigration; that summer, after receiving a copy of *The White Man*, he asserted that he "favor[ed] exclusion." In August, William R. Wheeler, former assistant labor secretary, sent the "Hindu" edition of the magazine to labor commissioner Charles Neill, a civil servant in Washington, DC charged with investigating labour conditions, to request that he influence IS policy on South Asian immigration. Wheeler, now representing the nativist San Francisco–based California Immigration Commission, reminded Neill that in the writer's former capacity as assistant secretary, he had "sustained the US Immigration officials stationed at Vancouver, BC in their refusal to permit to Hindus to migrate from BC to American ports," on the grounds that they were LPC. Wheeler informed

Neill that with South Asians now travelling directly from Hong Kong to San Francisco, the new labor secretary, Charles Nagel, "told me that he proposed to adopt the policy which I had inaugurated but which Secretary Straus had not favored after his return from his summer vacation in 1908." Using Fowler's sensationalistic claims in *The White Man* as evidence, he warned that "their general anemic appearance, their slavery to caste," and "the strong sentiment existing on the Pacific coast against their employment" made them especially likely to become public charges. He likened South Asians, who often camped on riverbeds while unemployed, to "the Gypsies who, on account of their nomadic life, have been excluded from Atlantic coast ports." He concluded that "*it seems to me that the Administration is justified in adopting any policy which will keep these undesirables out.*"[86]

Also in August, American Consul General to India William H. Michael redoubled his efforts to shape federal policy on the issue. After his superiors approved his previous efforts to discourage South Asian immigration to the United States, Michael advised them to bar a vessel of several hundred Punjabis en route to San Francisco. He reported that after interviewing the individuals who had applied at his office in Calcutta for medical inspection by a "medical attaché" to the consulate, he had "invariably rejected them," not for health problems but because he believed that most only intended to work in the United States for a year and not become permanent settlers; this was the same "sojourner" argument applied against Chinese immigration. When other prospective immigrants began to avoid requesting visas at his office, Michael advised steamship agents in Hong Kong to stop selling them tickets. He warned that California would soon be "overrun" with South Asians unless the government intervened. After receiving Michael's August cable from the State Department, assistant labor secretary Benjamin S. Cable announced "a policy of increased restrictions" for South Asian immigration, which would apply what the *Chronicle* called "a broader construction of the law than generally obtains" for other immigrants. The paper's editorial the following day commended Cable's policy of keeping out "the Hindoo coolies," who were "the dirtiest and most degraded of Asiatics": in fact, the editor argued, "compared with them the Chinese, and even the Japs, are angels of light."[87]

The rejections of South Asians at Angel Island increased again following Cable's instructions. By late August, PHS officers at the station were barring the majority of Indian immigrants as "physically unfit"; IS officials were rejecting others for being LPC. An Indian newspaper observed that the most recent ship from Hong Kong had returned 150 South Asians to

India, most of whom had been sent away from Angel Island after a twelve-day quarantine for "physical unfitness." In response to the escalating rejection rate, steamship companies, anxious about returning passengers, increased their own physical inspections of South Asians in China. In September, several coast newspapers reported that vessels destined for San Francisco now carried only a fraction of the South Asians who had wanted to purchase tickets; for example, the *San Francisco Call* stated that the SS *Siberia* had turned down all but twenty-two of the three hundred South Asians who had sought tickets in Hong Kong. It was also public knowledge that the IS had briefed its Angel Island BSI members on "the characteristics of the Hindoos, which, in the bureau's estimation, are likely to cause them to be public charges."[88]

On September 9, labor secretary Charles Nagel, Straus's successor, arrived in San Francisco to inspect the South Asian immigrants at Angel Island. The *Call* reported that the secretary had seen the "dark scum of Asia float unrestrained through the Golden Gate" when the SS *China* arrived at the station with dozens of South Asians on its decks. After meeting with H.H. North, Mayor P.H. McCarthy, and William Wheeler, Nagel told the *Chronicle* that he would consider issuing an order to his officers to "restrict such immigration as far as possible under the law."[89] But before he had the chance to draft these instructions, PHS physician M.W. Glover, Angel Island medical inspector, made a startling discovery that finally enabled the IS to do what it had strived for since 1906. On September 20, Glover announced that a large number of South Asians currently detained at the station had the "loathsome and contagious disease" of hookworm, a "Class A" excludable condition under the Immigration Act.

The preceding pages have shown how, in BC, the polyvalent deployment of the climate and disease theses – especially the latter – continued to influence both popular and official responses to South Asians in the period immediately following legislative exclusion. When the province's small South Asian community refused to move en masse to Honduras, thus challenging the climate theory that South Asians were inherently more comfortable in a tropical setting, BC politicians, labour leaders, press editors, and others renewed and expanded the association between South Asians and disease. This chapter has also demonstrated that South Asians' reputation for transmitting infection had been planted in the popular imagination by the repeated association of the group with a series of illness, including Oriental sore in 1908, "tropical disease" in 1909, and leprosy and beriberi in 1910, to name just a few. Although these allegations were never confirmed, they succeeded in singling out South Asian immigrants and would endure among several sectors of Pacific coast society.

American PHS officials diagnosed some South Asian arrivals at Pacific coast ports with "poor physique" – an assertion that was difficult to prove, as was the related contention that South Asians threatened public health. While the IS's LPC ruling was a stronger means of executive restriction, this pretext for exclusion could be challenged as a reason for barring an entire immigrant group. Since the American executive continued to stall on legislative exclusion for political reasons, what exclusionists (including those in the IS) needed was unassailable medical evidence that could confirm what a large number of Pacific coast residents already "knew" about the new arrivals, and, by extension, what they believed about the racial inferiority of South Asians to other groups. The next chapter will explain how American and Canadian officials alike championed the discovery of hookworm among South Asians at Angel Island as concrete proof that immigrants from India threatened population health and, furthermore, how this perception cemented South Asians as medical scapegoats for coast-area disease outbreaks, just as the Chinese of San Francisco had been scapegoated during the plague outbreaks of the previous decade.

4

Amoebic and Social Parasites, 1910–13

We don't want the standard of living of the Hindoo; we don't want his religion; we don't want his diseases; we don't want his filth.

> – *Vallejo, California, Trades and Labor Congress,*
> *September 13, 1913*

Although at first I was strongly prejudiced against them I lost this prejudice after thousands of them had passed through my hands ...
I refer in particular to the Sikhs and I am not exaggerating in the least when I say that they were 100 per cent cleaner in their habits and freer from disease than the European steerage.

> – *E.H. Lawson, MD, September 25, 1913*

IN SEPTEMBER 1910, DR. M.W. Glover, a PHS medical inspector at San Francisco's Angel Island immigration station, found hookworm ova in the stools of six anemic South Asians who had recently arrived on the SS *Chiyo Maru*. The physician then found the same ova in 60 percent of the other South Asian hospital patients, including several who exhibited no obvious symptoms of the disease. Press reports on the discovery used it to retrospectively diagnose the large numbers of South Asians whom the PHS had recently and mysteriously rejected for "poor physique." Journalists also speculated that the association of South Asians with hookworm, a "Class A" (medically excludable) disease, would effectively halt a wave of immigration that was already in decline since earlier in the year.[1] Previous chapters of this book detailed the germination and perpetuation of the "Hindu disease" thesis on the Pacific coast after 1906. The normalization of this thesis among all sectors of Pacific coast society prepared the ground for the massive popular and official reaction to Glover's discovery of this relatively minor (and curable) parasitic infection in South Asians.

Moving forward with this conclusion, this chapter makes three major claims: first, while US immigration officials were already in the process of shutting out South Asian arrivals at San Francisco, the IS used the hookworm finding to complete this process at that port and to close a loophole in executive restriction at all Pacific ports shortly thereafter. Second, Pacific coast observers interpreted the hookworm discovery as proof that the new arrivals carried dangerous "Oriental" diseases. Third, Canadian immigration officials mobilized Glover's finding at San Francisco to prepare to meet challenges to the Dominion's exclusionary legislation.

Historians suggest that South Asian rejections at San Francisco for "poor physique" in the months preceding Glover's discovery were largely a result of IS pressure to reduce immigration from India. Nayan Shah explains that Glover's bacteriological testing of the anemic South Asian passengers of the *Chiyo Maru* "had been spurred by an internal crisis over medical exclusion procedures," after IS officer Frank Ainsworth publicly accused Angel Island Commissioner Hart H. North of admitting South Asians despite the PHS certification that they were physically unfit to enter as immigrants. In an internal investigation into North's leadership, Glover testified that IS officials could not determine an immigrant's employability without a complete medical inspection. Thus, "in a move calculated to bolster the PHS's authority to determine physical fitness," Glover had used his microscope to expand his inspection capabilities and "provide specialized knowledge of an immigrant's capabilities and the precise cause of an immigrant's disability."[2]

Since Glover's initial sample size was only twenty-two individuals, sixteen of whom were infected, assertions linking most South Asians with hookworm represented the logical fallacy of hasty generalization. Yet Shah points out that inspectors at Angel Island – the last US Pacific port accepting South Asian arrivals before Glover's discovery – "emphasized the unassailable expertise of the medical examiner's diagnosis,"[3] and observers in the press attributed the recent slump in South Asian admissions to the disease. Utah's *Ogden Evening Standard* opined that "the average Hindu looks as though something had been gnawing at his insides"; since hookworm reduced the vitality of its carrier, Glover's findings made sense. The *San Francisco Bulletin* similarly asserted that the diagnosis was unsurprising as "the average Hindu, from time immemorial, has been peculiarly susceptible to many abhorrent physical afflictions." After San Francisco tropical disease expert Bruce Foulkes corroborated Glover's initial findings at the quarantine station, the *Bulletin* correctly predicted that soon "the turbaned natives of the Punjab will be a rarity at Angel Island."[4]

In his October report to Surgeon General Walter Wyman, Glover explained that his sudden rise to fame in San Francisco after his *Chiyo Maru* findings had resulted from newspapers making "undue sensation over anything that would tend to disbar the Hindu immigrant." Yet since 111 more South Asians had just arrived on the SS *Asia*, he would look for traces of the disease "in view of the popular interest" and "the expressed wish of the IS for a careful detailed examination of Hindus." He added that while he had found only the ova (not the worm) of the parasite in fifteen out of sixteen South Asians who carried the disease, in the Chinese patients he examined he had found hookworm, whipworm, and roundworm. Glover concluded by asking his superiors in Washington, DC for authority to employ temporary medical assistance for microscopic and other work at the station; this was granted.[5]

The fact that the Glover had extracted a large number of hookworms from the wastes of captive patients – a new procedure at the island – demonstrated his comfort with experimenting on his patients.[6] In her discussion of the expansion of PHS medical inspection procedures in this era, Amy Fairchild draws from Michel Foucault's theory of power, which posits that in either "a punitive or normative political economy of power," "it is always the body that is at issue – the body and its forces, their utility and docility, their distribution and their submission." For Fairchild, power at the nation's borders in Progressive Era America (1890–1920) meant enforcing a series of standards on how to be "not necessarily a good citizen, but a good *industrial* citizen." Although Foucault's critics point out that his theory of power sets aside the possibility of human agency, Fairchild convincingly argues that his ideas offer a useful framework for deconstructing immigrant medical examination, "where, from the time they left their homes until they arrived in America, immigrants could exercise very little autonomy" in a dramatically unequal relationship that Fairchild has described as one of "discipline, exclusion and power."[7] This was especially the case at Angel Island, where all Asians faced additional levels of medical scrutiny and detention even before the implementation of bacteriological testing for hookworm at that station.

Glover saw Angel Island, positioned as it was at the gateway between Asia and continental North America, both as a safeguard for public health and as an ideal research and training facility for testing for internal parasites from Asia. The ascendance of parasitology in Glover's laboratory after the *Chiyo Maru* discovery echoed a rise in eugenic theory in American public health, wherein medical students conflated germ theory with Galtonian theories of heredity to explain why germs appeared to spread more rapidly in certain groups, while others appeared immune. White California residents in particular believed themselves to be especially susceptible to tropical disease, to the extent that this vulnerability was seen "a sign of whiteness"; conversely, Asians and Mexicans were widely believed to transmit tropical disease to whites while largely resisting its effects themselves. Linda Nash argues that sustained anxiety about epidemics and the importation of disease "underscored the sense that California, despite almost three generations of white settlement, remained a kind of biological and environmental frontier." Leftover nineteenth-century concerns about the "fatal miasma" of warmer climates meant that the purported incursion of disease from Asia and Mexico incited concerns about "the possibility that a 'tropical' California might re-emerge from within."[8]

While scientific experimentation on non-consenting patients was a building block of the American health sciences, bacteriological screening for hookworm was virtually unknown in California or at any PHS station before 1910. Microscopic work later became "complementary yet subordinate" to visual inspection at Atlantic ports, where inspectors generally only used the microscope to confirm a visual diagnosis in a suspected case of tuberculosis or other infection.[9] However, after Glover found microscopic evidence of hookworm in healthy-looking South Asians whom he would not have suspected were infected, bacteriology became routine at Angel Island. This, according to Shah, represented a "critical reversal of the principal of the medical gaze." Shortly after Glover's discovery, bacteriological work at the station "supplanted physical observation of the epidermal body," especially in the case of hookworm testing.[10]

Organizers of the Rockefeller Sanitary Commission's (RSC) hookworm eradication campaign, which targeted the American South between 1909 and 1914, found that as many as 40 percent of Southerners carried the disease, which had existed in southern states for at least two centuries. Historian John Ettling explains that hookworm was so common there that people frequently "mistook the physical appearance of its sufferers for the peculiar badge of an unfortunate economic and social class." Many of the afflicted were unaware that they had the parasite in their small intestines, as hookworm infection, now called the condition of ancylostomiasis, occurred so unobtrusively, usually from fecal contact with toes. The cure, first devised in the 1880s, was simple: it involved drinking first thymol (a solution made from the herb thyme), or the plant chenopodium, or Male Fern, and then Epsom salts, a combination that, although risky for the patient, detached worms from the intestines and forced them from the body. In the early twentieth century, the treatment cost about 50 cents.[11]

After detecting hookworm in the stool of some of the *Chiyo Maru* passengers in September, Glover also found the parasite in fifty of seventy-five South Asians from the SS *Asia*. He reminded IS authorities that this finding offered the "great advantage of certifying undesirable aliens for a contagious disease," as the BSI ruling in the case of a "Class A" disease was final and prevented the "delay and embarrassment of appeals to Washington." While he doubted that many South Asians he had previously admitted carried the parasite, it was necessary to continue screening new Indian arrivals for hookworm, given the prevalence of "discussion and opinion among the mainland men of this city" on the topic; failure to continue testing might "influenc[e] popular feeling and action to the extent of embarrassing the Service."[12]

Shah clarifies Glover's final point by explaining that by October, "popular anti-Hindu politics and the IS controversy" had "emboldened Glover to demand time-consuming bacteriological exams of all Asian Indian immigrants." He discovered that 65.6 percent of the 218 South Asians he had examined had the parasite, compared with 54.1 percent of the 290 Japanese and 29.4 percent of the 762 Chinese tested. These findings quickly led to compulsory bacteriological testing of both South Asians and Chinese at Angel Island. Shah points out that the finding effectively "merged the two groups into the category of 'Asian'" and affirmed the idea that all Asians could have the disease, even when they exhibited no symptoms. Chapter 2 has shown that the epidemiological concept of the healthy carrier was a recent addition to germ theory, as Robert Koch and the US Army's Typhoid Board had theorized its existence in 1902 and 1904, respectively, in relation to typhoid transmission. Yet racial theory had long held that some groups were more diseased than others. Glover was particularly concerned that healthy-looking Asians, some of whom might live indefinitely with "dangerous portable pathogens" such as hookworm, could wreak havoc on white populations.[13]

The IS began rejecting large numbers of South Asians for hookworm infection in October. Despite the relative simplicity and low cost of the cure, only those who had the funds and who could prove they were not labourers (which would make them LPC), but businessmen, students, or those married to US residents, could avoid rejection. According to statements made by IS and PHS staff during a local Chinese association's tour of Angel Island in 1911, after being divided into groups according to race, and then undergoing primary medical inspection, oral interrogation, and fecal examination, those with hookworm were officially rejected and slated to be deported, unless they requested and the IS approved hospital treatment. IS Inspector Frank Steward informed the tour group that treatment "[did] not usually occupy more than from one to three weeks," and treatment required a deposit of $50 and IS approval from Washington, DC. Another official declared that the treatment was "rather heroic" for those who were granted permission and could afford it. However, other sources indicate that by late 1912 the IS had stopped offering this option in almost all cases at Angel Island, Seattle, Portland, and Vancouver.[14]

PHS records through December 1910 show that very few (if any) South Asians could take advantage of this arrangement in 1910, as virtually all were deemed LPC. In October, 75 South Asians with hookworm were rejected, and a later report indicated that most of the 126 South Asians sent back to Hong Kong on the *Asia* had been rejected for hookworm infection. By November, Glover and his staff had found 87 cases of hookworm among the 141 South Asians examined in the last three boats to arrive at the island, indicating a rate of infection consistent with that of the *Chiyo Maru*. A *Chronicle* reporter called the rejection of these passengers a "more potent" method of exclusion than "former efforts of the immigration officials." In Washington, DC, Charles Earl, acting labor secretary, expressed his relief over the high infection rate, reasoning that South Asians would soon stop trying to immigrate if "rigid inspection" continued at mainland ports.[15]

The hookworm finding also had important consequences for South Asian immigration along the US border with Mexico, where new arrivals from India began to enter after Angel Island was closed to them. PHS officials on the border at El Paso, Texas, rejected five South Asians because inspectors feared they carried hookworm. It is unclear whether officials actually collected fecal samples from these men; however, an El Paso station report from the following April indicates that PHS physicians had begun testing South Asians for hookworm by 1911, apparently on the instructions of Surgeon General Walter Wyman. The PHS physician in charge at El Paso stated that he had found eight cases of hookworm among the twenty-two South Asians examined for the disease. It appears that Mexicans were the only other ethnic group subjected to the hookworm test, as the inspectors extended testing to a group of thirty-four Mexican labourers who appeared to show symptoms of the disease.[16]

The discovery had the greatest impact in San Francisco, however, where the *Chronicle* dedicated a three-page report to Glover's "little laboratory on Angel Island." This article stated that the doctor had produced results that would "greatly mitigate, if not very nearly solve" the Hindu problem without the need for further legislation. The journalist used the disease to retrospectively diagnose the large numbers of South Asians whom the PHS had recently and "myster[iously]" been rejecting as "physically unfit."[17] Similarly, the city's AEL celebrated the timing of Dr. Glover's "new and astounding" discovery. The innovative bacterial testing in place at Angel Island appealed to local union leaders because it appeared to scientifically confirm what they had been saying since 1907 – that South Asians were diseased and undesirable.[18] At the AEL's October meeting, former leader A.E. Yoell declared that most medical authorities knew that "nearly all these Orientals carry with them the bacilli of various Asiatic diseases, such as cholera, bubonic plague, hook-worm, etc." Many Asians were immune to these infections but spread them easily, which, Yoell argued, explained a typhoid outbreak in California's Russian River valley near where South Asians had camped that summer. Although this claim was not substantiated by press reports or official accounts of any South Asian typhoid cases in California, the high rate of hookworm infection among the recent arrivals at Angel Island reinforced the popular belief that the group carried more serious diseases. For example, the editor of the *Los Angeles Times* congratulated Glover for using hookworm screening as a means to protect Americans against the more "loathsome oriental diseases" of "the Hindu tide."[19]

Other voices in the press used hookworm to explain India's continued occupation by Britain. The *San Francisco Chronicle*'s editor, who prided himself on being the first among his peers to predict the "sociological and political importance of Dr. Glover's discovery," asserted that in ancient times the population of India had been "warlike, and in their way, progressive." Yet India was now "a sleeping nation, held in bondage by a distant white power"; he reasoned that "science holds the hookworm largely to blame for their wretched condition," just as the disease explained the condition of "poor whites and Negroes," who were "the laziest people of the [US] South."[20] Although the editor concluded by calling for legislative exclusion, by late 1910 South Asian immigration had virtually halted at Angel Island, just as it already had at immigration stations at Seattle, Portland, and Vancouver.

By the end of 1910, the hookworm discovery, paired with the IS's vigorous and subjective application of the Immigration Act, had effectively ended South Asian immigration to the Pacific coast. The *Tacoma Times* and other exclusionist dailies heralded Glover and his mighty microscope for stopping the South Asian incursion. Glover's annual report for that year accurately observed that his demand for fecal tests on South Asians at his station had been "a large factor in stopping the influx of East Indians into this country." Station IS agent H. Edsell reported that while September had seen 210 South Asian arrivals and 92 rejections at the San Francisco station, since Glover began rigid hookworm inspection, 181 of 184 arrivals in October had been rejected; only three had arrived in November, and none of the fourteen on board the last three ships to arrive in December had been admitted. Although these numbers did not include immigrants travelling via Hawaii, he reported that those numbers were also decreasing and would "soon stop almost entirely when [the] Honolulu gateway [was] effectively handled."[21]

Edsell was referring to what Joan Jensen calls the "one serious loophole" remaining in America's "informal system of exclusion." Under 1907 immigration legislation, immigrants arriving from American territorial possessions (Hawaii and the Philippines) could enter the mainland without being re-examined medically or being interrogated by BSI members; Japanese immigrants had previously landed on the Pacific coast using this method. In mid-September, North warned Commissioner-General Keefe that South Asians were also beginning to use the same law to circumvent Angel Island's tightened screening controls. Since border authorities in Hawaii had not implemented the same executive exclusion in effect at mainland Pacific coast ports, a group of Indian workers living in Hawaii had obtained inspection certificates there and were currently en route to California. Admitting the subjectivity of the Angel Island inspections, North informed a contact in Hawaii that, for any South Asians still arriving without certificates from Hawaii, "all Hindu cases were held at this port for the Board of Special Inquiry and were denied upon very slight evidence." Yet he admitted all twenty-five South Asians travelling from Hawaii, even though they had been in Hawaii less than a month before leaving for the mainland.[22]

Keefe responded to this new development by working with the War Department – which was the agency governing the territory of Hawaii's affairs – to implement Rule 14, a regulation compelling all immigrants to pass a second inspection on the Hawaiian Islands, in order to get a new certificate to gain entry to the continental United States. This "nailed shut the door from Hawaii" for prospective South Asian immigrants from that territory, as the IS rejected all Indian applicants for being LPC. During a six-day voyage from California to Hawaii, Keefe personally investigated the "Hindu immigration" issue by interviewing South Asians and other Asians returning to Asia on his vessel. Honolulu's *Evening Bulletin* reported that Keefe was "in close conversation" with these passengers nearly every day of the trip, and on his arrival in Honolulu he informed reporters that he planned to recommend more stringent immigration restriction for all Asians.[23]

Yet two years later, a number of South Asians realized that "the loophole that immigration authorities had closed in Hawaii" in 1910 was still "open in the Philippines," where several thousand South Asians were working as policemen, agricultural labourers, or shopkeepers. South Asians could obtain a residence certificate after six months in the Philippines, which would allow them to circumvent examination at mainland Pacific coast ports. IS records indicate that some South Asians entered the mainland after spending significantly less than the requisite six months in the territory. Indeed, of the forty-seven South Asians admitted at Seattle from the SS *Minnesota* in March 1912, thirteen had resided in the Philippines for less than six months. This number was likely higher, as above-mentioned Indo-Canadian Oral History participant Imanat Ali Khan recalled – in 1912, he showed a Manila relative's papers to IS officials at Seattle in order to gain entry. Yet he had spent only three months in Manila en route to the United States. Khan's friend Kehar Singh Kailey, who also had spent just three months in the Philippines, also presumably entered using fraudulent means. After 139 more South Asians arrived later in March, Ellis DeBruler, Seattle's Immigration Commissioner, warned his superiors that "it now appears that the existence of this backdoor-entrance has become generally known."[24]

In July 1912, the acting labor secretary advised officials in the Philippines that, because South Asians had "poor physique[s]" and there was a "very strong prejudice" against them on the coast, "the policy of the IS for several years past has been to refuse admission to aliens of said race" unless they offered "very convincing evidence" that they could survive in the United States. The assistant war secretary, whose agency governed both Hawaii and the Philippines, agreed to help the IS's cause by securing legislation similar to Hawaii's Rule 14, although the interdepartmental collaboration required to pass the provision delayed its passage, and small shiploads of South Asians sailing from Manila continued to arrive at Pacific coast ports into 1913. In March 1913, DeBruler in Seattle reported with alarm that 130 such individuals had recently arrived at his immigration station, and a Philippines customs officer travelling on the same boat had informed him that 6,000 to 7,000 workers from India were in Manila awaiting passage to follow them. He added that he had been "anticipating a Hindu invasion from the Philippine Islands" for more than two years and that it now seemed certain "a horde of these East Indians will invade our shores." In his annual report to Washington, DC, he added: "I am open to argument on any debatable question, but to my mind there is no debatable ground so far as the admission of the Hindu is concerned." He observed that South Asians' customs and low standard of living made them unwelcome in society and on the labour market, and argued that "if his presence here can add aught but trouble, I am unable to see in what possible way."[25]

In Washington, DC, Keefe reminded labor secretary W.B. Wilson that it would likely be difficult to argue that recent South Asian arrivals on the coast had been LPC when they entered the Philippines, given that industrial and social conditions there were more favourable for the group than they were on the mainland Pacific region. Although officials in the Philippines had now tightened their admission requirements for South Asians, most of those already living on the islands would make "undesirable" additions to American society if they chose to immigrate. Wilson, seeking a long-awaited solution to this "grave situation," pressured Lindley Miller Garrison, the new war secretary, to find ways to prevent South Asian residents of the Philippines from coming to the mainland. While Shah, Jensen, and others have described the evolution of the Philippines issue and its eventual resolution in mid-1913,[26] scholars have overlooked Wilson's innovative, health-based remedy for the problem. Wilson proposed using hookworm screening, so successful for immigrant rejections at Angel Island, as a stopgap measure to further decrease the number of South Asians admitted at Manila, including those allowed to land under bond – a practice largely forbidden at Pacific coast ports. As he informed Garrison, the "prevalence of hookworm among Hindus" who had arrived at Pacific coast ports "may be of use to the Insular officials in their efforts to enforce the law in the Philippine Islands in the same manner as it is enforced on the mainland." By July, South Asians destined for the mainland were required to prove that they were free of both hookworm and trachoma at the time of their departure.[27]

Wilson's own staff implemented a similar policy at San Francisco in May 1913, when five South Asians arrived at Angel Island from Manila on the SS *Korea*. Instead of simply clearing them for entry because their certificates excused them from a second medical inspection on the US mainland, PHS physicians went against protocol by testing them for hookworm. After one of the men tested positive for the disease, Wilson, who had been warned that the Pacific Mail steamship line was planning to bring in more South Asians from Manila, decided to make the *Korea* passengers a "test case" by rejecting the infected individual for hookworm and the rest for being "undesirable." Accordingly, he issued a warrant for the arrest and deportation of all five men, arguing, with little support, that their certificates were invalid because they should have been identified as LPC when they first entered the Philippines.[28] Wilson eventually agreed to admit most of the group on their appeal of the LPC ruling, but these were among the last South Asians to enter the United States at Angel Island. In late June the new commissioner-general, California native Anthony Caminetti, announced a congressional amendment to the Immigration Act that would allow the reinspection and rejection of immigrants arriving from the Philippines. Caminetti also quietly met with representatives of American, Japanese, and Canadian steamship companies, who agreed to stop selling tickets to South Asians.[29]

In an opinion piece immediately following Caminetti's announcement, the editor of the *Washington Post* declared that the timing of the legislative amendment suspiciously coincided with a recent statement by Surgeon General Rupert Blue that leprosy was increasing in the United States. Wilson's decision to bar South Asians from the Philippines appeared to indicate a "recognition" that "closer supervision of aliens hailing from hotbeds of the disease is necessary." Hansen's disease, which existed in India, also routinely appeared throughout the US mainland and in Hawaii during this period. According to Michelle Moran, health officials saw it as the product of "broader patterns of national intervention in world affairs, particularly imperialist ventures." Physicians and congressional representatives alike "incorporated apprehension of foreign contamination into their characterizations of the disease." Shah adds that after San Francisco's health authorities first diagnosed a Chinese leper in 1871 and a small number of cases cropped up shortly afterwards, the leprosy issue was a key factor in the successful passage of the 1882 Chinese Exclusion Act.[30]

For the *Washington Post* editor, then, the existence of leprosy in India and the success of the "Chinese leper" argument in support of Chinese exclusion offered a useful basis for South Asian legislative exclusion. This attempt to transcribe an effective argument against Chinese immigration onto the newer Asian threat failed, however, since IS records indicated that South Asians were not arriving at Pacific coast ports with this bacterial infection. Meanwhile, other observers viewed the congressional decision to end South Asian migration from Manila as a move to contain the threat of other "Hindu" diseases. Shortly after Wilson closed the Philippines loophole, an American railway agent based in BC wrote Caminetti to congratulate his immigration service on the legislation. This agent stated that during his work in BC he had found that "these filthy human beings (if they can be called human) are not fit to mingle with even the Chinese, let alone white people." He concluded that "as a good American Citizen I here enter my vigorous protest against these low, disease ridden, filthy, people." Similarly, the *Seattle Star*, noting that despite the new Philippines legislation, South Asians were still technically allowed to immigrate to the United States because no law officially barred them, asserted that "all of the objections raised against the Chinese and Japs pale into insignificance when compared with those against the East Indians," as in India "*They Breed Like Rats, Live in Squalor, And Die By The Million Of Plague And Starvation.*"[31]

Two weeks after the legislative amendment, when Seattle officials detained a ship from the Philippines with South Asians on board, representatives of the *gurdwara* [Sikh temple] in Victoria, BC, held a meeting of protest, and cabled the British Foreign Office and US labor secretary Wilson for help in the matter. Caminetti agreed only to let in those who had left before the amendment, and Britain offered the South Asians virtually no assistance, although in August consular officials intervened when Angel Island IS agents attempted to deport, as LPC, a healthy second class passenger from the SS *Persia* who carried more than $500 with him. Into the fall, California labour leaders, like the *Seattle Star*'s editor, remained skeptical that the amendment and the IS's general policy of South Asian executive exclusion would hold. The Vallejo Trades and Labor Council resolved in a September letter to Caminetti that "we don't want the standard of living of the Hindoo; we don't want his religion; we don't want his diseases; we don't want his filth." The San Joaquin Valley's Central Labor Council similarly asserted that white society was "degraded and debased by the presence of these Hindus," who had "obnoxious habits and ill-smelling bodies and filthy appearance."[32]

Notwithstanding the anxieties of many journalists, labour leaders, and private citizens, who believed that South Asian immigration would resume unless Congress introduced "anti-Hindu" legislation, the closing of the Philippines loophole effectively ended South Asian immigration to the United States, a full four years before legislative exclusion in 1917. PHS officers at Angel Island continued to closely inspect the small number of South Asian arrivals for hookworm, although in the 1913 arrivals they found the disease in only around one in three South Asians. This proportion directly contradicted a statistic that Caminetti widely distributed that year to his IS officers at Pacific coast ports. The Rockefeller Sanitary Commission (RSC) had recently published the conclusions of a 1903 study on hookworm infection in the world's tropical and semi-tropical regions, which had found hookworm in most of the 547 Indians tested in the study. Using this study alone, RSC officials estimated that between 60 and 80 percent of India's population had hookworm. In November 1913, Caminetti circulated an abridged version of these findings, which were to be "be carefully perused and considered" by Pacific coast inspectors evaluating South Asians for admission.[33]

Samuel Backus, Angel Island's first official commissioner since H.H. North's removal for purported corruption and mismanagement in late 1910, opined that South Asian healthiness and "a good physical appearance" now meant nothing, as even South Asians who did not have hookworm, had paid the $4 head tax, and could show significant cash on entry were still LPC owing to regional feeling against them. Furthermore, as he explained in the case file of Sucha Singh, who arrived in November with four other South Asians on the SS *Hongkong Maru*, "while many of them appear in good physical condition, it is my judgment that the mental traits above referred to" – their "inherent characteristics of instability, lack of truthfulness, and nomadic tendency" – would "eventually lead to their becoming persons likely to become public charges." Backus in fact had "no recollection of any group of individuals, other than gypsies," who appeared "so uniformly condemned because of those undesirable characteristics."[34]

During Caminetti's absence from Washington, DC, in December 1913, F.H. Larned, his temporary replacement, observed in an internal memorandum that South Asian "racial characteristics" were a leading cause of the strong prejudice against them in the Pacific coast states. Larned pointed to the field reports recently completed by a San Francisco inspector, almost certainly Angel Island IS officer W.H. Chadney. After speaking with various California residents, Chadney, who had chaired several BSI hearings for South Asians arriving from the Philippines in the fall of 1913, concluded that the Indian immigrant was undesirable because he "does not try to conform to our customs," is "not cleanly in his habits," and is "religiously forbidden from adapting himself to American life." He added that "the morals of the Hindu are not good," as "Hindus are addicted to the use of intoxicating liquors" and, when in town, "frequent the cheapest saloons and lowest houses of prostitution." Overall, he reasoned, "the Hindu is a very objectionable alien."[35]

Although Chadney and other IS officers at Pacific ports now had the weight of the amended Philippines transmigration legislation behind them, this report demonstrates how IS officials continued to refer to South Asian religious practices, personal habits, and especially morality in order to prove that group could not assimilate. Eithne Luibheid explains that the financial and legislative obstacles to family migration that forced Asian males to live in non-traditional households evoked a "continuing cultural anxiety" over interracial sexual activity, marriage, and procreation.[36] For Larned and other IS officials, South Asian immorality – sexual or otherwise – was a key "racial characteristic" mitigating against the success and social acceptance of Indian immigrants, and a major reason to bar South Asians. Importantly, however, Larned's December briefing note also reveals how the ascription of "racial characteristics" to individuals explicitly caused their exclusion. In his description of the case of Nika Singh and thirteen other South Asians appealing deportation orders, Larned stated that while most were deemed "undesirable" for lacking sufficient funds, for physical "slightness," and, in five cases, for having hookworm, even those in the group who were healthy could not be admitted because of the generalized characteristics of their nationality.[37]

One particularly telling example was that of Argen Singh, whom the IS described as "above the average in intelligence and general appearance" and "of fairly good physique." Since Indians purportedly had problems finding employment due to their racial qualities and the negative public opinion of them, Larned ordered Singh's deportation along with that of all the other men in the group, arguing that "the Bureau feels that the special evidence" of Singh's case "does not outweigh the general evidence" about the undesirability of South Asian immigrants. The counsel for another South Asian, Bram Singh, who arrived in October on the SS *Persia*, appealed after his client received the same treatment, arguing that Bram Singh had not been given a fair hearing because IS agents introduced as evidence "a mass of irrelevant matter, referring not to this alien in particular," but to "expressions of passion and prejudice against the Hindu

people as a race." Similarly, the appeal of a deportation order for Battan
Singh, who had also arrived on the *Persia*, contended that since the appellant was classified LPC without any explanation, "it is fair to conclude
that the local prejudice against the Hindu People, exhibited more particularly by Officials of the Department than by residents of the State
otherwise, is the controlling factor in the decision."[38]

The case of Ottam Singh, a South Asian who arrived in September along
with Nika Singh on board the SS *Nippon Maru*, reveals how the IS misap-
plied general evidence on hookworm epidemiology to prove that an individual had been infected with the disease prior to landing in the
Philippines. This was an important area of contention, given that even
though admission certificates from the Philippines were now invalid at
mainland ports, IS agents strived to add legitimacy to their LPC classifications by showing beyond a doubt that a South Asian should not have been
medically certified to enter Manila. Singh, a twenty-five-year-old single
male who had spent four months in the Philippines after living two years
in China, tested positive for hookworm ova at Angel Island soon after his
arrival, although he showed a government certificate stating he was free
of the disease on leaving Manila in July. At the conclusion of his BSI interrogation, the IS issued a standard warrant for his deportation due to
his positive hookworm diagnosis, even though otherwise he presented a
healthy appearance and possessed the required funds. The explanation
for the order stated that hookworm was "a debilitating disease that is very
enerveating [*sic*]" and was classified as "dangerous contagious."[39]

Singh's BSI examiners reasoned that he should never have been medically certified to enter the Philippines, because hookworm's prevalence in
India made it likely that he had been carrying the disease within him on
his arrival in Manila. The IS argued that the disease must have escaped
detection when the Pacific Mail tested his stool before he left Manila, after
which "the possible gastric and intestinal disturbances incident" on the
transpacific voyage loosened the ova in time for Singh's reinspection at
Angel Island. Thus, by using the general Rockefeller statistic showing a
high incidence of Indians with hookworm, IS staffers were able to overlook
the distinct possibility that Singh could have picked up the parasite en
route from Manila by coming into contact with contaminated fecal matter
on the ship, especially as the incubation period for hookworm averages
fifteen days but can be as short as ten days, which was the length of the
journey between the Philippines and Hawaii.[40] This oversight had important consequences for the admission of others like Singh, for it was used

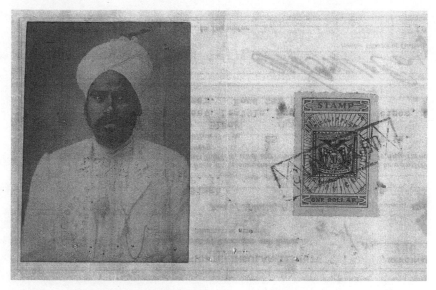

FigurE 3 "Alien Certificate (Insular Territory) for Ottam Singh," May 7, 1913, Manila. | (Front), RG 85, AICF file 12924/4–4 (case file of Ottam Singh), NARA Pacific Branch, San Bruno, California.

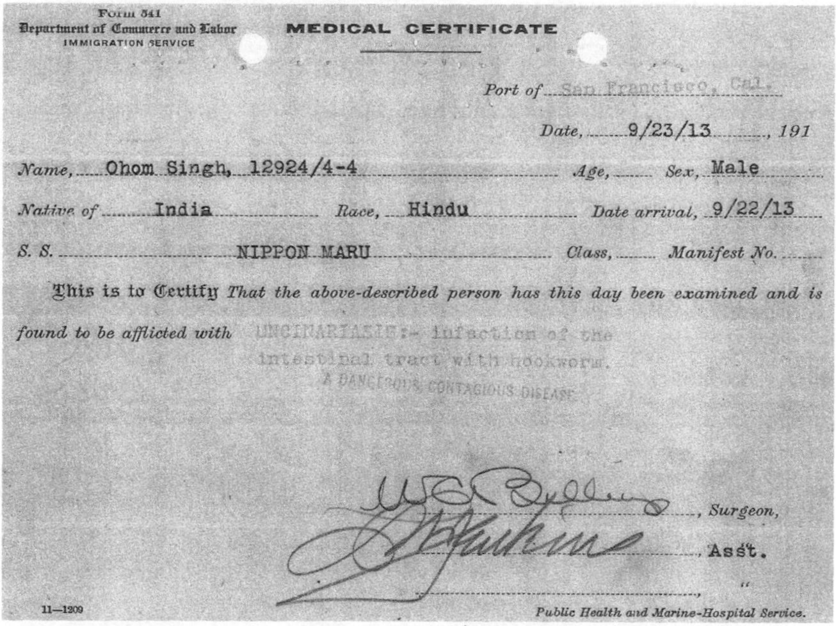

Form 541
Department of Commerce and Labor   **MEDICAL CERTIFICATE**
IMMIGRATION SERVICE

Port of ....San Francisco, Cal.

Date, ...9/23/13...., 191

Name, ...Ohom Singh, 12924/4-4........ *Age,* ...... *Sex,* Male

Native of ....India........ *Race,* ...Hindu........ *Date arrival,* 9/22/13

S. S. ....NIPPON MARU........ *Class,* ...... *Manifest No.* ......

This is to Certify *That the above-described person has this day been examined and is*

found to be afflicted with UNCINARIASIS:- infection of the intestinal tract with hookworm. A DANGEROUS CONTAGIOUS DISEASE

...., *Surgeon,*

...., Asst.

11—1209   *Public Health and Marine-Hospital Service.*

FigurE 4 "Medical Certificate for Ottam Singh, San Francisco," September 23, 1913." | RG 85, AICF file 12924/4–4 (case file of Ottam Singh), NARA Pacific Branch, San Bruno, California.

to prove that, since the immigrant purportedly had hookworm before leaving Manila, his exit certificate had been invalid. This meant there was no reason to extend the "grace period" that Wilson had allotted in August for South Asians with certificates issued before the congressional legislation came into effect.

Larned used this rationale to exclude the other South Asians at Angel Island with hookworm, referring directly to the precedent set "in the case of Ottam Singh." For example, the Philippines exit certificate of Joalla Singh, whose case was opened after Ottam Singh's, was ruled invalid because before arriving in Manila he had lived in Malaysia and Singapore, two areas where, according to the RSC, hookworm was also "prevalent." Yet if hookworm was as "dangerous" and "contagious" as the IS maintained, why were Ottam Singh and two other South Asians with hookworm released on bond into California within weeks of their arrival, where they lived with the disease while appealing their deportation orders over the course of the following winter? Ottam Singh's release on bail strongly affirms Shah's assertion that "government officials' confidence in hookworm's predictive value was dubious." It appears that IS staffers saw the parasite less as a threat to public health and more as a convenient tool for justifying South Asian exclusion. This certainly was the observation of Dr. Peter H. Bryce, who in 1911 had first learned that US officials rejected South Asians for hookworm, not out of fear of the disease, but instead "with a view to finding some new reason for excluding the Hindus from the United States."[41]

In his dual role as Chief Medical Officer of Canada's interior and (North American) Indian affairs departments since 1904, Bryce had been instrumental in the professionalization of federal health services and especially the adoption of germ theory and sanitary practices. Bryce, unlike Scott and other immigration officials, saw the association between immigrants and infectious disease as a consequence of environment, not genetics, and he applied this distinction in his efforts to protect public health. Megan Sproule-Jones has detailed Bryce's efforts to improve Aboriginal health in the prairie provinces, where children lived in cramped, dirty, and poorly ventilated residential schools. Church and state administrators had long explained away the high death rates in these schools by arguing that Native people were constitutionally weak or otherwise incapable of acclimatizing to Western living standards; Bryce, however, understood that the prevalence of tuberculosis in particular was largely due to direct transmission between students or their environmental exposure to infection. Bryce's 1907 report on this subject with a view to improving student health helped bring about some reforms in 1911, but it also ended Bryce's involvement with Indian Affairs two years later. Bryce continued to champion revisions to Aboriginal health administration long after this, and his 1907 and other reports together constituted Canada's first comprehensive study of Aboriginal health.[42]

Bryce came to his findings on American hookworm screening of South Asians in 1911 during his investigation of the disease in BC. The preceding pages have shown that the South Asian association with hookworm both affirmed and consolidated the executive restriction already in place at most US Pacific coast ports by late 1910. But Glover's discovery also had important consequences in Canada, where, for interior minister Frank Oliver and his medical inspectors at BC ports, the finding confirmed that Indians carried parasites, a key tenet of early-twentieth-century tropical medicine that Alexandra Stern explains was "deeply connected to the production of colonial and racial difference." Shortly after Glover released his findings from Angel Island, Oliver ordered Canadian border agents to reject any prospective immigrants of South Asian origin with hookworm coming from the United States, even though the Dominion's Immigration Act did not classify hookworm as an excludable disease.[43]

When Bryce visited the Pacific coast a year later, G.L. Milne, the department's immigration inspector at Victoria, recommended a more formalized inspection policy to check for the disease. However, after leaving the coast, Bryce learned at a Havana conference that hookworm could only be transmitted through direct exposure to infected fecal matter, something that was unlikely in North America and thus appeared to be questionable grounds for rejection. Yet since South Asian legislative exclusion in Canada meant that Canadian inspectors had not yet had the opportunity to test South Asians for the disease, he was insistent that the Dominion should verify that any future South Asian arrivals did not have hookworm. He thus permitted Milne to order, for the first time, a microscope and other equipment for the "*careful* examination of the bowel contents in Hindus or other immigrants whom you may deem suspicious."[44]

There the matter rested until April 1912, when William Charles Hopkinson, the department's immigration agent responsible for political surveillance of the province's South Asian population, received information that three to four hundred South Asians were bound for BC ports on the SS *Orterio*. Since the vessel was travelling directly from India, the potential immigrants could not be legally prevented from landing. In a telegram to the deputy interior minister, W.W. Cory, Hopkinson suggested that medical examiners at Vancouver and Victoria "confidentially" test the *Orterio*'s South Asians for hookworm, as this had proved "effective" in barring hundreds of South Asians at US ports. Cory approved, and ordered "a special Medical inspection" to ensure that all were "carefully examined," although given that no other ethnic group was subjected to this testing in Canada at the time, he added the proviso that "it is important that this matter should be kept private."[45] Immigration superintendent W.D. Scott's instructions to Milne and to Malcolm J. Reid, the immigration inspector at Vancouver, made it clear that this order was to apply only to South Asians; his terse telegram read: "Request Medical Inspector examine Hindu passengers 'Orterio' specially for hookworm. This is *confidential*." A week later, it was learned that the *Orterio* carried no South Asians.[46] Still, Bryce went out of his way to find Milne the first microscope to be used on the coast, which was specifically intended for use on future South Asian arrivals.[47]

Soon after the *Orterio* scare, Bryce went to Montreal to find Milne a "first class" microscope and, after choosing the best available type "used by most of the Montreal men," Bryce arranged for a friend at McGill University to select "perfect lenses" for it. With Cory's approval, the microscope was sent to Milne by month's end. The equipment cost $99, a significant expenditure roughly equivalent to an inspector's monthly salary.[48] The rationale behind the acquisition of this microscope – which was solely intended for screening members of an immigrant group already legislatively excluded from immigrating – must be understood in the wider context of early-twentieth-century North American conceptions of the racial theory of disease transmission. Although germ theory had been well established by the 1890s, and developments in bacteriology had shown that all national groups and social classes could catch and transmit infectious disease, colonial officials maintained the race–disease association because understandings about the "backwardness and pathology" of marginalized groups persisted. Shah points out that the emergence of bacteriological testing on the coast "collapsed the identification of a parasite organism within the body with the status of being a social parasite and dependent," because those infected would presumably require state aid. Amy Fairchild agrees that at Pacific coast ports in the prewar period, the practical application of germ theory had "both social and medical implications" as government officials argued that an immigrant's infection would likely impair his or her labour productivity. Just as pathogens caused disease in healthy bodies, diseased immigrants "infected the economic body."[49] While both Shah and Fairchild were specifically referring to the American situation at the time, these ideas offered convenient support in BC as well for the ongoing popular and official antagonism towards Asian and especially South Asian immigrants.[50]

By 1913, British Columbia's South Asian population had dwindled from the approximately 3,000 at the time of the 1911 census to fewer than 2,500.[51] Yet at summer's end, Superintendent of Immigration Scott expressed his concern that PC 920 and PC 926 were insufficient controls on Canada's South Asian community. In July, Hopkinson had informed the Immigration Branch that nine South Asians, five of whom were new to Canada, had arrived on the SS *Sado Maru* with pre-paid tickets purchased in Victoria in 1912. The five had "fully complied" with the Immigration Act by coming on tickets previously purchased in Canada, but they, unlike other immigrants in similar situations, were detained "a day or so at the Immigration Hall with a view to a strict medical examination – more especially for 'Hookworm.'" Yet all were landed at Victoria at the end of July. More troubling to the branch was a recent error by a Canadian immigration commissioner at Ellis Island, who had allowed eight South Asians arriving at New York to proceed to New Brunswick. E. Blake Robertson remonstrated against the agent at Ellis Island for failing to enforce the Continuous Journey Regulation, reminding him that "the attitude of the Department" was "so well known" that he could not believe that he had not realized that "all restrictive regulations against Asiatics are supposed to be rigidly enforced." For W.D. Scott, this oversight at New York indicated that a general and nation-wide order was necessary to keep South Asians out of Canada. Accordingly, he called for a new regulation "framed in such a way that it would apply without any question."[52]

The arrival of the Japanese steamer SS *Panama Maru* at Victoria in October triggered a brief immigration crisis.[53] Although federal officials rejected thirty-nine of the ship's fifty-six South Asian passengers for failing to meet the continuous journey provision of PC 920, the BC Supreme Court found a technical inconsistency in the wording of the order-in-council and allowed all but five of the passengers rejected for standard medical reasons (likely trachoma) to land. The decision dominated the province's newspaper coverage for almost a month, and federal MP for Vancouver H.H. Stevens and others wondered if the vessel was the harbinger of a broader Indian plan to circumvent the Canadian Immigration Act. What never made the newspapers, however, was that Milne and his assistant medical inspector, H.B. Rogers, had begun non-standard fecal testing on the detained passengers for hookworm – a test previously performed only on the South Asians of the SS *Sado Maru* – and had requested funds to hire a tropical disease expert.[54]

After examining a fecal sample taken from passenger Jewalla Singh, Dr. W.P. Walker of Victoria reported that there were no mature hookworms present but that he had found "numerous segmented non-opercular ova" that were "most probably" of the hookworm parasite. Walker could not be sure of these results, and noted that a mature worm specimen would only be passed from the body after the patient had taken an anthelmintic solution like thymol, which he recommended administering before taking another fecal sample.[55] In the end, Immigration Bureau staff were unable to prove that Singh had hookworm. The BC Supreme Court ruling on the *Panama Maru* came only a few days after Dr. Walker submitted his initial report. The immediate release of the vessel's passengers – paired with the fact that four of the five men ordered deported for other medical reasons had escaped from detention before deportation – deprived the specialist of the opportunity to retest the patient.

It is clear that Milne opposed the BC Supreme Court's decision. His letter to W.D. Scott later in December offers insight into his perspective as a gatekeeper of Dominion public health and, more importantly, into department-level policy approaches to South Asian immigration during the immediate prewar period.[56] Milne opined that "the more I consider the question of Asiatic immigration to this coast, the more am I convinced that the only really effective restriction would be obtained by thorough examination for hookworm disease." Yet in order to test future South Asian arrivals, Victoria's detention quarters required facilities for ensuring that passengers could be monitored during defecation. During the *Panama Maru* crisis, Milne had been unable to obtain fecal samples from most of the detainees because "the Hindus were rather rebellious, and it was rather difficult for us to segregate them." Milne's staff had secured Singh's sample only because he had been detained separately from the others while he recovered from a cold. Anthony Caminetti, the US Commissioner-General of Immigration, had informed Milne that US authorities along the coast were now checking every Asian immigrant for hookworm and wildly exaggerated that they were finding the parasite in about 90 percent of cases. Milne noted that, if Canada adopted the same practice,

I have no doubt that we would find 90 percent of Asiatics, and particularly Hindus, infested with this disease ... You will, therefore, see that if we were to proceed

on these lines, and were able to reject 90 percent of these people, the object of the Gov. would be attained. The rejection of immigrants under this cause would not be followed by so much criticism by the general public; in fact, on the other hand, it would appeal to them strongly as a measure for the protection of the public health."[57]

Replying to Milne, Scott agreed that "in view of the importance of the subject," he should continue to test any future South Asian arrivals for hookworm. Milne sent Scott the above-mentioned circular that Caminetti had recently dispatched to all IS agents, in which it was estimated that 60 to 80 percent of India's population had hookworm. Scott requested more copies so that he could "send them on to our Coast Agents" in BC. If the inspectors found that "any" Indian arrivals had the parasite, it would be "in order to hold up every individual Hindu until his case can be decided." Scott also informed Vancouver based immigration agent Malcolm J. Reid that Milne was "watching the matter" and would "take the first available opportunity" to make "a thorough examination" of a few cases.[58]

Shortly after the *Panama Maru* decision was handed down in November 1913, federal MP for Vancouver H.H. Stevens informed reporters that he planned to ask cabinet to hire a bacteriologist to study the health of Pacific coast Asians, whom he believed were "infested with several bacterial diseases," including hookworm, that had existed in Asia for hundreds of years. Like Milne, Stevens concluded that "the health side of the Asiatic problem is just as important as the industrial, racial and social."[59] However, Immigration Branch records contradict Stevens's contention that Asians were bringing hookworm to Canada. While US authorities had been finding the disease in some Asians at Angel Island since 1910, the only evidence of the disease in Canada was Milne's inconclusive finding with regard to Jewalla Singh. No further bacteriological examinations took place at this time, even though a visiting medical consultant recommended that all Asian arrivals at BC ports be inspected for hookworm. Reid in Vancouver, realizing that the issue could become a "political football," forwarded the suggestion to Scott, who took no action. Nor did Stevens follow through about making a request to cabinet, at least not in 1913; even after spending a month in central Canada, he informed reporters that he still planned to raise the inspection issue.

Stevens's continued use of the disease argument demonstrates how it prevailed even in the face of contradictory evidence. In 1913, Alberta physician E.H. Lawson informed the editor of the *Victoria Colonist* that, having served as ship's surgeon on CPR vessels during the height of Indian immigration to Canada before it ended in 1908, he had personally inspected many of the immigrants landing at BC. Lawson recalled:

> Although at first I was strongly prejudiced against them I lost this prejudice after thousands of them had passed through my hands and I had compared them with the white steerage passengers I had seen on the Atlantic. I refer in particular to the Sikhs and I am not exaggerating in the least when I say that they were 100 per cent cleaner in their habits and freer from disease than the European steerage passengers I had come into contact with. The Sikhs impressed me as a clean, manly, honest race.

Lawson added that his recent medical work with white labourers in mining camps, which were "rife" with immorality, had "increased my respect for the Sikhs." He concluded that he had "not yet seen one good reason why they should not be permitted to bring their families in as freely as the European immigrants."[60]

A Saskatchewan farmer brought Lawson's letter to the attention of the Prime Minister's Office the following year. David Ross stated that western farmers urgently needed 60,000 workers to harvest their grain. After hearing a rumour that more South Asians were destined for Vancouver, he asked the prime minister, Robert Borden, to "let western farmers sample the Sikhs, I beg of you. Let the coming ship-load of East Indians land after thorough physical inspection." After personally seeing South Asians at work, he emphasized that "*there are no finer men in Canada to-day than the Sikhs.*" He then quoted from Lawson's letter to show that "in regard to their cleanliness," most South Asians were socially suited for life in Canada.[61]

In January 1914, Dr. Bryce asked his supervisor W.D. Scott for permission to visit the Pacific coast to investigate the hookworm issue again first-hand. Quoting Milne's explosive December 12 memorandum, Scott at first rejected this proposal, stating that Milne's words indicated that Pacific coast inspectors were already well-apprised on the situation. He also pointed out that every BC agent now had Caminetti's IS circular on South Asians and hookworm. However, the Superintendent of Immigration quickly changed his mind after receiving Hopkinson's report that several Punjabis in Yokohama were purchasing tickets for steamship passage to Vancouver. While the timing of the report and the follow-up correspondence on the matter indicates that the still-unknown vessel in question was not the infamous SS *Komagata Maru*, Scott nevertheless revised his stance on hookworm testing shortly before that ship left was scheduled to leave Calcutta for Canada.[62]

Scott warned the British Consulate at Yokohama, the Japanese city rumoured to be a port of landing for the unnamed vessel that Hopkinson was expecting, that any Indian residents arriving there via Calcutta could have the disease. The Superintendent of Immigration also instructed Milne to "pay special attention" when screening the incoming South Asian passengers for hookworm. Without definitive proof that any vessel had actually been chartered to bring Indian passengers to Canada, Scott informed his superior W.W. Cory that, in light of the "probability of a number of Hindus applying for admission to Canada at Vancouver" in the near future, he recommended the use of a specialist to "detec[t] the parasite or ova of the Hook-worm in the case of Hindus or other immigrants from India." After Cory granted this request, Scott authorized both Milne in Victoria and Malcolm J. Reid, immigration agent in Vancouver, to hire tropical disease experts and to prepare "a properly equipped place" to detain any upcoming South Asian arrivals for defecation.[63]

Scott's instructions came in spite of the recent findings of Dr. W. Bapty of BC's Provincial Board of Health, who reported that the province had received no complaints that resident South Asians had or were spreading hookworm. Bryce had made a similar observation after his he visited BC in March to investigate South Asian health there. During his research trip he interviewed the medical teams of both Milne and A.S. Munro, the medical inspector of immigrants at Vancouver, and consulted with a physician attached to Vancouver's US PHS branch. Repeating a sentiment he first expressed to Milne in 1911, Bryce asserted that while hookworm infection was a serious health risk in India, where people often went barefoot and lived without proper sanitation, "it does not follow that we are to be satisfied that these are reasons why immigrants from these infected countries should be excluded from Canada, unless it can be shown that similar habits of life will be followed here, and that therefore the dangers through contamination through the spread of the disease are similar."[64]

Bryce was referring to the fact that hookworm is most often transmitted through fecal contact with bare feet. After entering through its victim's toe, the hookworm parasite travels into the bloodstream, then through the vascular system and bronchial passages and into the throat, where, after its victim swallows, it enters the gastrointestinal tract and hooks onto the lining of the upper intestine, where it begins taking blood.[65] The Chief Medical Officer knew that the chances of hookworm cross-infection were very low in Canada, where even "foreigners" lived more hygienically (by wearing shoes) than they did in countries where hookworm was prevalent. He added that none of the "prominent physicians in Vancouver and Victoria" he had spoken with had heard of any Asian individual with symptoms that could be "reasonably attributed to this disease," such as sallow complexion, anemia, or abdominal tenderness.[66] While, despite Hopkinson's information, no vessel carrying South Asians ultimately arrived until months later, when the charter vessel SS *Komagata Maru* anchored off Vancouver in May. By the time that this ship – which the following chapter discusses in detail – even left Asia for Canadian waters, the Immigration Branch had deferred its plans to test incoming South Asians for hookworm. Bryce's conclusion that Indian arrivals were unlikely to give Canadians hookworm apparently played no role in this decision, as Scott still intended to seek ministerial approval for wide-scale testing a full week after the Chief Medical Officer submitted his report. Three other factors appear to have quashed the formation of an organized hookworm testing program. The first issue was the plan's cost. Although both Milne in Victoria and Munro in Vancouver could collect stool from patients and do some microscopic work, they did not have the expertise to analyze the test results themselves. Dr. Walker in Victoria, the tropical disease expert whom Milne had consulted to test the stool of *Panama Maru* passenger Jewalla Singh, was the natural choice for the project, but when Walker was asked for a quote for testing a larger number of South Asians, Walker replied that "the proposed examination of Hindu or other immigrants from India" for hookworm would cost $2.50 per case for fifty passengers or more. At this price, the testing cost for an average-sized passenger vessel could be upwards of $1,000, which was over to half of an immigration inspector's annual salary.[67]

Walker may have inadvertently given the department a second reason to back off the hookworm strategy. In conversation with inspector Reid, he admitted that passengers could cheat the hookworm test by taking an initial dose of thymol while en route from Asia. Since, in his estimation, the timing of the dose would flush out worms but allow hookworm ova to remain clinging to the intestine in a later test, an immigrant with even a severe infection could disguise his condition because the ova would not come out in his stool.[68] There is insufficient evidence to prove the influence of this point on policy – especially since the presence of the eggs alone was insufficient grounds to prove hookworm infection – but a third factor definitely caused the department to defer its hookworm screening plan. On March 31, Order-in-Council 1914–897 passed, thus barring non-farming "artisans and labourers" from landing at BC ports. This was a renewed version of legislation the government had passed the previous December after hearing the rumour that a steamship line was considering opening a direct (and therefore continuous) service between India and BC. Chapter 5 will show that although plans for hookworm testing were not fully abandoned at this stage, Scott decided that "the provisions of P.C. 897 would appear to be sufficient to dispose of this matter for some time."[69]

The preceding pages have explored how, after M.W. Glover found hookworm ova in the stools of South Asians at Angel Island in September 1910, American exclusionists mobilized this finding as evidence that the majority of South Asians on the coast had the parasite and also carried more serious "Oriental" diseases. The hookworm discovery dramatically influenced inspection policies at Angel Island immigration station, the last US Pacific coast entry point open to immigrants from India. While South Asian admissions were already declining at the station by late summer, the introduction of mandatory hookworm testing virtually halted the entry of South Asians until some circumvented exclusion by arriving directly from the US territorial possession of Hawaii. Two years after that loophole was closed in 1910, more South Asians began to enter at mainland ports using exit certificates issued by US authorities in the Philippines, also an American territory at this time. Shortly after Congress closed this second loophole in 1913, IS officials met challenges to exclusion by arguing that hookworm infection among some of these arrivals nullified the validity of their Manila exit certificates, and more broadly proved that the entire group was LPC.

This chapter has also shown how Canadian Immigration Branch officials used the same discovery of hookworm to meet challenges to the legislative exclusion in effect at BC ports. After preparing for hookworm testing in 1912 on the phantom South Asian passengers of the SS *Orterio,* the branch quietly initiated testing in 1913 on South Asians from the SS *Sado Maru* and SS *Panama Maru.* Canadian officials began to develop a plan to use this testing method to ensure the rejection of South Asians in the event of the "probability of a number" of South Asians landing at Vancouver, although this avenue was revised and largely deferred in the spring of 1914. After discussing the ongoing polyvalent deployment of the disease arguments in BC politics and society, Chapter 5 will explore the arrival of the SS *Komagata Maru*'s passengers and their reception in the context of Pacific coast responses to South Asians in the prewar period. The chapter then discusses the 1914 congressional Hindu Immigration Hearings in Washington, DC, during which the Commissioner-General of Immigration, and others representing Pacific coast interests, used the same health arguments to lobby for South Asian legislative exclusion from the US.

5

South Asians, Public Health, and Eugenic Theory

*Probably the worst objection to them outside of the fact that they
are physically unfit for this country and are subject to tubercular
complaints, is the fact that they have some very objectionable religious
beliefs and some of the moral offences to which they are addicted are
quite unmentionable.*

– James McVety, BC Federation of Labour, March 10, 1913

*They are a dirty lot of fellows ... They smell, and sometimes a person
can hardly stand it ... You can not imagine anything more strange as
a human being than a Hindu.*

*– Denver S. Church, Member of Congress for California,
February 19, 1914*

THE 1914 *KOMAGATA MARU* incident continues to dominate the historical
and political narrative of the twentieth-century South Asian experience
in North America. On May 23 of that year, the SS *Komagata Maru*, a
Japanese-owned vessel chartered by Indian merchant Gurdit Singh, anchored off Vancouver's coast with 376 South Asians aboard. The ship's
arrival triggered a major crisis in the city and prompted serious concern
in Canada and the United States that India's "Hindu tide" would soon
overcome the new continental barriers to South Asian immigration. The
previous chapter has detailed how, following the example set by Angel
Island PHS officials in 1910, Canada's Immigration Branch began secretly
testing South Asian arrivals for hookworm in 1912 and 1913, and in 1914
began preparing a plan to test any incoming South Asians for the parasite.
While the Immigration Branch deferred action on this scheme, the following pages demonstrate how it reflected the Dominion government's
approach to the "Hindu problem" in the prewar era. In 1912, federal

legislators and the Immigration Branch used the "Hindu disease" thesis to address requests for a relaxation of the continuous journey provision. Public testimonials commissioned by the British Columbia government in 1913, along with a series of publications and reports that year, demonstrate that a majority of BC residents supported the continuation of legislative exclusion. In 1914, federal legislators revisited past health- and eugenics-based arguments in their response to the arrival of the *Komagata Maru*.

The following pages also discuss how, following Commissioner-General of Immigration Anthony Caminetti's 1913 closure of the Philippines loophole in US executive exclusion, American government officials pointed to the *Komagata Maru* crisis as proof that the United States needed the same legislative controls (if not better ones) as Canada had been using to bar South Asians since 1908. In the US, the ongoing polyvalent deployment of the "Hindu disease" thesis played a key role in the final transition to legislative exclusion; as will be made clear, the Immigration Service (IS) forefronted the health issue during a series of congressional hearings in 1914. Pointing to South Asian living conditions in California, federal representatives portrayed exclusion as necessary to prevent epidemic infection in Pacific coast populations; more generally, these politicians employed the disease thesis to legitimize the notion that South Asians could not assimilate into American society. These efforts influenced the introduction of legislative exclusion in 1917.

In 1911, Victoria's "Friends of the Hindu" organization brought together like-minded white and South Asian individuals opposed to the Dominion's policy of Indian exclusion, which had been in effect since the 1908 introduction of continuous journey legislation. The Friends petitioned the Imperial Conference in London on the issue, pointing out that married South Asian residents missed their wives in India, and that single men were unable to marry owing to the lack of potential wives in Canada. Keeping the men apart from women, they argued, could eventually cause immoral behaviour among the group, most of whom were males living with other South Asian men. Phanga Singh Gill, an informant for the Indo-Canadian Oral History Project, recalled that his cousin had coped reasonably well with communal living on farms near Surrey and Richmond before that year, but by 1911 he, like many others, desperately missed family members. To address this general situation, in June the Friends wrote to Governor General Grey to ask that the married South Asians in BC be allowed to bring over their wives and children.[1]

Most BC residents, however, opposed any further immigration from India, and that year saw a revitalization of the now well-established public health–based argument against the South Asian presence in Canada. Three main factors account for this. First, American journal articles, especially sociological studies of South Asians in the Pacific coast states, supported the main lines of the argument. Second, Immigration Branch officials continued to report on the public health threat of South Asians. Many of these reports were private; even so, they helped buttress the purportedly scientific justification for political posturing on the issue. That posturing was the third reason for the resurgence of the disease argument. Dr. G.L. Milne in Victoria articulated these sentiments in July in a confidential report to Scott in which he asserted that

> the Hindu it is true has made some money since coming to British Colum-
> bia but he has failed to assimilate himself with the Europeans especially his
> mode of living and etc ... Nor are they a race fitted for a wet climate such
> as portions of British Columbia or the cold climate of eastern Canada. One
> Hindu went home on the last Empress and another is sought to be deported
> by Victoria City authorities, both of these for tuberculosis. Taking all in all
> they are not the best sort of immigrants for this country.[2]

Milne's observations regarding the assimilative potential of the new arrivals reflected the fact that, like the province's Chinese community, South Asians were only partly integrated into BC society at this time. Although labour connected the new immigrants with whites in "a network of formal, impersonal relationships," and although South Asian residences were never as segregated as were Chinese houses in Chinatown, Peter Ward notes that "hosts and guests shared no significant bonds." Yet the personal accounts of some BC residents indicate that this was not universally true. Indo-Canadian Oral History participant Norman King of Golden, BC, recalled that in the first decade of the century, his parents had a friendly relationship with the Sikhs working at the Duncan mill. Every King family member visited the small Sikh temple the workers had built in the town by 1910, and when the mill closed down, some South Asians gifted the Kings with Indian clothing. Similarly, in a 1960s interview for the Imbert Orchard Oral History Collection, Ellen King of Union Bay (apparently no relation to Norman) recalled that when she was a child around this time, she and others interacted with South Asian labourers, some of whom even taught the locals "Hindu" (probably Punjabi) words.[3]

Ward is correct, however, that most British Columbians at this time resisted Indian integration into their communities. This popular opposition was rooted partly in established assumptions regarding earlier Asian arrivals, but that on its own does not explain the enduring stereotyping of South Asians. The "distinct Indian image" widely held by BC residents drew heavily from popular constructs of India as an overpopulated servant nation plagued by dirt, disease, and "exotic, peculiar customs" that firmly anchored the populace in an archaic way of life. Importantly, the presumption that the Indians were diseased – a "well-established Oriental stereotype" – continued to dominate media coverage, popular sentiment, and official discourse well after Indian exclusion.[4] This was especially evident in the Dominion's response to the Friends' request that the continuous journey provision be relaxed for compassionate reasons.

In late 1911, Superintendent of Immigration W.D. Scott informed his supervisor, assistant deputy interior minister W.W. Cory, that "personally I do not look with favour on the immigration of Hindus"; he contended that "it would be a great mistake" to reopen Canada's gates to South Asian wives and children. Scott had significant power to regulate South Asian admissions; for example, in November he decided not to provide Indians with certificates proving their previous domicile in Canada, which essentially dictated whether or not an immigrant could re-enter the country.[5] When the superintendent cancelled the deportation of the family of Vancouver resident Hira Singh, who had not arrived by continuous journey from India, he did so only on the direct order of Laurier himself. After this "act of grace," Hopkinson reported to Scott that many of Vancouver's South Asians were "flooding" the city's CPR office with requests to buy tickets for their own family members.[6]

In early 1912, young Frederick C. Blair, a rising star in the Immigration Branch, arrived in Vancouver to investigate the possibility of admitting the wives and dependent children of the approximately 2,500 South Asians remaining in BC. Blair is best remembered today for his anti-Semitism as assistant deputy immigration minister in the 1920s, and especially for serving as Canada's immigration director after 1936. According to Irving Abella and Harold Troper, Blair's famous 1939 statement that, with respect to Jewish refugees, "none is too many" for Canada typified his broader approach to the Jewish refugee crisis. The authors point out that Blair's personal anti-Semitism heavily influenced Canada's willingness to accept Jews; in the event, very few Jews desperate to escape Europe around the time of the Holocaust were able to enter Canada.[7] Blair is less known for

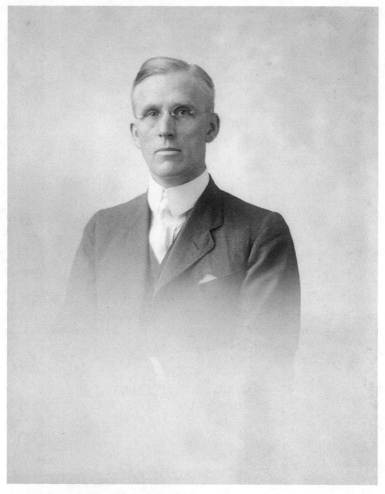

FIGURE 5   Portrait of Frederick C. Blair. *"Mr. F.C. Blair in 1920," Ottawa.* | Topley Studio/LAC / PA-208773.

the influential stance he took against South Asian immigration in the earlier years of his career.

His well-publicized mission to BC was the Immigration Branch's sixth official inquiry into Indian immigration – a remarkable sum, considering that BC's South Asian population had never numbered more than 5,000 by that time. After meeting with the mayor, city health authorities, members of the Board of Trade, and others, Blair predicted that Canada would not grant the family concession to the South Asian immigrant community. He argued that the group would never assimilate and that it did not matter if "a Hindu has fought for the Empire and the flag in India," because, for BC, "it is enough that the Sikhs are not white." He added that any South Asians missing their families should simply return to India.[8] Blair submitted his report on his Pacific coast mission in January 1912. While he acknowledged that "their habit of living" allowed the men to save their earnings, and admitted that "in some cases they are well housed and live under sanitary conditions," he asserted that "the Medical Health Officer of Vancouver says that these people live under conditions ... which are a disgrace to any human being, that they are uncleanly in their habits, are afflicted with tuberculosis, are addicted to drink and that the City cannot enforce its health regulations in many instances.[9]

Blair was likely referring to the recent findings of city health inspector Robert Marrion. In early January, Marrion delivered a special memorandum to the Health Committee detailing local sanitary conditions. He described cleaning up Chinatown and other areas, and he recalled finding overcrowding and unhygienic conditions among Asians and impoverished whites. In his discussion of the city's South Asians, he declared that "from a sanitary point of view I consider them worse than the lowest class of Chinamen." He added that "it is impossible to conceive a more filthy condition that the manner in which these men live in any old dilapidated building they can manage to rent." These statements were well-publicized; the *Vancouver Province* used the headline "Declares Hindus Are Filthiest" to summarize Marrion's report, even though most of that document criticized Chinese and Italian domestic hygiene and devoted only two sentences to South Asians.[10]

Blair ended his own report by arguing that Indian social customs would prevent "good women" from immigrating and that "moral conditions" were "infinitely worse" in India, a nation with high rates of "sodomy, buggary [*sic*] and prostitution." He concluded that he "would not recommend an immediate decision as to open the door."[11] Unlike W.L.M. King's 1908 Royal Commission report, Blair's memorandum was never published. This was partly because it was an internal memorandum, but also because W.D. Scott informed his superiors that "there are things in it which I think should be carefully kept from the public."[12]

Most British Columbians, however, would have agreed with Blair's conclusions. A *Province* editorial cartoon in February 1912 depicted a man with "BC" on his hat, sitting on a log with "The Hindu Problem" written on it. The man held a snake and was playing a flute like a snake charmer, while a nearby beaver said "The suspense is awful!" The same month, the new *Vancouver Sun* newspaper described in detail the anti-Indian declarations made at a recent meeting of Vancouver's Ward Seven Conservative Club. The meeting's consensus was that the city's "white women and children" would be at risk from infectious disease if more Indians were allowed into BC. Many of the city's South Asians lived in Ward Seven, and some whites who lived close to them complained that "the filth and squalor of the colony is worse than that existing in the slums of London." James Reid, president of the local taxpayers' association, doubted that allowing in South Asian wives would improve their husbands' living conditions. "If such was the case," he asked, "how do we account for the inherent filth of the men?" He reasoned that "if in nature they were cleanly, they would be so under any circumstances." Another resident declared that he avoided letting his children play close to South Asians, because "who can tell whether in their childish innocence, they might not wander into the hovels of these people and contract some fearsome disease?"[13]

Other Pacific coast groups made similar assertions. While the Victoria chapter of the Council of Women sided with the Friends of the Hindu by requesting that the Dominion welcome South Asian family members, the organization's Vancouver chapter sided with Blair. A *Province* article about the lack of women in northern BC offers an interesting example of the double standard inherent in this opposition. The paper reported sympathetically that many men in the remote Cariboo were "Ready and Willing to Marry" but had not "seen ten white women in thirty years." Instead of expecting the men to move to the cities, residents campaigned to bring women to the men.[14] It seems that whites earning their living in the remote interior were entitled to companionship, but non-whites who had travelled to Canada for similar economic reasons did not merit the same privilege.

Like the Ward Seven Conservative Club and the Vancouver Council of Women, Henry Herbert Stevens, the federal Conservative MP for Vancouver City since late 1911, strongly advised against allowing the families of resident South Asians to enter Canada. In his widely circulated 1912 pamphlet "The Oriental Problem," he argued that even if keeping South Asians from their wives caused homosexuality or other "immoral" behaviour, it would be worse to allow any more of the group to immigrate. "The Hindu is in every way different from us," he asserted, including in his "race," "morals," and "physical attainments." He further alleged that all Sikhs in BC were liars, a quality that was "so deep-rooted" that it was impossible to "shake them in this ingrained deceit."[15] A few days later, Stevens told the Toronto Women's Canadian Club that, in his former capacity as chairman of Vancouver's Health Board, he had seen for himself that the new immigrants lived in the "most *revolting conditions.*" He contended that perhaps the greatest argument against relaxing the continuous journey legislation for families was that the issue represented a struggle for "the establishment of a race, morality and tradition fit to carry on the great work" of building the Dominion. Canada could only succeed, he argued, "by keeping our race pure and clean."[16]

Nayan Shah asserts that Stevens saw the campaign supporting the immigration of South Asian wives as "the opening salvo in full-thronged demands for social, legal, and political equality in Canada." If this concession was granted, immigrants from India would leverage residential rights into the "political rights" of voting and holding public office.[17] Stevens's private correspondence from February certainly reflects this fear. Acting well outside his capacity as a junior MP, he wrote to the attorney general of New South Wales, Australia, asking for information about that state's White Australia Policy and suggesting the possibility of a conference between Canada, Australia, New Zealand, and South Africa to draft a joint policy on immigration from India. The conference never materialized, although Stevens publicized the idea in his speech to the Toronto Women's Canadian Club.[18]

Enakshi Dua points out that white Canadians like Stevens, and South Asian men as well, largely sexualized South Asian women and the effect their presence would have in the province. If admitted to Canada, these women would not be pioneers, economic migrants, or nation-builders; instead, they would be the wives of South Asian men and/or the "creators of ethnic communities" through their reproductive potential.[19] Whites and South Asians both also expected that bringing women to Canada would maintain the purity of the South Asian *and* white races. The Indian nationalist *Ghadar* and *Hindustanee* newspapers, both of which circulated widely among the province's small Indian population, often referenced a "fear of interracial sexuality in Canadian society" and made the case that allowing the wives into Canada would help perpetuate racially homogenous ethnic populations. Yet if some South Asian men asserted that Indian women in Canada would help keep the races separate, western labour unions advocated total Asian exclusion as means to preserve the country's white homogeneity. White labour unions vehemently opposed the entry of women from India because they believed that these migrants would only further entrench South Asians in society.[20]

The ruling Conservatives finally decided the issue on February 27, 1912. After ousting the Liberals from office in October 1911, Prime Minister Robert Borden, like Laurier before him, had attempted to "find a course through the perilous shoals of provincialism and racism," although Donald Avery points out that Borden ultimately maintained his party's position, in effect since 1907, that BC should remain white.[21] Using only Blair's January report to justify his approach, interior minister Robert Rogers announced that he would not relax the immigration regulations to allow any of Canada's 2,500 remaining South Asians to bring in their wives. Rogers identified Blair only as "a special officer" and paraphrased all of Blair's key conclusions, including his estimation that the police found many of the South Asian men in BC "troublesome" and, perhaps more significantly, that Vancouver's health officers found them undesirable. These arguments appeared to be enough for interior affairs critic Frank Oliver. He changed the topic, and the House did not revisit the family reunification issue until 1923.[22]

That Borden's government defended its decision to maintain South Asian exclusion using one agent's unsupported generalizations about South Asians demonstrates two things. The most obvious point to be taken is that the federal cabinet continued to subscribe heavily to racial stereotypes, which it translated into gatekeeping policies designed to sustain a particular vision for Canadian society. Yet by deferring to the arguments that South Asians uniquely threatened the nation's health and morality, and that the introduction of Indian wives and children would exacerbate this threat, Ottawa also reinforced and affirmed the widespread belief in BC that South Asians were inherently (and immutably) apart and below other races in Canada, including the Chinese and Japanese. While some Chinese and Japanese residents won access to their families – through the head tax and quota provisions respectively, that allowed a certain number of wives and children into Canada – South Asians did not. This fact re-affirms the need for a major course correction in scholarship on nativism in BC and Canada generally in the prewar period. The established view is that Chinese and Japanese immigrants were the major victims of nativist portrayals of Asians as racially inferior and diseased,[23] when in fact by 1912 South Asians were more vilified than any other group for those reasons.

Other issues, including the "immorality" argument, saturated discourse on BC's South Asians. A few months after Blair submitted his report to Ottawa, Victoria's mayor John Beckwith told reporters that BC's South Asians were "immoral" and a "source of trouble" in the community. These remarks incited a flurry of letters to newspapers. One writer declared that "every one knows they are very peaceable, law-abiding and industrious," while a South Asian writer accused the mayor of libel and threatened legal action if he did not retract his statements. When Beckwith refused, a group of Victoria's South Asians launched a libel suit. Vancouver immigration agent Malcolm J. Reid remarked glibly to reporters, "You have to be careful what you say about immigrants into Canada these days."[24]

Beckwith's statements, like those of H.H. Stevens, offer an interesting example of official opinion in the province in the prewar period. Angus McLaren has shown that the rise of Canadian eugenics in this era, like the spread of Francis Galton's hereditarian theory in the United States and Britain, "symptomized a shift from an individualist to a collectivist biologism" on the part of those wishing to prevent societal degeneration and immorality. Many exclusionists who argued there was a link between social degeneracy and the new immigrants currently meeting BC's labour demands supported their position with "a virulent mix of nativism [and] racism." Intellectuals like J.R. Conn, who argued in *Queen's Quarterly* that Canada should bar immigrants representing the "lower types of life," drew from British imperial concerns about maintaining racial separation. Sir Alexander Morris Carr-Saunders, a leading demographer of the period, similarly held that countries with small numbers of European-origin citizens (such as Canada and Australia) needed to restrict non-white immigration to keep control of their territories and maintain social morality.[25]

These sentiments on racial separation reflected popular thinking among a broad swath of BC society, including workers and employers, and among others who were not directly affected by Asian labour. Testimony from the province's 1913 Royal Commission on Labour, which investigated BC working conditions, indicates there was anti-Indian sentiment among most of these groups.[26] These testimonials can be grouped into the categories "Business Owner/Manager," "Union Representative," and "Other." Small business owners, the only respondents speaking on the topic who favoured relaxing South Asian exclusion, found the immigrants to be "pretty intelligent" and "satisfactory workers." Two respondents even favoured South Asian workers over other Asians and many whites; one Chilliwack mill owner declared that "I should hardly say it but as a matter of fact we find Hindus worth as much as the white men, and in some instances worth more." Another mill owner stated that he felt a "good white man" made a better citizen than a "good Hindu," but to this he added, "I think if anything they are a little more cleanly than the whites in their personal habits. Of course, if you get a bunch of Hindus together they have an odor, but I suppose they can notice an odor from us too." He also found that "when the Hindus get a dose of liquor in their system they can't control themselves any better than the whites," which showed that "they are adopting our vices." To overcome this, he had placed one South Asian employee on the "Indian list" (prohibiting alcoholic purchases) the previous year, and reported that this man was "staying sober this summer."[27]

Not surprisingly, all five "Union Representatives" firmly opposed Asian immigration and labour, and BC Federation of Labour leader James McVety specifically targeted South Asians in his testimonial. McVety, a leading Socialist Party of Canada member at this time, generalized that South Asians were "the most useless of all the Asiatics who are here":

> The poor Hindu is more to be pitied than blamed ... His body is in no way suited to the rigours of this northern plane ... They are longer [than Chinese] yes. I would not say bigger. Probably the worst objection to them outside of the fact that they are physically unfit for this country and are subject to tubercular complaints, is the fact that they have some very objectionable religious beliefs and some of the moral offences to which they are addicted are quite unmentionable.[28]

McVety's use of the climate argument, and his assertion that South Asians were especially susceptible to tuberculosis, parroted the earlier statements of G.L. Milne, Vancouver's health officer Frederick T. Underhill, and others. However, McVety's connection between South Asians and immorality, which echoed Victoria mayor Beckwith's statement the year before, reflected the ongoing evolution of BC popular opposition to Indian immigrants. Nayan Shah explains that during this period, western labour advocates and newspaper editors were beginning to associate Indian immigrants with sexually deviant behaviour, especially homosexuality. This contention emerged, at least in part, because South Asian populations in BC and the Pacific coast states were almost exclusively male until after the First World War. However, Shah asserts that racist sentiment was a major reason why the idea endured in popular discourse.[29] Like the argument that South Asians threatened public health, the purported concern that South Asians were given to vice was often a guise for labour concerns about South Asian workforce participation.

Respondents to the Royal Commission who fell under the "Other" category represented neither capital nor labour. Eight decidedly opposed all Asian immigration and labour. An accountant for a Salmon Arm mill asserted that "personally I don't like the idea of Chinamen or Hindus." Barber C.F. Burkhart went further, declaring that "I would go without any clothes at all before I would have a Chinaman wash them." He stated that "lots of them have leprosy," recalling that two whites had contracted the disease from Chinese laundries in Los Angeles. Here, Burkhart was likely referring to an unproven case of leprosy in Santa Ana in 1906.[30] One respondent who had lived in India observed that males in that colony had several wives and cautioned that "that's the custom they're bringing in here." "If they're allowed to come," he added, "it will be just the same as if the Pacific Ocean overwhelmed the whole of Canada. We will be submerged." Duncan mayor Kenneth Duncan reasoned that South Asians caused societal decay and dominated industry. In the past year, Vancouver Island's small Indian community had controlled Victoria's dairy sales because South Asians could operate farms more cheaply than other farmers.[31]

E. Lukin Johnston, editor of the *Cowichan Leader*, delivered the final and most philosophical criticism of the South Asian presence in BC. In his 1913 testimony, he opined that Indian immigration was detrimental to the Empire, because the return of South Asians from Canada to India would "undoubtedly" destabilize British control over India. After arriving in Canada, South Asians realized that white men there did not have the same "pride of a Britisher." Johnston, who put forward similar ideas in a 1929 *Canadian Magazine* article, told the Commissioners that this pride, an Indian "pride of race," was in fact "the whole thing that keeps India in subjection at all." Johnston was the only informant to discuss the South Asian immigration issue in its broader imperial context.[32]

Victoria-based journalist E.R. Gosnell took a different approach in his 1913 article in *Annals of the American Academy of Political and Social Science*. Gosnell, like Johnston, opposed further Indian immigration, but he did not feel the same obligation to support British rule in India. He believed that BC was within its rights to demand that whites and South Asians remain "within [their] own biological spheres," for intermixing would be "disaster to one or both races.[33] At a Vancouver community meeting, Stevens similarly argued that, if Britain was to maintain a positive influence on India, then "its 'heel' on Indians must not be softened by the admixture of alien blood among the people to produce lower types of humanity than the lowest of either race." Stevens's correspondence files show that at least some of his constituents shared this opinion. For example, a financial broker in Vancouver informed Stevens that having lived for eight years in India, he was one of the "strongest backers" of the Vancouver MP's efforts "to eliminate entirely the immigration of the Hindoo." The writer asserted that the South Asian was "undesirable and one of the most dangerous weapons to have in our midst in connection with Empire matters."[34]

Although this and other discussion and correspondence on the issue was largely moot after the government's February 1912 decision not to relax the continuous journey provision for the families of resident South Asians, the Immigration Branch still intervened when local papers published criticisms of Canada's treatment of the group. After the *Vancouver Sun* printed G.D. Kumar's 1912 editorial "The Hindu Grievance" about local anti-Indian racism, and the *Vancouver Province* published Kumar's rejoinder to a speech by H.H. Stevens, Stevens personally instructed Malcolm J. Reid, who owed his job as head of Vancouver's Immigration Branch to Stevens, to see if "some of these stories could be nipped" from city papers in the future. Reid accordingly met with the editors of the *Province* and the *Vancouver News-Advertiser*, the two papers "friendly" to the Immigration Branch; both promised not to publish any more of Kumar's letters. The *News-Advertiser* even agreed to screen future editorials from South Asians whom Reid and W.C. Hopkinson considered troublemakers.[35]

Reid's and Hopkinson's interference with the Vancouver press offers an excellent example of Hugh Johnston's assertion that 1913 was an important year for the government's surveillance of South Asian activities. Especially in the later months of the year, Hopkinson's monitoring activities became invaluable to the Immigration Branch, which gave him permission to travel extensively between BC and the Pacific coast states gathering information. The province's South Asian population continued to dwindle from the under 3,000 noted in the 1911 census; but even as it did, the small community attracted attention by lobbying for better treatment in Canada, especially in June 1913, when a delegation went to India to petition their colonial government to ask for a reversal of Canadian legislative exclusion.[36]

Liberal senator Hewitt Bostock, founder of the *Vancouver Province* and a staunch defender of BC interests, criticized this mission to India during a Senate debate, declaring that W.L.M. King's 1908 report had shown that the group could not handle the climate and were not suitable for Canada.

In contrast, Liberal senator James Douglas of Saskatchewan argued, as he had in 1908, that "the reception they have met with in BC was unworthy of the Dominion as a whole." After meeting an Indian delegation in 1910, he sympathized with the group, whom he called "a vigorous race," and felt they would leave on their own if they could not cope with the cold. Directly addressing what he felt was at the core of resistance to South Asian immigration, he reasoned that "climate is one thing," and "probably the view that they are pagans" was significant too, but "the real question at issue is the labour problem." He pointed out that after Indians had found jobs on their arrival in BC, "the more work they got to do, the more was said against them." He ended by stating that "we have made a great mistake in the way we have treated the Sikhs ... The fact that they have done the same thing in the US is no reason why Canadians should have followed a bad example."[37]

Douglas, however, was in the minority on the issue, just as he had been in 1908. In a July 1913 address to Vancouver's Canadian Club, H.H. Stevens reflected the dominant view when he declared that South Asians in Canada could not expect better treatment because they were "subjects, but not citizens, of the Empire" who had "done nothing for civilization." Two Anglo-Indian visitors to the city shared these sentiments, following in the footsteps of Rudyard Kipling and others who fit the pattern of Kornel Chang's description of imperial "conduits for racial knowledge."[38] J.M.G. Davis, the son a Calcutta bank owner, and personally notable as a survivor of the recent SS *Titanic* disaster, told the *Province* that "Canada made a serious mistake when it ever permitted Hindus" to enter Canada. Davis opined that the Dominion "should lose no time in adopting a policy of exclusion like the Australian Commonwealth and New Zealand." Major W.J. Ottley, husband of a "well known Vancouver girl," and himself a combatant in the Indian army's 34th Sikh Pioneers, told the *Vancouver World* that after commanding South Asian army contingents for years, he found that when a South Asian left India and the "disciplinary influence of the army," he became "lazy" and "a very unsatisfactory citizen." If Britain left India, "the virile races of the North" would conquer "the effeminate people of the South," causing the nation to devolve to where it had been when Britain first assumed leadership.[39]

Ottley's assertion of Indian effeminacy was firmly rooted in colonial perspectives of India, which held that a marked difference in skin colour and cultural norms between the peoples of the different hemispheres pointed to a dramatic divide in inherent physical characteristics, including sexuality. White colonials in the Indian subcontinent during this period argued the "passive, feeble and generally 'unmanly' nature of the Indian." Richard King offers the example of a late-nineteenth-century text used by white Indian Civil Service trainees, which claimed that "the physical organization of the Bengali is feeble even to effeminacy ... His mind bears a singular analogy to his body: it is weak even to helplessness for purposes of manly resistance." Here, as King points out, "we can see the ways in which notions of gender race and nationality impinge upon each other in the colonial context." Western observers often asserted a close resemblance between Indian men and Western women, and "just as the myth of India has been constructed as the 'Other' (i.e., as 'not-West') to the West's own self-image, women have been defined as 'not-male' or other in relation to normative patriarchal paradigms." In the colonial context, the very arguments that omitted "the feminine" from the "realms of rationality, subjectivity and authority" were also employed to exclude the non-Western world – in this case, India – "from the same spheres of influence."[40] Beyond the Indian Subcontinent, concepts of Bengali effeminacy were often transformed into a generalized theory of Indian effeminacy.

Ottley's remarks to the *World* more generally demonstrated the province's enduring opposition to South Asian immigration, a sentiment heightened significantly in 1913, when a report surfaced that a steamship company planned to be the first to offer direct passage from India to Canada. Stevens, apparently unaware that since 1912, the Immigration Branch had implemented hookworm screening as a "back-up" means of restriction, feared that Canada would now have no means of stopping the "Hindu tide." He quickly advised W.J. Roche, who had replaced Robert Rogers as interior minister in late 1912, to enact an order-in-council that explicitly barred new immigration from India. Roche reassured his colleague that if the steamship rumour was true, "something will have to be done by way of amendment to the Act to prevent this state of affairs." In late August, Prime Minister Borden issued PC 2218, a copy of which was sent to India's government, stating that any Indians arriving by "a regular service, or by individual and occasional boats," would "greatly excuse and even inflame public opinion in important portions of this country." Canada could not allow entry to Indians as a "race, unfitted alike by their constitution, temperament and habits." Borden hoped that India would intervene before Canada was forced to enact further (more direct) legislation that might embarrass India.[41]

Chapter 4 detailed how, in November 1913, passengers of the SS *Panama Maru* successfully disputed the validity of PC 920, the continuous journey order, and PC 926, the order requiring Asian arrivals to show $200 on arrival. Shortly after these acts of legislation were overturned, and after Roche learned that South Asians might soon have access to direct travel from India, Borden issued PC 1913–2642, an order-in-council barring all "artisans and labourers" from entering BC save at the port of Alberni. In a letter to US Commissioner-General of Immigration Anthony Caminetti, Malcolm J. Reid of the Immigration Branch at Vancouver stated that "of course it is needless to inform you that this is directed against the Hindus, although it appears on the face of it to include all nationalities."[42] The India Office responded to the new order by admonishing Canada for continuing to bar the families of resident South Asians. An India Office staffer declared that South Africa's continued discrimination against its Indian population had produced tensions in India that were "already so grave" and that would be aggravated by Canada's continued refusal to grant concessions to its South Asian community. In the same vein, Ontario writer Isabella Ross Broad protested against the order, suggesting that the Dominion's treatment of Indians was "un-Christian." However, another Ontarian, Agnes Laut, presented an opposite view in her 1913 pamphlet on the broader issue of South Asian immigration, which she prepared after *Saturday Night* sent her to BC to study labour problems in the wake of a 1912 railway worker strike.[43]

Mark Leier explains that, although Laut purported to be an objective observer of BC race relations, she largely "justified anti-Asian sentiment based on stereotypes and notions of the 'essential nature' of Asians," employing views on racial hierarchy that "reflected the world view of many Canadians who supported the British Empire."[44] It is difficult to isolate Laut's personal opinions within the text, for she interspersed her own conclusions with her summary of BC sentiments on the "Hindu" issue. Overall, however, her discussion was strongly anti-Indian. Although Laut called the continuous journey legislation "a sort of subterfuge ... rigged up in our immigration laws to keep them out," she also contended that Canada should not have to accept India's large population. The notion that South Asians would adapt to local conditions was "no reason for Canada's accepting as her burden the heritage of another country's cess-pools of crime." The local social environment, she argued, "hasn't *yet* modified the negro." Although an Anglo-Indian living in BC had told her that "*the Hindu is the negro problem multiplied by ten plus craft,*" Laut opined

that Indians were also particularly dangerous because they were "intellectual and spiritual as well as crafty and sensuous." According to a BC
mill owner, these qualities derived from "generations of vice" and "birth
from immature mothers." Laut concurred, adding that even "Chinese
vices" were not "a stench to Heaven as the Hindus'." Addressing South
Asians as a group, she concluded that "*what we do fear, and we are determined
to shut out are your Asiatic vices.*" She added that "we are sorry for you, just
as we are sorry for any plague-stricken region; but we do not welcome the
plague among us because of that pity."[45]

Many provincial residents supported Laut's assertions. A November
1913 *Saturday Sunset* editorial decried eastern Canada's "maudlin sympathy" for the South Asians in BC; echoing the statements of Victoria mayor
John Beckwith in 1912, the editor declared that the South Asian "takes
to trouble" just as "a newly landed Irishman takes to politics in New York."
The difference between the two was that Indians could never become
citizens. Referring to the major Asian groups in BC, he asserted that "of
the three races the Hindu is the greatest drinker and they indulge in orgies and debauches such as I have never observed among either Chinese
or Japs. The Hindu is crafty, unscrupulous [and] only fear of the whites
will keep him straight in his relations to them." A few weeks later, the *New
Westminster News* similarly declared that "nothing tickles" a South Asian
"quite so much as an opportunity to project his smelly carcass into the
limelight where he will be the centre of public gaze."[46]

In January 1914, Borden's cabinet reinstated the PC 920 and PC 926
orders-in-council as PC 23 and PC 24. This final version of the continuous
journey provision would remain in effect until it was made redundant by
1930 legislation that excluded all "Asiatic" immigrants.[47] The ruling Conservatives passed the 1914 orders with no debate, although future prime
minister W.L.M. King confided in his diary that he had "urged that the
Liberals" debate what he saw as the ruling government's "incapacity to
handle" imperial diplomacy. Borden followed the reinstatement of the
continuous journey provision by again denying India's request that Canada
admit South Asian wives and children. The prime minister justified this
position by stating that Indians had a lower standard of living than whites
and could not assimilate; moreover, the "susceptibility of this class of
people to tuberculosis" and their "inability to withstand the rigors of the
climate" meant that exclusion was in the interests of the South Asians
themselves. These statements had been taken directly from E. Blake Robertson's 1913 briefing note, which conflated ideas from Robertson's own

1906 memorandum linking South Asians with tuberculosis, King's 1908 report on the climatic barrier to South Asian success in Canada, and F.C. Blair's 1912 affirmation of the tuberculosis argument.[48]

Chief Justice Hunter's overturning of PC 920 in November had shown Borden and Roche that the BC court could strike down the continuous journey stipulation, even in its revised form, if another technical inconsistency was found. So on March 31, Borden issued PC 1914–897, a renewed version of December's temporary order-in-council barring non-farming "artisans and labourers" from landing at BC ports.[49] Chapter 4 showed that although the Department had prepared for hookworm screening in 1912 on the South Asian passengers of the SS *Orterio,* and had initiated testing in 1913 on South Asians from the SS *Sado Maru* and SS *Panama Maru,* Roche's faith in the reliability of PC 897 caused immigration officials to deprioritize hookworm testing a month before the SS *Komagata Maru* reached Canada. However, while the Immigration Branch ultimately turned to PC 897, along with two other non-medical "anti-Hindu" provisions, to bar the passengers' entry into BC, Scott kept the bacteriological testing option in his back pocket as a fail-safe means of exclusion even after the vessel's arrival.

Scholars have discussed the two-month *Komagata Maru* incident at Vancouver in greater detail than any other chapter in the story of South Asian immigration to Canada. Hugh Johnston's newly revised 1979 study is the authoritative text on the topic, although other historians have discussed the event in the broader contexts of politics, immigration, labour, and Indian nationalism. Peter Ward points out that event showed the "deep and permanent racial cleavage" between Asians and a white majority. Ian McKay describes the incident as "a play, in large part, about race," which "threw into sharp relief the paradoxically fluid identities of Canadians." In 1914, "the constructed image of the 'Hindu' was that of a harbinger of a monstrous wave" that threatened to "sweep all the cherished things of everyday British life into a vast tsunami of disorder and ruin." Many felt that while Canada was still strongly connected to the Empire, physical and cultural characteristics prevented South Asians from being regarded as imperial equals. Ali Kazimi adds that the incident "set a precedent" for Canada's refusal in 1939 to offer asylum to almost 1,000 European Jewish passengers on the SS *St. Louis* who were attempting to escape Nazi persecution.[50]

This infamous 1914 debacle began with the above-mentioned arrival of 376 Indian passengers aboard the Japanese charter vessel SS *Komagata*

Maru. Punjabi merchant Gurdit Singh had chartered the ship and booked passengers to challenge the continuous journey order. The *Komagata Maru*'s anchoring in Vancouver's Burrard Inlet on May 23, 1914, triggered a flurry of activity in that city and in Ottawa, where Scott and his boss, assistant deputy interior minister W.W. Cory, had been scrambling since April to arrange the incoming passengers' exclusion. While both believed that the government's use of PCs 897, 23, and 24 would render hookworm testing unnecessary, on April 29 the superintendent wrote that "an effort is [still] being made to ascertain definitely whether it is a fact that East Indians applying for admission to Canada are really suffering from this disease."[51] Indeed, after the vessel's arrival a few weeks later, Dr. A.S. Munro at Vancouver proposed special testing for this purpose. Since only 15 percent of the passengers had failed the initial shipboard medical examination for eye diseases, Munro asked permission to conduct a more thorough, hands-on inspection "with each immigrant stripped in order to eliminate others on account of diseases only discoverable by detailed special examination." Since this type of exploratory screening was impossible on the cramped deck of the vessel, immigration agent Reid, writing to Scott on behalf of himself and Munro, suggested removing the passengers "under guard in batches of ten" and returning them after the inspections; they accordingly asked permission to hire tropical specialists "to have those not rejected on account of other diseases examined for hookworm."[52]

While Scott did soon grant Reid permission to hire a hookworm specialist, the superintendent wrote that he "would rather depend for exclusion on civil examination" using the orders-in-council, and instructed that the medical *and* civil screenings be held on the ship. Fecal testing would have been nearly impossible on board; however, Munro conducted more stringent physical inspections between May 26, when he failed approximately fifty-six men for trachoma and other eye conditions, and June 6, by which time he had failed thirty-four more for undisclosed reasons. Reid reported on May 31 that "the medical examination is still being carried on – the men being stripped and thoroughly examined by Dr. Munro."

It is possible that some in the latter group were rejected merely as a delaying tactic, given that Reid confided to Scott that "under pretext [of] medical examination still in progress," all "outside individuals" such as J. Edward Bird, the passengers' lawyer, had been prevented from boarding the vessel for at least five days after it dropped anchor.[53]

Despite these medical rejections, most of the remaining passengers never had the opportunity to be officially rejected in a civil examination

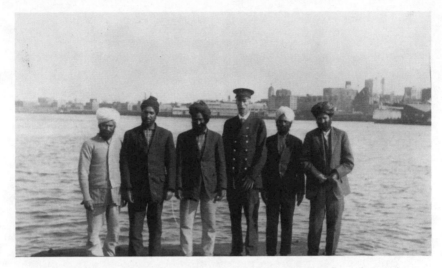

FIGURE 6   Five SS *Komagata Maru* passengers with Immigration Branch security guard James Quinney on July 6, 1914. | Accession No. 13161, Vancouver Public Library.

hearing. After Reid and other Immigration Branch officials refused to allow any of the vessel's passengers to leave ship except the ship's physician, his family, and twenty returning immigrants, the government delayed holding individual Board of Inquiry hearings for the remaining passengers as a means of stalling the immigration proceedings. The passengers thus surprised officials in June when they refused to leave the harbour and overpowered the vessel's Japanese crew. Prime Minister Borden's correspondence with Vancouver residents during the summer of 1914, when the vessel remained in Vancouver's harbour until late July, shows that many locals strongly supported the government's refusal to admit the passengers. An anonymous Vancouver writer informed Borden:

> I admire the firm stand you have taken in connection with the Hindus, as do all other true Canadian citizens. The Hindus are an immoral, and here I speak from personal experience, "evil-smelling" lot. In travelling in the cars, one has either to remove or have them removed to the other end of the car. I presume their condition is due mostly to the fact they mostly live in small shacks and seldom bathe.[54]

This common observation was not lost on South Asians. Bishan Singh Aujla, an above-mentioned informant for the Indo-Canadian Oral History

Collection, shared stories he had heard from the first wave immigrants who lived in Vancouver in the prewar years. He recalled hearing that

> we always think why [the white man] hate us [sic]. Sometimes, suppose our people were working in the cow barn and you get on the street car along or with the same clothes on, the people who used to go to their offices they did not know that smell was due to work in the barn, but they hate us [because they believe] that smell was not from the barn but from the Hindu ... It is our own fault too, how to stay clean and how to travel.[55]

Many municipal politicians made similar observations about South Asian cleanliness. When the *Komagata Maru* first anchored off Vancouver, North Vancouver's councillors petitioned Borden, asserting that "unsanitary conditions" in Indian camps made it "impossible for any one [*sic*] with any self-respect to live with them."[56]

In fact, every city council in the greater Vancouver area petitioned Borden on the issue, broadly connecting South Asian cleanliness and

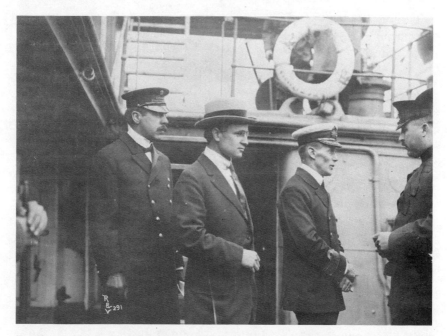

FIGURE 7   Malcolm J. Reid (left) and H.H. Stevens on the SS *Komagata Maru*. Also pictured is Captain Walter J. Hose of the HMCS *Rainbow* (centre right). | LAC, PA-034016 Box OS 0075.

unassimilability with the *Komagata Maru* controversy. When Vancouver mayor T.S. Baxter called a public meeting on June 23 to discuss the passengers' refusal to leave, 1,200 city residents crammed into a local auditorium to hear speeches by Baxter, H.H. Stevens, and former MP Ralph Smith. The *Vancouver Sun* reported that the crowd "unanimously" favoured sending the ship away. Tensions were so pronounced at the gathering that US immigration officials stationed in Vancouver thought another riot was possible. Meanwhile, the Vancouver General Hospital's board of directors sent Stevens a memorandum stating that they "view[ed] with alarm the proposal to admit more Hindus into Canada," since the hospital had not received payment from several South Asians for previous treatments. The *Sun* later explained that local South Asians were refusing to pay because at home, the Indian government paid their medical bills.[57]

Some Canadians living outside Vancouver were also concerned about the vessel anchored there. A Quebecer asked Borden if it could be "arranged that these people be segregated on some island in the Pacific or even sent to the W. Indies," where an Indian government official could "be placed in charge of them" until "this problem be definitely settled by the several Imperial dependencies." This writer suggested seeking advice from men like Rudyard Kipling, who were "well versed in handling the peoples of the Indian Empire," to help "impress upon" Indians that "their own Country and Climate is best suited to their needs." The *Vancouver Province* reported that former Vancouverite William Waterson, who now lived in Johannesburg, had "watch[ed] that cargo of Hindus with great interest" and was "glad" that Ottawa had not admitted them. He added that South Asians were "an absolute pest once they get a footing in a white man's country."[58]

Canada's parliamentarians, still in session in Ottawa in June, voiced their dismay at the arrival of the South Asians. The outcry crossed party lines, with members from the ruling Conservatives and the Liberal opposition agreeing that Canada should reject the passengers. The interior minister, W.J. Roche, declared that "we are going to stand by the immigration law in its fullness," notwithstanding Liberal Frank Oliver's criticism that the government had been slow to resolve the situation using the Immigration Act. Oliver also opined that excluding South Asians was necessary protection against a "population that shall hamper and deter" the nation's "ideals of civilization"; he reasoned that it was "under those principles that, for my part, I desire to see this law administered."[59] This reaction typified Oliver's own approach to immigration, which, as

Chapters 1 and 2 showed, he had implemented as interior minister between 1905 and 1911. His precept that South Asians were wholly at odds with Canadian society reflected the prevailing view on Parliament Hill in both parties in 1914.

This mode of thinking, which lay at the heart of all social, economic, and political arguments against further South Asian immigration in general and the admission of the *Komagata Maru* passengers in particular, stands as a near-perfect demonstration of Edward Said's now-classic theory of Orientalism. This theory holds that Europeans saw and treated Asians from a firmly Western perspective because of a pervasive "ontological and epistemological distinction made between 'the Orient' and 'the Occident.'" By arguing that South Asians were incapable of assimilation, Oliver and his colleagues were perpetuating an imagined demarcation between white society and what Said described as the "Oriental," by which he meant the Asian "people, customs," and, above all, "mind," all of which early-twentieth-century politicians and theorists perceived as an intractable philosophical affront to the values of Western civilization.[60]

Returning to the standby of public health protection, Roche replied to Oliver that the *Komagata Maru*'s passengers had been "undergoing a very critical medical examination" and that "a good many of [them]" were infected with trachoma and other eye diseases. Norman Buchignani, Doreen Indra, and Ram Srivastava argue that the government's discovery of trachoma at Vancouver was "an old trick" designed to "make deportation certain" by "finding non-existent disease in prospective immigrants." However, the authors offer no evidence to support this claim, and aside from telegram reports there are no detailed records of the initial medical examinations of *Komagata Maru* passengers in Vancouver. This is likely because, although on-board inspections continued for as long as two weeks, none of the rejected passengers were allowed to disembark for testing, save for one Santa Singh, who on June 1 was removed from the ship during an asthma attack and brought to Vancouver General Hospital, where he died four days later. But this appears to have been an isolated case, as there were no further reports of passenger disease.[61]

When the *Komagata Maru* first arrived, a *Province* reporter had declared that the men "seemed in good health," "were certainly clean," and were, "as a body, a particularly fine looking lot of men."[62] In July the *Sun* stated that "it is a wonder that she has had so little sickness aboard," given the cramped and unsanitary living conditions. Further evidence of the men's good health could be found in the ship physician's requests for medical supplies to restock his pharmaceutical stores. Dr. Raghunath Singh, who forwarded this list to Reid before disembarking, requested a standard selection of diuretics, painkillers, expectorants, and antiseptics necessary for treating the minor ailments of more than three hundred people as they made the long return journey to India. Conspicuously absent from the list (which included potassium citrate, syrup of ipecac, camphor, and other early-twentieth-century herbals and pharmaceuticals) were thymol/chenopodium/male fern for hookworm, arsenical drugs for syphilis, and tuberculin skin-test kits for tuberculosis. Had the passengers carried these communicable diseases, it is highly likely that Singh would have requested these diagnostic and curative items for his medicine chest.[63]

So the overall health of the passengers was good. However, the ship's facilities were such that they could not stay clean, given that the vessel had been equipped to bring them to Canada, not house them for two months after their arrival. The *Province* illustrated this in a June editorial cartoon that depicted the men as dirty, sweaty, and dishevelled; meanwhile, the *Sun* described the ship as a "fragrant marine home" for its "unwashed humanity." That newspaper later demonstrated its hypocrisy in criticizing the men's hygiene. When the men were preparing to recross the Pacific in late July, a journalist ridiculed them for asking for hair oil, toothbrushes, and combs for their journey. He described them as "Hindu dandies" and "simpering popinjays" for being "particular about their personal appearance" and requesting these goods.[64]

In the end, and despite the fact that Munro's staff may have found that some of the men aboard the *Komagata Maru* had trachoma, disease was not a determining factor in the crisis's outcome. This is shown in July 1914's BC Court of Appeal decision to reject passenger Munshi Singh, who had launched a test case in an attempt to gain admission to Canada. The Court of Appeal ruling upheld the government's finding that Singh was excludable, not for health reasons but because he did not meet the provisions of PCs 23, 24, and 897. The government's November 1914 report on the incident confirmed that Singh had been deported for the sole reason that he had failed to satisfy the stipulations of these orders-in-council.[65] Shortly after this decision, the remaining passengers – who were never formally deported because, unlike Singh, they had not undergone immigration hearings – decided to abandon their mission and return to India on their own accord.

As the crew of the *Komagata Maru* prepared to leave Canadian waters, a rumour circulated in the press that a shipping company planned to transport other South Asians to Halifax via the Suez Canal. Borden asked his justice minister, C.J. Doherty, to investigate. Borden warned that South Asian immigrants brought direct to Canada's east coast "could not be excluded under existing Orders-in-Council." The prime minister's reasoning was correct. Under current legislation, Canada would have to land all healthy South Asian immigrants who arrived by continuous journey, providing they could show $200; the recent order prohibiting unskilled workers and artisans only applied to BC.[66] The Suez plan never materialized, but Borden's response to the rumour demonstrates his firm opposition to any further immigration from India. On July 23, the day after Borden issued his warning, the Canadian navy's HMCS *Rainbow* escorted the *Komagata Maru* from Canadian waters. A major tragedy occurred when the vessel reached India at the region of Budge Budge, near Calcutta. When police officials attempted to arrest Gurdit Singh on his arrival, a riot ensued and twenty of the *Komagata Maru*'s passengers were killed, while others became political prisoners. Jane Singh writes that popular indignation in India over the treatment of the vessel's passengers strengthened the position of independence activists in India. For South Asians living in BC and the Pacific coast states, the tragic outcome of the *Komagata Maru* affair was a reminder of the enduring opposition to their presence on the continent.[67]

American immigration authorities had closely watched events at Vancouver that summer. Shortly after the vessel's arrival in May, John H. Clark, the IS agent in charge of US immigration at Canadian west coast seaports and the Canadian border, cautioned that Canada's handling of the Vancouver incident would have "a material effect" on American South Asian immigration. South Asians were already surreptitiously entering Washington from BC; if Ottawa admitted the *Komagata Maru*'s passengers, they could covertly cross the border as others had done; if Ottawa barred the group, the Indians already in BC might protest by leaving Canada for the United States. Either scenario would be detrimental to American society because, Clark argued, Indians as a group were wholly "undesirable" to a nation whose mission was to "assimilate and build up one strong virile people." Thus in June, Commissioner-General of Immigration Anthony Caminetti advised the labor secretary to ask President Woodrow Wilson to change his position on the need for South Asian exclusion. While the labor secretary, W.B. Wilson, surmised that "I do not think the problem is yet in the shape where it ought to be taken up with the President," he did raise the issue with the chairman of the Congress's Immigration Committee, John L. Burnett.[68]

Caminetti's recommendation reflected the IS's enduring position on the "Hindu menace." Between 1907 and 1910, his predecessors Daniel J. Keefe, F.H. Larned, and Frank P. Sargent had overseen the collection of data for the "Reports of the Immigration Commission," a forty-one-volume government study produced by a commission chaired by Senator William P. Dillingham. Senate Asian restrictionists like Dillingham and Henry Cabot Lodge, together with other exclusionists, represented one-third of the commissioners. David Tichenor writes that the research of the Dillingham Commission was unprecedented, even "by the standards of Progressive era fact gathering and social engineering." Given that the commission's chief expert on race was Jeremiah Jenks, who asserted that the "physical characteristics of races" influenced their "temperament and [level of] civilization," it is not surprising that the study called for tighter controls on immigration from Asia and especially India. The commission also recommended limiting the settlement of southern and eastern Europeans; and it called for a higher head tax, a national origins quota system, and the introduction of a mandatory literacy test.[69] Mark Haller points out that the main outcome of Dillingham's report was "to fix the stereotyped distinction between the desirable, easily assimilated old immigrants [from the UK and Northwestern Europe] and an undesirable, inassimilable new." These findings offered key theoretical support for exclusionists and, more importantly, influenced government policy over the next decade. In particular, the findings facilitated the passage of the 1917 "Barred Zone" legislation and the 1920s Quota Acts.[70]

The commissioners had surveyed 36 different groups (mainly non-Indian community organizations) and close to 400 South Asians in California, Oregon, and Washington State, where they found a combined total of 5,000 South Asian labourers. The commission's agents determined that these workers were not strikebreakers and were filling a need for labour in resource extraction and agriculture; however, they added, the South Asian "dress, religion and manner of living" mitigated against their industrial success in the Pacific Northwest, and their declining numbers in that region's mills were due "primarily to the hostile attitude of the white workmen."[71] Commission agents found fervent anti-Indian sentiment in each Pacific state, but especially in California, where most of the new arrivals now lived, and where they were "almost universally regarded as the least desirable race of immigrants thus far admitted to the US." Although California's South Asian employment rate was high, and the group appeared to be resistant to malaria (a traditional source of labour disruption), the commissioners nonetheless adopted the popular view on the coast, adding that "the poverty and peculiar character and position" of this "filthy, ignorant, and despised race" was "likely to make them a public charge at any time."[72]

The commissioners concluded that the United States should negotiate an agreement with Britain similar to the 1907 Gentlemen's Agreement that restricted emigration from Japan. Just as Clark and Caminetti would assert three years later in 1914, the commissioners determined that exclusion was necessary because "the assimilative qualities of the East Indians appear to be the lowest of any race in the West," for "the strong influence of custom, caste, and taboo, as well as their religion, dark skins, filthy appearance, and dress, stands in the way of association with other races." Moreover, since Pacific coast communities strongly resented the South Asian presence among them, Indian immigrants would not be given the chance to assimilate and thus would "find no place in American life save in the exploitation of our resources." Although the commissioners admitted that the number of South Asians entering the country "has been affected somewhat by the attitude of the immigration authorities against them," they reasoned that "the more severe interpretation of the law has met with almost unqualified approval."[73]

While the commissioners were correct that most Americans in the west coast states approved of the executive restriction now in place at all US Pacific ports, British consular officials privately criticized the IS for discriminating against South Asians. In March 1912, A. Carnegie Ross, the British Consul General in San Francisco, complained to British ambassador James Bryce that two Indians were being detained on Angel Island for being LPC, even though they had $154 between them – significantly more money than the usual $50 that immigrants were informally expected to have – and had offers of local employment. When Ross telephoned the station to investigate, IS staffer H. Edsell informed him that "it was not enough that they should have $50" each, as South Asians were likely to lose it and then "beg at backdoors and scare white women by their appearance and threats." Ross recalled that "it was quite evident" that Edsell was "prepared to use any reason or excuse not to let Indians into the country."[74] In a letter to British foreign secretary Edward Grey, Ambassador Bryce, who did not recommend that Grey take any steps to change the situation, similarly complained that

the manner in which the US Immigration authorities utilize the Immigration law for the purpose of excluding Indians is already known to you. It is not denied by the Department that the power given to them by the law to exclude those who are "lpc" is used, not because there is any serious ground for thinking that the Indians would become a charge, but merely as an excuse for their exclusion.[75]

Paired with exclusions for hookworm infection, LPC certifications ensured a South Asian rejection rate of 25 percent over the next two decades at Angel Island. That was nearly 20 percent higher than for the next most rejected group (Mexican, at 5.15 percent).[76] IS translator S.N. Guba, a Berkeley medical student who also presumably had some knowledge of the hookworm treatment process from his work on Angel Island, offered Ross an interesting perspective on the IS policy of deporting South Asian labourers with the parasite. Ross recalled that in an interview, Guba had told him that IS officials were using hookworm as an excuse for South Asian exclusion, even though "Hook worm [*sic*] could be cured in a week and was therefore not a serious matter." This was an accurate statement. While treatment might take up to three weeks, an IS agent at Angel Island admitted in 1911 that the parasite could be expelled in just one week. Ross, who identified himself as "an Anglo Indian" who "considered [it] my duty to do all that I could for all subjects of Our Sovereign," had thus sympathized with Guba's quest to help the small number of South Asians who continued to arrive after the introduction of hookworm testing at Angel Island in the fall of 1910.[77]

Shortly after Ross and Bryce criticized IS practices at Angel Island, western Congressional representatives began to argue that this manner of executive exclusion was insufficient protection against the "Hindu menace." In Washington, DC, Congressman Denver S. Church, a Democrat from Fresno, introduced an Indian exclusion amendment to the Immigration Act, only two months after his state had passed the California Alien Land Law (or Webb Act), which in 1913 effectively barred all foreign-born Asians from landownership. His contention in October that "[South Asians] have no more love for this country than a rattlesnake has for a young turkey" preceded similar statements made in December by Congressman Albert Johnson from Tacoma, Washington. Johnson, a Republican member of the House Committee on Immigration and Naturalization, which was struck after the Dillingham Commission to consider an immigrant literacy test, declared at a committee hearing that "the State of Washington is not going to stand by and see its area filled up with Hindus, Japanese and Chinese without a protest." He conceded that "the Hindus are healthy," but he also insisted that they had "a different system of living, apparently, from ours, and a standard to which I hope no part of the United States will ever be reduced." At the same hearing, John E. Raker, a representative from Modoc County in northern California and a committee member, added that "physically and mentally, even their method of living, their method of dress, is repulsive to an association and to becoming a part and intermarrying with our American people."[78]

The recurring theme of South Asian unassimilability dominated several pages of discussion at the next committee hearing, a week later in December 1913, during which Raker prompted lobbyists from American ethnic associations to demarcate an imaginary line with immigrants from Europe on one side and "Hindus" on the other. Although congressmen J. Hampton Moore of Pennsylvania and James Manahan of Minnesota opposed this position, other committee members pontificated on the dangers of white–South Asian miscegenation, especially after Raker and Johnson equated "assimilation" with "inter-racial marriage." When New York resident Charles Sulzburger, a representative of a Jewish organization, argued that assimilation might be possible for South Asians if the term simply meant "grasp[ing] the nature and character of our institutions," Johnson used *reductio ad absurdum* statements to ridicule this position. Johnson asked, for instance, "if you lived in the West, and you heard of a business plan to bring thousands and thousands of Hindoos and line them along the Canadian line on both sides, would you not protest?" Sulzburger ultimately conceded that he would not like his child to marry a "Hindoo," and supported the regulation of South Asian immigration.[79]

For scientists, politicians, and others, the biological tenets of eugenic theory, which drew heavily from recently "rediscover[ed]" Mendelian inheritance laws, offered a cautionary tale against race mixing. Gregor Mendel's finding that plant hybridization produced a "weaker" generation easily carried over to the new sciences of biology and social studies in early-twentieth-century America, just as they did in Canada. The 1907–10 Dillingham Commission had affirmed the purported danger of interracial marriage, which David Palumbo-Liu has shown was "one of the most commonly articulated fears" at this time, when nativists exploited fears that "interbreeding" would precipitate both the "dilution of American blood" and the "demise of the nation." For nativist legislators like Raker and Johnson, immigration regulation dictated and upheld a "primordial 'natural' law" that reduced the risk of racial hybridization.[80] New Mexico Republican George C. Curry demonstrated this position when, in a congressional debate over immigration amendments in early 1914, he expressed his regret that there would be no time to debate the "Hindu" and "Asiatic" exclusion bills recently introduced by Church and Raker. Describing the American West as the "frontier between occidental and oriental civilization," he declared that intermarriage between South Asians and whites would produce "a hybrid mongrel, mentally, morally, and physical inferior to both races."[81]

Curry's remarks are important for three reasons. First, they exemplify what Palumbo-Liu views as having been an anti–melting pot groundswell in the "overall discourse of the highly rationalized project of American modernity." Second, Curry's position demonstrates what Higham has described as Southerners' sympathy for Pacific coast Americans' anxieties over Asian immigration. He explains that the dangers of the "yellow peril" "touched a responsive chord in the South," whose inhabitants "sensed the general, nativist significance" of the Japanese issue in particular, although this was caused by "long-standing 'ethnophobia'" precipitated by the black issue that "stirred southern anxieties" about maintaining "white supremacy" in America. Third, Curry's words also embody what Karen Leong describes as the prevailing "Orientalist perceptions" of Eastern decadence, exoticism, and racial "otherness" that permeated American discourse about Eastern civilizations. If, as Michael Hunt asserts, American foreign and domestic policies in the early twentieth century were rooted in a "process of nation building" and "ethnic and class division," Leong explains that American orientalism also reproduced American ideologies of "gender, race, class and nation," wherein Asians embodied and transplanted the immoral, hypersexual, and uncivilized essence of their home countries.[82]

Shortly before Curry warned Congress about the spectre of Anglo-Indian miscegenation, Commissioner-General Caminetti, a California native, reminded Pacific coast residents about the "Hindu peril" of hookworm transmission. During a tour of western inspection stations in December 1913, shortly after the Philippines loophole was closed, he informed reporters in Portland that the damp soil of Oregon and Washington was especially adapted to preserving and spreading the parasite, which was "far more prevalent and dangerous than most people believe." Since much of India's population supposedly had the disease, South Asian immigration presented a threat "greater even than that of the 'yellow peril.'" Although the *Los Angeles Times* brushed off Caminetti's warning, arguing that "we do not love hookworms or Hindus, but we are not seriously alarmed by either," other observers of South Asian immigration echoed

his anxiety. In the same week as Curry's remarks, Daniel J. Keefe, Caminetti's predecessor, wrote from Japan to warn a friend in the IS that a
small number of South Asians had just left there for San Francisco. Seeing
eight South Asians aboard the outbound SS *Nippon Maru*, he remarked
that "I don't know just how they will look when they reach the coast, but
they certainly were a dirty looking outfit, and were being treated daily for
trachoma and hookworm."[83]

By 1914, South Asians had become the particular targets of Asian exclusionists in Congress. Chinese and Japanese labourers were already
restricted through Chinese exclusion and the American–Japanese Gentlemen's Agreement; that being so, Church, Raker, and others now sought
"South Asian–specific" legislation that would remove the need for executive restriction. In February 1913, the House and Senate passed a bill
requiring immigrants over sixteen to pass a literacy test. This bill, a product
of the Dillingham Commission, would have barred most Indians, but
outgoing President William Howard Taft vetoed it before leaving office.
In March, shortly after taking office, Democratic president Woodrow
Wilson and his secretary of state, William Jennings Bryan, pressured Congress to avoid legislation that expressly targeted Japanese nationals, and
requested that the Senate not pass a Japanese exclusion bill, as these things
would reignite diplomatic tensions between Japan and the United States.
Since Britain had long been reluctant to defend the interests of South
Asians in America, and India thus had little geopolitical "pull," Wilson
made no similar pleas regarding South Asians. Congressional exclusionists
thus had free rein to campaign for the group's exclusion, but their insistence on conflating South Asian and Japanese immigration stalled progress
in this matter.[84]

Meanwhile, IS officials were deeply concerned that the Indian issue
remained unsettled, despite the dramatic drop in admissions from India
since 1910. As Chapters 3 and 4 indicated, this drop was the product of
what Jensen calls the IS's "aggressive application of general immigration
laws to South Asians," which was more effective than the "use of race-based
policies for other Asian immigrant groups."[85] While more South Asians
left the country than entered it in 1912 and 1913, Caminetti remained
concerned that the current barriers to Indian immigration would fail
before Congress officially barred the group. South Asians were no longer
entering the country via the Philippines. Now, more than half the nation's
recent Indian arrivals had landed at New York, where, unlike at San Francisco, officials did not designate these immigrants LPC, because the local

public feeling against them was less of an issue in the east. Caminetti also knew that South Asians in Panama and Cuba were attempting to enter the United States through southern ports. And Caminetti realized that the courts on the Pacific coast could easily reverse their current support for the IS's subjective application of immigration laws, and that transpacific shipping companies could renege on their recent policy of refusing to sell tickets to Indian arrivals.[86]

In January 1914, Caminetti's supervisor endorsed the need for an "anti-Hindu" law in a letter to the Speaker of the House of Representatives. Jensen describes labor secretary Wilson's letter, which was written at Congressman Church's request, as the "the most elaborate argument by an official for the exclusion of Indians."[87] Wilson recommended that the government use Bill 102, a general Asian exclusion proposition then being considered by Congress, to "dispose of the entire matter of Asiatic immigration in one measure" and thereby remove the need for the IS to continue its informal rejection system of "expedients and makeshifts." The IS was barring South Asians for physical reasons and for being LPC; the problem was that "numbers of the Hindus ... are not physically defective in the sense of the existing statute, if at all." Furthermore, excluding them as LPC for their "clannishness, caste ideas, superstitions, and habits of life" and for the local opposition to them was too oblique an approach to maintain "something which ought to be brought about by direct methods." If Bill 102 failed in the House, and if the two South Asian exclusion bills introduced in 1913 by Church and by Washington's William Humphrey also failed to pass, Wilson recommended "raising the physical standard of immigrants" to the level required for US Army recruits. Failing this possibility, Wilson favoured Church's idea of using a blanket geographic stipulation to bar Asians by country.[88] Fortuitously for the labor secretary, the 1914 Hindu Immigration Hearings offered his agency the chance to warn congressional representatives about the "urgent and imperative problem" of South Asian immigration.

The Standing House Committee on Immigration and Naturalization, chaired by Alabama Democrat John L. Burnett, opened a series of special hearings in February 1914, two weeks after the House passed Burnett's revised version of the literacy act, to investigate a bill on the Indian immigration issue. Two members from California, Raker and Everis A. Hayes, were joined by fellow exclusionist Albert Johnson; the rest of the committee was a bipartisan mix of representatives from thirteen other states. Despite Indian requests for help from Cecil Spring-Rice, the new British

Ambassador to the United States, British testimony was not heard in the proceedings. While it is tempting to infer this absence as evidence of British collusion in American exclusion efforts, it is unclear whether British representatives had been invited to testify. At the first hearing, Dr. Sudhindra Bose, a Calcutta native who taught at the University of Iowa, attempted to reassure committee members that South Asians were healthy, boasting that "in the last 10 years since I have been here never have I been sick." A widow of the former American Consul General at Calcutta followed Bose with similarly positive statements about the South Asians she had met in India. She maintained that most Indians bathed frequently, were generally clean, and had "made a study" of health.[89]

Commissioner General Caminetti, representing the IS, attended the hearing armed with his recent circular on the prevalence of hookworm in India. As the final speaker at the hearing, he countered Bose's testimony by observing that Bose had described a different type of Indian than those on the Pacific coast. Speaking personally as a California resident, he cautioned that his state had a climate warm enough to encourage almost "unlimited" immigration from India and Japan. While fewer than 9,000 South Asians had immigrated to the entire United States, he asserted (incorrectly) that an additional 20,000 to 30,000 had illegally entered and were now in California. He reminded the committee that the Rockefeller Sanitary Commission had estimated that 60 to 80 percent of South Asians carried hookworm. The following day, a Washington, DC daily announced that the Commissioner General had contravened Secretary of State Bryan's order that he not mention the need for Japanese exclusion. The press speculated that Caminetti's remarks would cost him his job, but he surprised reporters by coming back a week later to speak at the committee's next meeting.[90]

Public health protection was the dominant theme of the second hearing as well. Raker reintroduced a claim he had made at the previous meeting that "the Hindus [carried] an intestinal disease, that is ... very, very destructive, much more so than the hookworm, and once fairly lodged in this country, it would be very difficult to wipe out." He supported this statement using a recent magazine article by Charles T. Nesbitt, a well-known physician and public health director in North Carolina. Nesbitt argued that just as the former slave had "revenged upon [whites] for his enslavement" by introducing hookworm and malaria to the American South, Asians had brought these same diseases to the American West. He reasoned that Asia was "the fountain from which has flowed the most destructive pestilences that are recorded," including plague, smallpox, cholera, and typhus. Applying Robert Koch's theory of the healthy carrier, he theorized that Asians were now "unconscious carriers of virulent infective organisms" and as such were likely to be "centers of infection" everywhere they went.[91]

These ideas about infection and susceptibility reflected recent developments in epidemiological research in Asia and especially India, where "the first priorities of colonial state medicine" centred on explaining why some racial groups appeared immune to malaria and other diseases. David Arnold explains that British Indian physician Ronald Ross and others saw disease as "a site [of] racial decay" and a means of explaining why some Indian castes thrived while others did not. Nesbitt's broad reference to these theories demonstrates that the "complex intermingling of ideas of race and ideas in colonial India" held important consequences for Western medical knowledge.[92] Exclusionist speakers at the committee hearings, especially those from California, drew heavily from this race/disease connection in their discussions of Indian labour productivity, morality, and health. Church, who claimed that his district had more South Asians than any other in the country, testified that many were alcoholics and that some engaged in sodomy. Mainly, however, he argued that they were unclean, which was a key precursor to disease. "They are a dirty lot of fellows," he declared. "You can see the grease and dirt on them whenever you see them ... They smell, and sometimes a person can hardly stand it." He concluded that "you can not imagine anything more strange as a human being than a Hindu."[93]

When Caminetti returned to the committee in mid-April, he failed to assuage Massachusetts representative Augustus P. Gardner's suspicion that the IS wanted South Asian exclusion simply to divert attention from the political minefield of Japanese immigration. Since the IS had won every South Asian court challenge to restriction in the past year, Gardner asserted, and Pennsylvania's Joseph Moore concurred, that Raker's bill was simply "politics" and "an excuse to show the folks in California that people are hustling around for California." Caminetti's warning that South Asians in the Philippines were now contesting their exclusion ultimately failed to convince the committee to support the bill's adoption. Since, as noted earlier, Woodrow Wilson, like both Taft and Roosevelt before him, understood the international consequences if he sanctioned any further controls on Japanese immigration, the connection that Caminetti, Raker, Church, and Humphrey made between Japanese and South Asian exclusion influenced the immediate outcome of the "Hindu Hearings." President Wilson refused to endorse any anti-Indian legislation that might emerge from the hearings, and he prevented his Democratic Party from raising the matter again that year.

After these hearings failed to bring about an exclusion bill, Caminetti continued to lobby for exclusion. In his annual report on immigration for 1914, he warned that Indian independence activism on the Pacific coast, which was "as yet in its infancy," could become serious if the country failed to bar those "who can not be readily and healthfully assimilated by our body politic." Then in June he warned (as noted earlier) that passengers from the *Komagata Maru*, by then in Vancouver's harbour, might sneak across the border into Washington State.[94] Shortly after he made this prediction, labor secretary Wilson advised Chairman Burnett that "a large number" of South Asians had recently entered illegally through Canada; later in the year, the US consular assistant at Newfoundland informed secretary of state Bryan that Syrian residents of that colony's Bay of Islands community had paid a local fishing boat captain to smuggle at least one South Asian, apparently an "imbecile" with trachoma, to Massachusetts. The *Los Angeles Times* later reported that similar events were taking place on the nation's other border. In October a group of "mysterious and unidentified" South Asians, along with several Japanese, were arrested at Calexico after walking from Mexico, where half of the party had died in the desert.[95]

While Caminetti's agents continued to prosecute and deport South Asians accused of surreptitious entry, the precedent set by a landmark court decision in early 1915 threatened the legitimacy of the IS's exclusion policy at Pacific coast ports. In February of that year, a lower court in Oregon overturned an earlier ruling that had allowed Portland officials to exclude a group of Russian immigrants on the grounds that they would be unlikely to find work on landing. Earlier chapters have shown that IS officials at Angel Island, Seattle, Portland, and Vancouver had long employed this argument to justify South Asian exclusion, and a series of recent court challenges had ruled in favour of exclusion for the reason that South Asians were LPC due to industrial and social conditions on the coast. Indeed, in 1914 Angel Island's chief commissioner reflected that "one of the most satisfactory developments" in the South Asian issue was the "unmistakable attitude of the district court" in refusing to challenge the IS's position that virtually all Indians were LPC. After the Russian ruling, Caminetti and others, including a prominent former district attorney in San Francisco, predicted an increase in Indian immigration while exclusionary legislation stalled in Congress.[96]

When, in February 1915, President Wilson vetoed the Burnett literacy bill, Denver S. Church warned the House that the continuing lack of congressional exclusion left the nation vulnerable to South Asians, who were the "greatest plagues we have in the west." He added that some who now lived in his native state of California always gave "the appearance of slothfulness, stupidity, and pity" and lived in filthy conditions.[97] Evidence from "Hindu" camp inspections suggests that some South Asians, like new immigrants from other ethnic groups, did live in unsanitary accommodations that considerably impaired their social standing among established populations along the coast in this era. For example, in early 1916, a California State Board of Health inspector found that a large South Asian agricultural work camp near Sacramento, which housed up to forty men in high season, was kept in a "filthy condition," mainly because the camp's owner had provided substandard housing for his workers. The same inspector found that a separately owned camp on Bacon Island in the Sacramento–San Joaquin river delta was in good shape except for the South Asian kitchen and dining room. At a Stockton camp with up to one hundred South Asians, Japanese, and Mexicans, the South Asian kitchen building was in "dilapidated and filthy condition," as was the kitchen at a separately owned South Asian and Italian work camp on Staten Island near Stockton. Given that these camps were managed by different owners, it is not unreasonable to surmise that at least some South Asians were keeping their meal preparation areas in poor condition. This was not universal, however; a camp owned by a prominent Japanese businessman in the San Joaquin valley, the inspector found that the South Asian quarters were kept clean while the Japanese and Mexican-occupied house was not. As was the case with camps owned by whites, unsanitary living conditions could probably be blamed as much (if not more) on the managers than on the workers themselves.[98]

In his 1915 Stanford University thesis on South Asian immigrants in North America, Joginder Chandler Misrow, a former interpreter for the IS and labour camp investigator in California, argued that these sorts of living conditions prejudiced Western populations against South Asians, but that the prejudice was also "partly an unreasoned color phobia, based on the primitive instincts of fear and hate." The fact that most of the immigrants had travelled so far for work indicated that their living standard was "dynamic," not static, and would over time "continually tend to conform to the locally prevalent standard." Like other labourers along the coast, South Asians "endure[d] all the hardships of inadequate lodging," especially the bunkhouse, which was often "a menace to health and morals" but often represented the only housing available to them.[99] State Board of Health documentation indicates that inspectors generally attributed unsanitary bunkhouse conditions not to the camp owners but to the immigrants themselves, especially since, as the board's assistant secretary wrote to a white farm manager, "certain nationalities" required "constant supervision" by camp managers.[100]

Most white populations saw the South Asians who lived in rural work camps in the 1910s as "sojourners," a term designating migrants who take up temporary residence in a new land and who, according to Paul Siu's 1952 study, "resist both cultural change and any form of integration." Siu, who researched Chinese immigrants in the United States, argued that "the essential characteristic of the sojourner is that he clings to the culture of his own ethnic group as in contrast to the bicultural complex of the marginal man." Overall, the sojourner is "psychologically ... unwilling to organize himself as a permanent resident" in his new land; when he finally does this, "he becomes a marginal man." Siu's term is in many ways a relic of the now outdated 1950s melting pot theory of assimilation, which presumes that immigrants replace traditional values and activities with new ones. Thomas Archdeacon's recent application of the sojourner label offers a more useful lens for understanding how Asians, the group who "bore the brunt of nativism's outbursts," initially planned their migration to the Americas as a temporary measure and thus lived a nomadic life, separate from other groups.[101] Certainly this describes the situation of most first wave Indian immigrants. In 1916, most of the roughly 5,000 Indians who remained in the Pacific coast states lived in camps where they were often housed separately from other ethnic groups. However, Bruce La Brack points out that the label does not fit all South Asian settlers, in that most of them over time underwent "varying degrees of culture change" and altered their "ideological and structural patterns," even if many continued to live apart from whites.[102]

In his discussion of bunkhouse living in the American West, Nayan Shah explains that the "intensive cultivation" demanded by agricultural production, especially of fruit, cotton, and rice crops, necessitated worker flexibility. Consequently, ranch managers often subleased their land or hired labour contractors, who then sought tenant labour to plant, maintain, and harvest produce. Often, groups of males and/or families were hired to work together and were sheltered temporarily in cabins, barns, or houses or at tented campsites. South Asian work gangs formed through connections within families or castes or with home communities, and later by necessity through shared work and commuting demands. Living largely apart from women and spending virtually all of their working and recreational time together, these male work bands cultivated very strong relationships. Ties between unrelated labourers were "recast with kin-like terms," such as brother, which "affirm[ed] the intimacy of the relationship." A bunkhouse could house several men, and sometimes the manager shoehorned more in by having two share one bunk. Outside observers of these sleeping arrangements, which diverged so radically from traditional family housing, often associated them with immorality, especially sexual impropriety.[103]

Overall, public and official tolerance of the presence and living situation of South Asian workers in the West continued to decline even after the group's exclusion, and especially by 1916, by which time public opinion was increasingly divided nationwide over the war in Europe. Attitudes on the broader immigration issue also changed, and Asian exclusionists, who had long been protesting Indian labour competition and the deplorable conditions at some South Asian labour camps, soon generated wide appeal for their cause. Western newspaper editorial pages abounded with anti-Indian diatribes, and many of these reflected the ways in which, as Alexandra Stern writes, the "biases" of tropical medicine, "social Darwinism," and "Victorian anthropology" had "insinuated themselves into the race betterment movement during its incipient formation, eventually leaving imprints on eugenics, especially in the American West." For example, a Portland resident warned Pacific coast newspaper readers that "if the yellow man is a peril, the brown man is a calamity," because despite the best efforts of India's British leaders, generations of incest and child marriage had produced an Indian populace both "stunted in growth" and "diseased in body." He concluded that while Americans were largely protected by the nation's "rigid quarantine measures against the dreadful diseases of India ... no quarantine measures will avail against the centuries of hereditary paganism and immorality that are born in every son of India."[104]

These remarks typified the eugenicists' argument that both infection and susceptibility were heritable. Stern describes the early twentieth century as a "transitory" time when "neo-Lamarckian" principles of hered-ity and the miasmatic, sanitarian theory of disease transmission were giving way to more rigid concepts of bacteriology and genetics. Developments in bacteriology had shown that "microbes and their vectors happily trans-gressed all social and national lines," yet colonial theory maintained the race/disease association, even after the shift from miasmatic to germ theory, because "assumptions of the backwardness and pathology of col-onized peoples remained largely intact," although they were now under-stood as the consequence of unsanitary habits and an inherited disposition for infection.[105]

This was not a denial of germ theory; rather, the idea was that better breeding could produce better resistance and even immunity. The link between bacteriology and eugenics was being employed to determine the health of certain races and to demand the exclusion of various immigrant groups, including South Asians.[106]

Eugenic theory dominated the 1916 congressional debates over the general immigration bill, which John L. Burnett had reintroduced after Wilson's 1915 veto. The bill now included generalized citizenship tests, literacy requirements, and a strategic geographic provision that would bar Asians from immigrating. Burnett informed the House that in drafting the bill, the "committee wants to say flatly that we intended to exclude Hindus." However, the committee later accepted Illinois Republican James R. Mann's recommendation that in order to prevent "bitterness" in India, the bill use language that excluded South Asians without identifying them specifically.[107] Denver S. Church, whom Jensen describes as "instrumental" to the Act's Indian exclusion provision, delivered a special address on the "Hindu crisis" shortly after the bill passed the House and was sent to the Senate. Church, like Burnett, argued that it was in the nation's interest to exclude Indian workers. He described India's population as "a plague" and "a swarm of hungry flies" anxious to take white American jobs. He predicted that if the Senate did not pass the bill, South Asians would soon crowd California with their "heathen shacks and shanties." He concluded passionately:

I wish you had seen the Hindu and knew him as I do ... his swarthy, ragged form ... his lifeless, shuffling walk and drooping, downcast head ... I say it is constitutionally wrong for these strange people, who have slept and de-generated through the ages, to wait until the last great prize of civilization,

America, has been discovered and won, and then ... fall upon us like hateful birds upon the first fruits of spring.[108]

Church's lobbying on the Indian issue, which clearly drew heavily from the "Hindu disease" thesis, came to fruition in December, when the Senate passed a version of the Burnett bill that included the Indian Subcontinent within its Asian immigrant "barred zone." The Act was in fact a compromise between those who wanted to explicitly exclude all Asian immigrants, and President Woodrow Wilson's desire to keep Japanese nationals out of the legislation for reasons of diplomacy.[109] When Wilson rejected the bill, the House and Senate passed it over his veto; thus, the Immigration Act of 1917 became law on February 5, 1917. Most Chinese immigration had been prohibited by the Chinese Exclusion Act of 1882; now, for the first time, South Asians and other Asians and Pacific Islanders were officially excluded. Japanese nationals, whose immigration was still governed by the 1907 Gentlemen's Agreement, were exempt from this legislation, as were Filipinos. The Barred Zone provision of the 1917 legislation decisively ended Indian immigration, which in practice had ceased several years earlier, soon after the IS began barring the group by executive action. Seven years later, the "Asian Exclusion Act" provision of the Johnson–Reed Act would exclude India's residents by name.

This chapter has shown how health-based anti-Indian logics and policies established early in the movement of South Asians to North America, including governments' resort to hookworm screening, were employed to defend the propriety and legitimacy of South Asian exclusion. In Canada, the Department of the Interior used a 1912 report connecting South Asians with tuberculosis to justify the decision not to allow the families of resident South Asians to immigrate. Federal legislators also used health and eugenic arguments to defend the decision to reject the passengers of *Komagata Maru* in 1914. American observers of the *Komagata Maru* affair warned that it might threaten American executive exclusion and set a precedent for other Indians to increase their efforts to migrate to the continent; for this reason, US federal officials emphasized the urgent need for exclusionary legislation. Taking up the cause, congressional representatives from Washington State and California contended, like their counterparts in Canada, that South Asian health, living standards, and genetic stocks precluded their assimilation into Pacific coast society. Finally, Congress passed the 1917 Immigration Act, which designated South Asians as residents of a geographic area barred from immigrating to the United

States. The following chapter will address the consequences of this legislation for South Asian rights in America. After first exploring how Canadian officials used health-based arguments to respond to South Asians' requests for citizenship during and after the First World War, the focus will shift to the Pacific coast states, where, after legislative exclusion, American officials used similar reasoning to address the franchise issue in that country.

6

Franchise Denied

I cannot work up my mind to view with favor the situation of the franchise to a body of men 90% of whom are low caste Hindus, filthy, morally and physically, and entirely ignorant with respect to our political ideas and with no "vision" as Canadians.

– *Charles Herbert Dickie, MP for Nanaimo, BC, 1921.*

IN 1921, THIRTEEN YEARS after the introduction of Canada's continuous journey provision, the leader of the federal Opposition party explored introducing the franchise to the Dominion's fewer than 3,000 South Asians. The following pages show how the bipartisan political reply to this idea was rooted in vociferous anti-Indian sentiment that had endured in Canada throughout the First World War and, in 1919, had intensified when federal officials allowed the families of resident workers to emigrate from India. In the United States, several South Asians had become American citizens in the first two decades of the century, but in 1923 a landmark court decision revoked their national status and decreed that South Asians could no longer become citizens. The second part of this chapter explains how the US government maintained this policy by resorting to the argument that South Asians, who had been legislatively excluded in 1917, could not assimilate because of their health practices and morality.

In an article published shortly after the resolution of the *Komagata Maru* crisis in July 1914, the Dominion's Superintendent of Immigration W.D. Scott reminded Canadians that the nation's South Asians were susceptible to "pneumonia and pulmonary troubles," which had already claimed the lives of "no small number" of them. Echoing the similar assertions of Immigration Branch agent Frederick C. Blair and interior minister Robert Rogers in 1912, he reasoned that "it is doubtful whether with their constitutions, suitable for the country and climate from which they came, they will become thoroughly acclimatized in Canada."[1] In a private letter to a Vancouver doctor, H.H. Stevens, federal MP for Vancouver, similarly asserted that South Asians were inassimilable because, while all Asians were "most trouble-some from a sanitary standpoint," "the worst sinner of all is the Hindu." Stevens concluded that the "Asiatic diseases" of small-pox, cholera, hookworm, and plague made the group a "distinct menace" to the Pacific coast. Science had proved that some Asians were immune to the effects of these diseases but that those same illnesses caused "epidemics of the most violent character" among whites. Perhaps the greater danger, however, was the possibility of intermarriage between whites and Asians, which would "invariably" produce children of inferior genetic stock.[2]

Theories about the pitfalls of race mixing dominated Canadian and especially British Columbian popular and academic discourse at the time. According to Sherene Razack, BC's nineteenth-century colonial administrators and religious leaders worried that race mixing would "confuse the racial hierarchies they were constructing" and obstruct the "illusory goals of a homogenous and respectable white settler society." After BC joined Canada, the demarcation along racial lines had become vital to nation-building on the Pacific coast.[3] While some theorists had begun to question Galtonian theories of race categorization, Ian McKay points out that virtually every element of the Canadian Dominion, including its "institutions, intellectual theory, popular culture, and the law," all "resonated with the idea and practice of race" in this era. These observations help explain Stevens's warning about the perils of white–Asian intermarriage.[4]

In October 1914, a murder captured evening newspaper headlines across Canada. Vancouver resident Mewa Singh killed Immigration Branch agent W.C. Hopkinson in a Vancouver courthouse where the immigration inspector was defending Bela Singh, one of his informants. Hopkinson's five years of surveillance work had dramatically affected the province's South Asians; he had become a visible representation of British repression and a convenient focal point of anti-imperialist sentiment. His attempts to repress Indian activities had, as Hugh Johnston explains, "helped to politicize and factionalize the local Sikh community." This had led to his death and to a string of related murders. Overall, he had become "as much an author as an investigator of the agitation on the Pacific coast."[5]

After Hopkinson's death, interior minister W.J. Roche decided that the Immigration Branch would not hire another agent to continue the inspector's work. In part, this was because no more than 3,000 South Asians remained in Canada. Federal officials attributed this to the physical unsuitability of the recent arrivals to Canada's climate and labour conditions. It is likely, too, that many were unable to find work in 1913 and 1914, when unemployment in the province was high. Some South Asians were returning to India because their families were prohibited from joining them in Canada. Also, beginning in 1914, many left to join India's independence movement.[6] However, Malcolm J. Reid, who became the Dominion Immigration Agent for BC in 1915, took over some of Hopkinson's old duties by meeting his informants and forwarding information to imperial authorities. After the 1915 Singapore Mutiny, during which several hundred South Asian sepoys rebelled against their British officers, Reid secured federal press censorship of all telegrams among South Asians in BC and became, in Johnston's words, "the key intelligence figure" in the province, running a special surveillance agency within the Immigration Branch. Reid may also have worked with Britain's Intelligence Service until 1936.[7]

In August 1915, H.C. Clogstoun, a retired India Office staffer commissioned by Robert Borden's government to investigate the aftermath of the *Komagata Maru* incident, reported a major health crisis among the province's South Asians. His extraordinary conclusion that many of them were alcoholics – for which there was limited evidence – offers another example of official anti-Indian racism in the province. According to an inspector whose testimony was appended to Clogstoun's report, two Duncan employers claimed that their "Hindu" workers regularly drank to excess, which "seriously impaired their usefulness." The daughter of an Indian Army officer living in the province reported that she had been shocked by remarks made by "a number of Hindus sitting under a tree drinking beer" in Nanaimo. The author surmised from these accounts that the South Asian in BC, with his "sensitive nature and excitable temperament," had misinterpreted the West's "peculiar mixture of familiarity and equality, together with much subtle rascality" (i.e., alcohol use). Clogstoun memorably concluded that "under reasonable control the native of India is amenable and capable of such good." But "in its absence he is as troublesome as an undisciplined child, with the capacity for mischief of a man."[8]

Norman Buchignani, Doreen M. Indra, and Ram Srivastava assert that excessive alcohol consumption due to loneliness was one of the few "social and psychological problems" that resulted from the "Spartan life" of BC's

South Asians, who were living apart from their families. The authors contend that heavy drinking spiked among the group in the 1920s and that some men were "consumed by it," although most drinking occurred in private and resulted in few arrests. One participant in the Indo-Canadian Oral History Collection, whose father was Gurdás Singh, a champion wrestler in Canada, reported that he (the son) became an alcoholic and served jail time for related behaviour during this period. He attributed his alcoholism to cheap beer relative to the high wages in BC's lumber industry, and recalled that drinking was a central social activity of his life as a young man. The *Toronto Star Weekly* later reported a Vancouver Island missionary's belief that the "drink traffic and its attendant evils" had rendered the region's South Asians immoral. Interestingly, however, in his 1913 public statement defending South Asian health, former CPR physician E.H. Lawson had testified that Sikhs' "use of alcoholic liquors" was more moderate than that of Europeans.[9]

In 1916, shortly after Clogstoun submitted his report, the India Office finally convinced Scott to recommend that Canada now assuage the loneliness of resident South Asians by waiving the continuous journey order for their wives and dependent children. Scott conceded that this move was necessary, in light of India's contributions to the ongoing war effort in Europe and Africa, along with the "unfortunate" political fallout in India from the *Komagata Maru* affair and the Budge Budge tragedy of 1914. The war – and significant wartime unemployment in BC – delayed interior minister W.J. Roche's action on the issue, although in the meantime the minister informed the cabinet that the immigration of more male South Asian labourers should be discouraged since "disease has made considerable inroads upon East Indians." After the India Office raised the family issue again at the 1917 Imperial Conference in London, Borden agreed to consider it, and finally, in March 1919, he introduced an order-in-council allowing resident South Asians to send for their wives and dependent children. However, many BC residents vociferously opposed the 1919 order. For example, John Wallace de Beque Farris, the provinces' attorney general, spoke out against it, as did the editor of Vancouver mayor Louis D. Taylor's newspaper *The Critic*.[10]

In June, Reid forwarded to Ottawa what he called the "rather remarkable letter" of Canadian Lieutenant-Colonel Charles Flick to the *Vancouver Sun*. Given its contents, it is perhaps surprising that Flick became one of Vancouver Island's most vociferous opponents of Japanese internment during the next war. Writing from Karachi in 1919, Flick recalled that in

his work with the Euphrates defence forces in the First World War, he had
personally convened courts martial on several Indian soldiers accused of
sodomy "either with man or beast," and warned that "it is to men of this
perverted nature that Canada wishes to open her western door." He asserted that the "belauding [*sic*] of the Indian soldier" was misleading many
Canadians at home about Indian morality and loyalty. He had seen very
few South Asian regiments fight admirably for the British Raj, especially
in Mesopotamia, where Allied forces would send in Indian soldiers only
after Turkish morale had been "broken" by white forces. Flick concluded:
"I may say that were Sikhs or Hindus allowed free access into western
Canada there would arise in cities like Vancouver and Victoria native
quarters that [in] filth and bestiality would put the worst slums of Chinatown into the shade."[11] Nayan Shah explains that in Canada, as in the
United States, legislation in place since the nineteenth century had strictly
prohibited homosexual behaviour. There was some question about how
to define "male volition, consent, and violation" between adults, but the
courts generally treated sodomy as an act "against nature."[12] Flick therefore
had made a very serious assertion.

   Flick's contention that Canada's South Asians were homosexual was
incorrect; the majority of them were heterosexual married men who would
be able to reunite with their immediate families after 1921. Most of the
family arrivals were healthy, given that before leaving Asian ports, steamship passengers were now required to pass at least one medical inspection.
However, Indo-Canadian Oral History Project participant Kartar Singh
Ghag recalled that some contracted trachoma while en route to BC. Ratan
Kaur Thauli, another Project informant, who arrived in 1924, reported
that she had had to undergo three months of treatment for the same
disease in Hong Kong before continuing to Canada. Surviving files of the
Department of Immigration and Colonization, the agency that took over
the Department of the Interior's responsibility for immigration in 1917,
indicate that nine South Asians were detained for observation and/or
treatment out of the close to seventy arriving in 1921, and the same number were held for these reasons in 1922. Some of the detained were male
minors classified as "schoolboys"; the balance were dependents or returning labourers, whose names appeared after long lists of Chinese
detentions.[13]

   The new arrivals joined members of the province's South Asian community, who generally were at least as healthy as other Asian immigrants
in the province. Victoria's Chief Medical Officer reported that only one

South Asian in the city had died from tuberculosis in 1920 – the first year that the city published tubercular deaths categorized by ethnic group – compared to eighteen whites and eight Chinese. In 1922, Dr. Frederick T. Underhill, who was still Vancouver's Medical Officer of Health, reported that while municipal mortalities from the disease had steadily declined over the past three years, Chinese rates were "very high" – an astounding 1 in every 2.5 Chinese deaths was linked to the disease. Although BC and Canadian officials continued to connect South Asians with tuberculosis, no members of the group died from it in 1923, while Chinese deaths accounted for 31.3 percent and Japanese deaths counted for 26.9 percent of the city's 143 tuberculosis deaths that year.[14] Overall, throughout this period, South Asian mortality rates in Vancouver remained at approximately the same level as the rates for other groups.[15]

In 1921, Hon. V.S. Srinivasa Sastri, Indian politician and League of Nations delegate, reminded the Imperial Conference in London that despite the Canadian government's concession on the "family immigration" issue, Canada and every other white UK Dominion continued to discriminate against resident South Asians by denying them the franchise. Canada's Conservative prime minister Arthur Meighen responded by stating his hope that Canada would soon take steps to grant citizenship rights to the nation's South Asians, who now numbered only about 1,200 in BC. Sastri visited the country the following summer during an imperial tour to promote Indian rights in the Empire. Prime Minister W.L.M. King, who had defeated Meighen in the December 1921 election, arranged for Under Secretary of State Sir Joseph Pope to accompany Sastri on his speaking tour of BC in July, which forced Pope into the awkward position of serving as Sastri's chaperone *and* public relations moderator. Before the mission, King warned Pope that Canada's "official position" was that any past grievances had been resolved and that relations between whites and resident Indians were now "wholly cordial." Sastri could incite "serious agitation on the Pacific Coast" if his visit revealed that "any grievances existed" or that any "rights should be permitted which [were] being denied." King also advised Pope to discourage Sastri from saying "anything that might encourage more South Asians to want to settle in Canada," later adding that it would be unwise for Sastri to disrupt "the satisfactory state of things" by drawing public attention to any injustices against South Asians in BC.[16]

To King's relief, Sastri was relatively well received on the Pacific coast, where his moderate speeches at Vancouver's Canadian Club and other venues called only for a reconsideration of South Asian voting rights, not the resumption of South Asian immigration. When Pope travelled with Sastri to Victoria to meet with BC's premier John Oliver, he found that the premier had left town in advance of his arrival. The under secretary of state privately observed his disappointment that no one in the provincial government was on hand to meet the "cultivated East Indian" who "speaks English perfectly," and his secretary, G.S. Bajpai, who was "also an Indian, but an Oxford man."[17] At Pope's request, Premier Oliver eventually returned to Victoria to meet with Sastri, but he offered no concrete help on the franchise issue. On his return to Ottawa, Sastri asked King to consider modifying the Dominion Elections Act to allow residents to vote in federal elections even if they were denied the right to vote in BC, which was the current barrier to the Dominion franchise for the group. Sastri reminded King of Meighen's 1921 promise, and offered examples of times when Parliament had "not strictly adhered to" provincial requirements for the federal franchise.[18]

King and his cabinet decided, after "personal discussion," not to honour Meighen's 1921 pledge to seriously consider introducing the franchise.

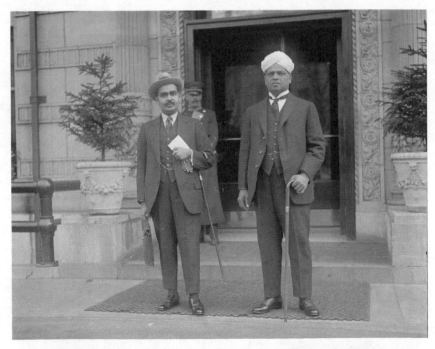

FIGURE 8   V.S. Srinivasa Sastri (right) in Washington, DC, 1921. | Digital File No. LC-DIG-npcc-05297. National Photo Collection/US Library of Congress, Washington, DC.

This was for three reasons. First, King's Liberals had a House majority of only one MP and could not guarantee the success of a franchise measure. Second, it was against the party's "tradition and policy" to oppose a provincial government on election matters; in order to grant South Asians voting rights without overhauling the Dominion Elections Act, King would have to convince BC legislators to grant the group the provincial franchise before they would be allowed to vote in federal elections. Third, and most importantly, the cabinet felt it would be "tacitly unwise" to initiate debate on a policy that "would probably array all the conservative forces in the country against it." In a 1946 memorandum on the issue, however, a staffer in the Department of External Affairs recalled that Sastri had shown "the hollowness of these arguments" by pointing out that the Liberals had the support of the Progressive Party, which held the balance of power in a minority Parliament, and that Meighen, still the Conservative leader, "might be trusted to persuade his own followers to agree" on a franchise bill.[19]

Likely unbeknownst to King and his cabinet, opposition leader Meighen launched a similar discussion within his own party in the fall of 1922. The former prime minister had befriended Sastri after the 1921 Imperial Conference, had travelled to Vancouver to see him during his visit that summer, and had introduced him to the Meighen family. Meighen's biographer Roger Graham argues that for Meighen, "love of country [meant] more than love of Canada alone" – that Canada was "inconceivable except as a partner of that old land he had never seen but to which he was devoted for its traditions, achievements and nobility of character." Likely for this reason and for his feeling of imperial obligation, on Sastri's request Meighen asked his Conservative MPs from BC for their advice on whether he should introduce an Indian franchise measure in the House. He told them that despite the "small political danger" involved in raising the issue with Liberals, who were "liv[ing] up to their usual tactics and show[ing] no attitude at all" on it, Canada might someday "deep[ly] regret" denying Sastri's appeal, which was of "very real consequence to the Empire as a whole."[20]

The replies of five of the seven Conservative MPs from BC are a treasure trove of personal and candid opinions that reflected the general views of their constituents. Each MP asserted that Meighen should not raise the franchise issue in the House, nor take any initiative on the matter. Interestingly, Asian exclusionist H.H. Stevens was the only one to agree without exception that resident South Asians should have the vote, likely because

Sastri had personally assured Stevens that India would not ask Canada to reverse its exclusion policy. However, Stevens felt that the "proper course" was for Canada to convince BC to modify its Elections Act, a duty that "rests wholly upon Mackenzie King and John Oliver and you and I are not called upon to relieve them of this responsibility."[21]

Vancouver South MP Leon Ladner, who had written his riding's recent petition for a general Asian exclusion law, replied that after Sastri's summer address at the Canadian Club, the Native Sons of BC, an organization planning speeches to a "large number of public bodies on the Lower Mainland" with the goal of "forming public opinion against extending the vote to East Indians," invited Ladner to speak to them. When he spoke about the possibility of granting the franchise, he found that most audience members were "willing to sacrifice their prejudice in the interests of the Empire," although since "90% of the Hindus here are ignorant, uneducated and unacquainted with our form of Government," he predicted that most residents of his riding would be against an Indian franchise concession. However, he agreed with Meighen that "the interests of Imperial unity must determine the minds of those of us in public life."[22]

Two weeks later, Ladner retracted this admission in a follow-up letter. After reportedly interviewing "all classes of the people" in Vancouver South, he now believed that "it would be politically unwise for our party to take the initiative" on the matter. There was a "deep rooted objection to the Oriental, both to his presence and to the extension of any rights," and residents worried that granting the vote to South Asians as British subjects would, by extension, grant the vote to naturalized Japanese. New Westminster MP William Garland McQuarrie was "very much opposed to granting the franchise to East Indians" for this reason. Ladner added that Victoria City's MP Simon Fraser Tolmie had "retained his original view that he was entirely opposed" to the Indian franchise. In his third and final letter on the subject, Ladner reported that in a meeting with thirty-five members of his riding's executive council, "some of the best heads in the gathering" had stated that prevailing racial sentiment in the district would prevent Vancouver South from accepting Indian voting rights. Overall, Ladner recommended that, as "a matter of good judgment and practical politics," Meighen should "let the Government carry the whole matter through if possible without a division and without our people being brought into a debate."[23]

Nanaimo MP Charles Herbert Dickie, the most vociferous opponent of Meighen's proposal, reassured his leader that "our East Indians are prospering" and "not laying awake nights because of franchise restrictions." He added:

> I hardly know how to answer your request as to my views respecting enfranchisement of our East Indian population. Viewed "by and large" these people should be given full citizenship, but I cannot work up my mind to view with favor the situation of the franchise to a body of men 90% of whom are low caste Hindus, filthy, morally and physically and entirely ignorant with respect to our political ideas and with no "vision" as Canadians ... Any small concession we can make would do but little to allay discontented discussion when wild eyed orators are at large among those credulous, inconsistent and not altogether lovable people.[24]

In October, Meighen informed Sastri of his decision not to raise the matter in the House, but promised to raise the matter again with his party, as "the vital interests of the Empire as a whole" depended on it.[25]

When the House debated a different amendment to the Immigration Act in February 1923, J.A. Robb, King's trade and commerce minister, suggested that the Dominion's 1,200 South Asians be enfranchised because the Canada–India trade relationship was growing. Samuel William Jacobs, a Quebec Liberal like Robb, and an influential figure in Montreal's Jewish community, agreed, adding that many Indians had volunteered to fight in the Great War. However, several BC Liberals privately told King that they "strongly opposed" this concession. King thus concluded, as had Meighen the previous year, that "it will never do to go to [*sic*] oppose wishes of BC electors in this matter." In his diary, King also reasoned that "we had done enough for the Empire and its problems without endangering our own position as a Gov for something that is really not a sound grievance," and that the "empire citizenship business can be overdone," as each colony had the right to control its own citizenship. When the House revisited the matter in a twenty-seven-page discussion in June, Jacobs likened Meighen's remarks at the 1921 Imperial Conference to US president Woodrow Wilson's signing of the 1919 Treaty of Versailles, which pledged that America would join the League of Nations – a promise the Senate later refused to endorse. In a startling about-face from his 1912 remonstrations against South Asians, Labour MP James Shaver Woodsworth of Manitoba sided with Jacobs, recalling that he had been greatly impressed with BC's Sikhs after visiting a Vancouver *gurdwara*.[26]

Jacobs and Woodsworth represented the minority opinion. Progressive MP Thomas George McBride of Cariboo, BC, countered in the debate that "we in BC want no more Hindus," and added that "never did I value Canada and the laws of Canada more highly" than when the nation turned away the "boat-load of Hindus" in 1914. Not surprisingly, Nanaimo's C.H. Dickie added that "for the Hindu of low caste we have still less room than for others of the oriental races." He elaborated that "you cannot comprehend the eastern mind unless you have lived among the people," because "these Hindus are not men such as we are; they have the mentality of children without childhood's innocence." Once enfranchised, the group would obediently vote for whomever their seditious leaders felt would support their cause. King closed the discussion by declaring aloud what he had written in his diary in March – that Canada could not force the matter since BC so strongly opposed it, and that it could be resolved in the House alone and not "at any Imperial Conference." Members voted to delay action on the issue, and it rested in the House until 1936.[27]

Although BC's federal politicians provided the loudest and most passionate opposition to the South Asian request for the franchise in BC, the Department of Immigration and Colonization's Frederick C. Blair also played an important, and largely overlooked, role in maintaining the barriers to the Indian franchise and further immigration. The continuous journey order, PC 920, could only be revised or repealed by parliamentary decree or through another order-in-council, but I have shown that in 1912, interior minister Robert Rogers had used Blair's field report to justify maintaining the exclusion of wives and children from India in the prewar period. Shortly before the 1923 House debates on the franchise, King prepared for discussions on the issue using another Blair report that repeated the immigration agent's arguments from 1912. In a lengthy and confidential memorandum to Sir Joseph Pope, who reported directly to King, Blair maintained that "the climate of British Columbia," was the "chief" cause of the South Asian "exodus from Canada" over the years. Blair later added that Canada continued to bar South Asians for climatic reasons, and also because the group could not be quickly assimilated into society.

After King successfully deflected debate on the voting in June, Blair continued to perpetuate the climate argument when he replaced W.W. Cory as assistant deputy immigration minister in 1924. In that year, Blair stated that it would not be "a kindness" to reopen Indian immigration because South Asians were "accustomed to a tropical climate." Blair would

maintain this viewpoint almost twenty years later when he became immigration director. In 1943, when the Immigration Branch of the Department of Mines and Resources, the agency then responsible for
immigration, faced increasing opposition in central Canada to the continued exclusion of South Asians, Blair defended the now thirty-five-year-
old Indian exclusion policy as "necessary in the interests of East Indians
themselves, as well as of Canada in general and British Columbia in
particular."[28] Blair's position on the issue helped delay the South Asian
franchise until 1947, five years before Canada reopened its borders to
South Asians using a small annual quota of 150 Indians, 100 Pakistanis,
and 50 Ceylonese.

The protracted quest for South Asian suffrage in the United States was
similarly stalled by racial sentiment in the first half of the century. Unlike
their counterparts in Canada, some émigrés from India living in the United
States had won the federal franchise before and after legislative exclusion
in 1917; by 1923, around sixty had successfully applied for US citizenship
in the lower courts of several states using a 1906 law that granted naturalization rights to eligible "free white persons" and those of "African nativity and descent" who had learned English. In Progressive Era America as
today, "race" and "ethnicity" were fluid and ambiguous categories, con-
sciously constructed and employed in order to differentiate between
groups within American society.[29] This explanation holds true in the case
of South Asians, who were variously seen as "Asiatics," "blacks," "low caste
Indians," and "Aryans." For British Indian social scientists, caste divisions
represented racial differences, and physical distinctions between castes
demonstrated the varying levels of race purity between the Dravidian,
Mongoloid, and Aryan "types" that had been carefully maintained by what
Arnold describes as "the race-consciousness of the fair-skinned Aryan
[northern invaders of India from millennia ago] and the taboos on marriage enforced through caste endogamy."[30] "High caste" (mainly Brahmin)
South Asians transplanted these ideas in the United States by pointing
out that Indians and Europeans were ethnologically linked through a
shared Aryan heritage, and also by equating "Aryan" with "Caucasian."
Using this argument, several "high caste" individuals convinced American
lower court judges that they were, as members of the Mediterranean
branch of the Caucasian race, "white."[31] It is worth noting that no South
Asian applicants for US citizenship argued that they were "black" and/or
that their darker skin tone indicated ancestral ties to Africa, which, under
the above-mentioned 1906 Naturalization Act and the Fifteenth

Amendment of the US Constitution in 1870, was the other option available to them.[32]

Eugenic theory featured prominently in the public and official responses to these "high caste" naturalizations, just as it had in the push for South Asian exclusion in the decade preceding the 1917 "Barred Zone" Act. Hernan Shah explains that the American courts, the press, and Congress together "manipulat[ed] the meaning of the term white to ensure that the rights and privileges of citizenship could be limited to those designated white." Prior to the US government's arrest of philosopher Har Dayal for propagating anarchist literature in 1914, "high caste" Brahmins garnered relatively little press coverage compared to the "low caste Hindus" who formed the majority of those who had settled on the Pacific coast. After Dayal was arrested and fled to Switzerland, "high caste" Brahmins were no longer seen as agents of social change but as anarchists and terrorists, an association cemented by press coverage of the 1917 "Hindu conspiracy trial" in San Francisco. In that trial, several South Asians, including Ram Chandra, C.K. Chakravarty, Bhagwan Singh, and former IS translator Taraknath Das, along with Franz Bopp, the German Consul in San Francisco, were tried for violating American neutrality laws, as well as for conspiracy for plotting to incite a revolution in India using German arms. Extensive press coverage of the court proceedings, the dramatic assassination of Chandra in the courtroom, and the guilty ruling at the trial's conclusion all served to downplay that Germans had orchestrated the plot, and the prosecutor emphasized that only whites could be patriotic, civic-minded "true Americans." Shah convincingly argues that this depiction of non-white "radicals and revolutionaries trying to undermine the colonial empire of a US ally" led to "the crystallization of the image of all Asian Indians as undesirable for citizenship."[33] This was reflected in voter correspondence with US immigration authorities. For example, in 1922 a Mrs. I. Malone of New York warned that "high caste Hindu" spiritual teachers in the United States "take out citizenship papers for a bluff, go over to India every once and a while to stir up and know they can leave their country with out [sic] trouble as American citizens."[34]

When Bhagat Singh Thind, a US Army veteran of the First World War, applied for naturalization three years after the trial, a federal district court judge in Oregon granted his request, ruling that Thind's classification as a "Caucasian," along with that the fact that the 1917 "Barred Zone" immigration act did not affect the residency eligibility of South Asians already in the United States, meant he was eligible for naturalization. Treating the *Thind* decision as a test case, the IS appealed to the US Supreme Court with the argument that being "Caucasian" was not the same as being white. Shortly before the *Thind* appeal came to trial, Supreme Court Justice George Sutherland ruled in *Takao Ozawa vs. US* (1922) that Japanese nationals were aliens ineligible for citizenship because they were not Caucasian and were therefore not white. This decision rendered Japanese nationals as aliens ineligible for naturalization. While many South Asians believed that this ruling affirmed their right to citizenship, when Thind's case came to trial in 1923, Justice Sutherland decided that although ethnographers identified South Asians as Caucasian, the immigrant group did not fit the definition of whiteness held by the drafters of the Naturalization Law of 1790, who had referred exclusively to those from the British Isles and northwestern Europe. Sutherland decided that while other European groups (e.g., Italians) were also eligible for naturalization because they were similar to the original "free white persons," "the physical group characteristics of the Hindus render them readily distinguishable from [those] commonly recognized as white." Referring to the 1917 "Barred Zone" legislation, Sutherland added that "it is not likely that Congress would be willing to accept as citizens a class of persons whom it rejects as immigrants."[35]

At the heart of the decision was the idea that skin colour trumped phenotypic features and ancestry. For Sutherland and his supporters, an admission that South Asians were white because they shared ancestral ties with Europeans would open up the possibility of naturalization to "low caste" Indians and "the dusky Ceylonese or Afghan," two other "Aryan" groups deemed unfit for naturalization and therefore not admissible as white.[36] Sutherland's ruling, which prevented new South Asian naturalizations, led, over the next three years, to the denaturalization of around sixty South Asians, who were retroactively considered ineligible at the time of their application, and cancelled the citizenship of the small number of American women who had married some of these men. In an interview for a social study shortly after Sutherland's verdict, El Centro resident Inder Singh, who stated that "I have applied for American citizenship but this has been denied me," bitterly remarked that "were I in the immigration service in India, when an American would apply for entry I would refer him to his Consul, and that would be of no avail."[37]

The *Thind* ruling effectively ensured the continuation of immigration exclusion the following year, when the 1924 Immigration Act (also known as the Johnson–Reed Act) stipulated that "no alien ineligible to citizenship shall be admitted to the United States."[38] Besides reaffirming the exclusion of new immigrants, the *Thind* case affected the entry eligibility of returning residents. For example, when, in 1925, US Army veteran and previously naturalized citizen Joginder Singh attempted to re-enter at Angel Island after a year overseas, his BSI examiners barred him from entry because "validity of applicant's naturalization is the issue." The *Thind* decision meant that Singh, despite his past military service to the nation in the First World War, had not been eligible for the naturalization he had received before 1923 because he was not white. Since the 1924 Immigration Act barred South Asians and others who would not be eligible for citizenship, he was thus excluded "as being an alien ineligible to citizenship not in possession of an Immigration visa sustained as required as Section 23 to Act of 1924" (which renewed the Indian exclusion first stipulated in 1917 and renewed in 1921).[39] Denaturalized South Asians who lived in California were also stripped of any landholdings, as that state's 1913 Webb–Haney Act, renewed in a more comprehensive form in 1920, restricted landownership to residents eligible for citizenship. Since Chinese and Japanese residents were ineligible under federal legislation passed in 1882 and 1906 respectively, naturalized South Asians were the last Asians to own land in California.[40]

In 1926, Senator David Reed of Pennsylvania submitted a resolution to protect the citizenship status of naturalized South Asians and their American wives. The Senate Immigration Committee, chaired by Hiram Johnson, who along with Reed had authored the 1924 Immigration Act, heard testimony from many of the same interest groups as had been represented at the 1914 "Hindu Immigration" hearings. Several naturalized South Asians made statements in favour of Reed's bill, including philosopher Taraknath Das and chemical engineer V.R. Kokatnur, inventor of strains of mustard gas supplied to the US War Department. Just as Commissioner-General of Immigration Anthony Caminetti had spoken out against continued immigration from India in 1914, Raymond F. Crist of the Commission of Naturalization criticized South Asian efforts to regain the American franchise.[41]

V.S. McClatchy, secretary of the nativist California Joint Immigration Committee, argued in 1926 that an "unfortunate precedent" would be set if Congress recognized "illegal Hindu naturalizations." Although close to half of the 838 Japanese residents of Hawaii who had joined the US forces in the recent war had initially gained their citizenship, the group lost their citizenship in the 1925 decision *Toyota v. United States.* If Congress allowed South Asians to remain citizens, these US war veterans from Hawaii would expect the same treatment. Overall, McClatchy concluded that "the present and future of the nation should be carefully considered when in conflict with the interest or desire of individual aliens."[42] Since, as Gary Hess explains, most members of the Senate committee "shared McClatchey's fears that an uncomfortable precedent would be established," Reed's resolution was tabled after the second hearing. The Commissioner of Naturalization did advise the cancellation of pending South Asian denaturalization cases the following year, but only after a lower court decided in favour of California barrister Sakharam Ganesh Pandit in his high-profile denaturalization hearing.[43]

McClatchy's view was by no means universal on the coast. Baptist missionary Dr. Theodore Fieldbrave of California reflected the minority opinion that "to recall citizenship from those few Orientals to whom this honor was willingly granted and with all good faith years ago, seems unfair, un-American and un-Christian." Similarly, southern California resident Willard A. Schurr declared that "it seems most unfortunate that citizenship should be taken from a man after it has been granted to him. This is almost like an ex post facto law, and I must oppose such action even though it be taken by our courts."[44] There is no question, however, that a majority of California residents generally opposed the naturalization of members of any Asian group and especially the continuing Asian presence in the state. Two state publications from the period immediately preceding Thind's original application for naturalization demonstrate the primacy of the public health argument in the continuing popular aversion to the approximately 4,000 South Asians remaining in the state. These reports, the California Commission of Immigration and Housing's 1918 "Report on Fresno's Immigration Problem," and the State Board of Control's 1920 "California and the Oriental," have been almost entirely omitted from the historiography of South Asians in America. This is unfortunate because they offer useful examples of official and popular attitudes towards South Asians compared to immigrants from other groups, and also demonstrate that the "Hindu disease" thesis superseded all other objections (economic or otherwise) to South Asians in this period.

The California Commission of Immigration and Housing (CCIH), created in 1913 after a dedicated campaign by Progressive Era philanthropist Simon Lubin, began as an investigation into the well-being of immigrants in California. The resulting state agency helped new arrivals from other countries look for work and helped private, charitable, and other organizations match employers with workers. "Americanization" was a key tenet of the agency, whose members provided immigrants with programs to assist in their social and industrial assimilation. The CCIH's principal mandate was the inspection of every work camp in the state to help "protect" immigrants from poor conditions, although it fell to the state's Board of Health to force camp owners to keep work and living areas clean. The CCIH's actual power was limited because, according to Richard Street, "certain immutable political realities impeded most other Progressives from demonstrating much concern for bindlemen [transients] and other migrant workers." The most significant of these was the vote of rural residents, as country districts held a key position in governor Hiram Johnson's progressive electorate base. So, besides conducting camp inspections and helping immigrants directly, the CCIH influenced policy, mainly by compiling a series of survey reports on social and industrial labour conditions.[45]

The CCIH's 1918 report on Fresno's immigrant "problem" included a general assessment of employment in and around the central California city, a synopsis of current race relations there, and a series of testimonials by white community leaders and other residents. While the report covered immigrants from across Europe, Asia, the Philippines, and Mexico, investigators found that "Hindus" lived in the worst conditions in Fresno, where they rented Japanese-owned houses near Chinatown in the summer. Here they "caused the most trouble to the housing inspector." A local resident stated that the city's Asians "become just what we make of them," as white employers placed them in "poor shacks" they had not chosen "and curse them because they 'live like hogs.'" Not surprisingly, area farmers who employed South Asians defended their worth: a former president of the Raisin Growers Association stated that while they lived in rustic conditions, they were still in some ways "vastly better" than white workers. C.A. Degnan, the commission's secretary, was less understanding. He reported that many Chinese residents illegally rented out their cellars as rooming houses, and in one such "hole" inspectors had recently found six consumptive Chinese men using the space as a "death chamber." "The Hindus coming into Fresno," Degnan reported, "frequently sleep in these places and mingle intimately with the Chinese and become infected." A policeman in the city's "Chinatown Squad" added that "the Hindus are the laziest fellows of all the Orientals and they need some one [*sic*] to drive them"; he concluded that "they are a dirty, beastly lot."[46]

In September 1919, California governor William D. Stephens tasked the State Board of Control with investigating the need for a new Alien

Land Act that would update the 1913 Webb–Haney law prohibiting aliens "unable to obtain citizenship" from owning land. Since, as was shown earlier, a small number of South Asians had gained US citizenship before legislative exclusion, until 1923 these individuals would continue to be exempt from the state's alien landownership regulation. Asian farmers, including South Asians without citizenship, had initially circumvented the provisions of the Webb–Haney Act by signing long-term leases of up to three years. In response, Stephens commissioned the Board of Control's investigation to determine whether a new bill could close this and other loopholes in the 1913 act. The board submitted and published its resulting report, "California and the Oriental," five months before 75.1 percent of state voters cast their ballots in favour of the new bill in the November 1920 general election. The bill was largely intended to curb the Japanese acquisition and control of farmland. Yet like the CCIH report on Fresno, "California and the Oriental" also offers fascinating insights into popular opinion on Asian immigrants, in much the same manner as did the federal "Reports of the Immigration Commission" (Dillingham Commission) in 1911.[47]

After extensively surveying California's "Asiatic" problem in the immediate postwar years, the State Board of Control commissioners concluded that the state could never successfully assimilate Asians because it was "manifestly impossible" for the two races to mix successfully, neither in ideas nor in "blood fusion." Californians were determined to avoid the "mistake" that Hawaii had made in allowing significant Japanese landownership in that territory. South Asian land control in California was, in fact, a minor issue compared to the one that arose over Japanese or Chinese leaseholding. South Asians leased or held crop contracts for 2,099 acres in the entire state, while Japanese and Chinese settlers controlled 388,287 and 65,181 acres, respectively. Furthermore, only 2,600 South Asians remained in California, for many had left before the war. Despite the small size of this resident population, the commissioner of the State Bureau of Labor Statistics found that the South Asians were the state's "most undesirable" immigrants due to their "lack of personal cleanliness," "low morals," and "blind adherence to theories and teachings."[48]

Edward A. Brown, the CIHC's sanitary engineer, offered the most vociferous argument for abolishing South Asian land leasing. Brown's authority with regard to "Hindu" hygiene is highly questionable, given that he supported his position by claiming that his agency had received "numerous" complaints by American employees of South Asian farmers alleging unsanitary working conditions. The CIHC's extensive "complaint" files, which are largely complete, show that even by 1922, two years after Brown's report, workers had submitted only four such complaints about farm or ranch managers with the last name "Singh," which was by far the most common name among California's South Asians. Yet Brown argued that the South Asian standard of living was "so vastly different from ours that it is difficult to present it properly." He elaborated that since "any kind of a shack will serve as living quarters for Hindus," it was very difficult to compel Indian farmers to keep their camps clean, and most of their camps had "unscreened kitchens," "open toilets," "very crowded" sleeping areas, and overall "filthy" camp grounds. However, four CIHC camp inspectors offered a contradictory view by painting a fairly positive picture of South Asian housing generally. Fresno's city health inspector reported that the ten or so Indian settlers in Bakersfield "lived in fairly respectable houses." A camp inspector described the homes of South Asians living around Sacramento as better than Japanese abodes in that area, while another found that Indian tenants usually installed "Hindu baths" to help workers stay clean.[49] Recalling similar bunking arrangements in Vancouver during the 1920s, one Indo-Canadian Oral History participant shared that while his camp was about as clean as those of the whites and Chinese working in the area, his group may have kept themselves cleaner because they insisted on decent bathing facilities and because bathing was "the first thing [an] Indian would do when he comes from work."[50]

While the statements contained in the Fresno and State Board of Control reports and the CIHC papers likely had no bearing on the 1923 *Thind* decision, they do indicate that, on the Pacific coast (and especially in California), sustained associations between South Asians and dirt and disease offered the most compelling support for the idea that the group as a whole could not assimilate into American society and was thus unworthy of immigration or citizenship. As Chapter 5 showed, this argument featured prominently in the political hearings and debates that resulted in legislative exclusion in 1917. Like Canada, the United States granted citizenship rights only after the Second World War; in 1946, President Harry Truman signed the Luce–Celler Act, which allowed those born in India to naturalize and set an annual quota of one hundred South Asian immigrants. However, like other "Orientals," naturalized South Asians in California could not purchase land until the state's Supreme Court overturned the alien land law in 1952.

The previous pages have demonstrated that both national governments responded to the South Asian appeal for suffrage by resorting to the argument that South Asians could not assimilate – in part because their health, hygiene, and morality precluded their admissibility as citizens. Anti-Indian sentiment in the US Pacific coast states, predicated on the enduring idea of South Asian otherness, influenced the 1923 *Thind* decision that members of the group were not "white." That decision revoked the citizenship eligibility of South Asians in that country, and stripped many individuals of their citizenship. California state organizations, especially those with an interest in land allocations in the state, used health-based arguments to broadly support the legitimacy of the *Thind* decision and ongoing legislative exclusion, for these policies ensured that previously naturalized South Asians would lose their landholdings. As a result of these efforts, South Asians were prohibited from (re)claiming citizenship rights until 1946, the year the United States gave them the vote and instituted a token annual Indian immigrant quota. In Canada, Arthur Meighen's 1921 promise of better treatment for the nation's South Asians came to nothing, as BC delegates of the country's two main political parties used public health and other arguments to censure Sastri's franchise campaign. Moreover, W.L.M. King, who in 1908 had criticized Wilfrid Laurier's denial of the franchise to South Asians, refused to revisit the voting issue when he himself became prime minister. As a result of these developments, South Asians in BC did not gain the federal, provincial, and municipal franchise until almost thirty years later, in 1947. Not until 1952 did Canada follow the United States in setting a small South Asian immigrant quota.

Conclusion

THIS TRANSNATIONAL STUDY OF the first wave South Asian immigrant experience in British Columbia and the Pacific coast states has shown how bureaucrats, union leaders, physicians, members of the press, elected officials at all levels of government, and the general public used public health concerns to justify South Asian exclusion and disenfranchisement. While all Asian groups living on the Pacific coast faced opposition to their immigration and settlement, a sustained western North American association of South Asians with disease, and India's subordinate status within the British Empire, uniquely positioned discourse on the new immigrants at the intersection of medicalized nativism, colonial theory, and Orientalism. Many white residents sincerely believed that Indians endangered public health, made poor workers, lived in unsanitary conditions, and engaged in immoral behaviour, but the popular charge that South Asians were racially predisposed to disease was also motivated and sustained by widespread anxiety over South Asian labour competition for white workers, as well as concerns about the establishment of another "Oriental" group on the continent.

The previous pages have also addressed the following central questions: How were South Asians racialized and associated with disease in a manner different from other Asians? And how did the disease argument influence the popular reception of South Asians and bring about their executive and legislative exclusion and disenfranchisement in both countries? Health- and eugenics-based arguments against Indian immigration and settlement helped perpetuate the widespread belief that South Asians were the least likely among other national groups to assimilate into Pacific coast communities; this in turn propelled the group's executive and legislative exclusion and delayed the growth of South Asian communities on the continent. This manuscript has focused on the vitally important early stages of this process between 1906 and the early 1920s, during which the foundation was laid for the exclusion of immigrants from India;

however, popular, academic, and official discourse maintained elements of these arguments well after this period.

As a comparative case study, this project has contrasted the obstacles that the first South Asian immigrants encountered in BC and the Pacific coast states during the opening two decades of the twentieth century. There were some differences in the two cases: the United States legislated South Asian exclusion nearly a full decade after Canada, and the "climate" argument never took root in American discourse or policy as it did in Canada, nor did the related assertion that South Asians were especially prone to and likely to spread tuberculosis. Furthermore, the Canadian government's response to the initial arrival of Indian immigrants was influenced, albeit modestly, by the country's imperial ties to Britain and India, and the restrictive legislation in place for over forty years was the product of a careful diplomacy not required in American legislation on Indian immigration.

However, there were more similarities than disparities between the two national situations. In both countries, the disease argument prevailed even in the face of contradictory evidence presented by a wide range of sources, including physician accounts, health inspector reports, municipal health reports, provincial death certificates, and state and federal reports on resident South Asians. Furthermore, although the Japanese immigration issue caused the American executive to delay legislation on Indian immigration, Immigration Service (IS) executive restriction, firmly in place by 1910, achieved nearly the same end as Canada's legislative exclusion. Elected federal representatives from BC and the Pacific coast states and their respective bureaucrats used the disease argument in similar ways to further their exclusionist campaigns. Since members of the IS and the Canadian Immigration Branch occasionally corresponded and met on the "Hindu" issue, each agency influenced the policy of the other, especially after the discovery of hookworm at Angel Island in 1910. Finally, although the Asiatic Exclusion League (AEL), which was affiliated with the American Federation of Labor, was far more active in the United States than in Canada, AEL anti-Indian literature had much in common with Canadian Trades and Labour Congress publications, in that both asserted that South Asians threatened public health and morality in west coast communities. Moreover, American AEL participation in the 1907 Vancouver riot exacerbated racist sentiments in BC and indirectly helped bring about South Asian exclusion in Canada.

Other policy and practice on the "Hindu" issue also transcended the 49th Parallel. Cross-border collaboration occurred between government officials, physicians, politicians, members of the press, and the general public in BC and the Pacific coast states. For example, after Canadian exclusion in January 1908, American politicians and the press alike argued that the fact that the Canadians had already excluded their fellow British subjects meant there were no diplomatic or political reasons why the United States should not follow suit. Pacific coast press coverage of South Asian immigration widely portrayed it as a transborder issue. The South Asian reaction to anti-Indian activism was also transnational, as the new immigrants frequently travelled between the two countries, sometimes surreptitiously, to find work or to attend community meetings or protests against the treatment of their countrymen in North America. Indian independence activism also routinely crossed the border, as people and the revolutionary literature of the Ghadar (Indian mutiny or freedom) movement circulated widely between Vancouver and Seattle and San Francisco.

In BC, widespread popular opposition first erupted in response to the South Asian presence in lumber camps and cities, especially after 1906, when the Trades and Labour Congress of Canada, and later the Vancouver chapter of the San Francisco–based AEL, added the new immigrants to the list of Asian groups they protested against. A highly publicized allegation that South Asians had gang-raped a white woman in Vancouver exacerbated the issue, as did negative reports from Vancouver's civic health officer and the province's federal MPs, who asserted that Indians were unsuited for Canada's climate. These officials explained that the cramped and unsanitary living conditions of South Asian workers were products of their inherent dirtiness, not their poverty or the local housing shortage. Vancouver's City Council, local labour unions, members of the press, and others further alleged that South Asians carried "Asiatic" and venereal diseases. In the Pacific coast states, where first wave Indian immigrants appeared slightly later than in Canada, Public Health Service (PHS) examiners at Pacific coast ports responded to public pressure and official IS policy by rejecting large numbers of the new arrivals on the tenuous grounds that their "poor physique" made them physically unfit for work in the United States.

In both countries, 1907 was a pivotal year for South Asians. After two race riots on the coast and the arrival of a large number of immigrants from India only days later, Canada's Immigration Branch initiated executive exclusion at BC ports. W.L.M. King's 1907 investigation of the "Hindoo problem," which would help bring about legislative exclusion the following year, embraced the contention made by Vancouver city health officers that South Asians were particularly susceptible to tuberculosis. At IS stations at Vancouver, Seattle, and Portland, and later San Francisco, IS agents took advantage of a 1907 revision to the US Immigration Act by rejecting South Asians for having "poor physiques" or being likely to become a public charge (LPC). The widely reported views of an American consular official stationed in Calcutta, who argued that vessels transporting Indians across the Pacific to San Francisco carried largely "undesirable" immigrants, supported the IS position on the matter. Although the climate argument gained little currency in sunny and warm California, the major destination for most South Asians arriving in the United States, municipal, state, and federal representatives eagerly adopted the disease theory to argue that South Asians presented a significant threat to American public health. Orientalist arguments about the nature of life in India and the inherent traits of South Asians further supported the disease theory, as did the assertions of popular writers and others who erroneously linked South Asians to meningitis and bubonic plague outbreaks along the Pacific coast.

After Canadian legislative exclusion in early 1908, continuing tensions between white BC residents and the fewer than 5,000 South Asians living in the province compelled the Dominion to investigate the possibility of moving the group en masse to a British colony in South America. While this plan – and subsequent attempts to deport indigent and sick South Asians – failed, BC residents and international visitors alike continued to champion the miasmatic argument that South Asians were only suited to working in tropical climates. After the Vancouver, Seattle, and Portland IS offices used LPC and polygamy charges to bar South Asians, exclusionists in California in 1910 became increasingly frustrated that Hart Hyatt North, commissioner of San Francisco's newly built Angel Island Quarantine Station, was refusing to adhere to the IS's policy of executive restriction. The Commissioner-General of Immigration intervened by ordering that South Asians at Angel Island be rejected as a group for being LPC; however, this was not a sufficient "catch-all" means of exclusion, for it was legally vague and susceptible to court challenge.

So IS staffers rejoiced when, in the fall of 1910, a PHS doctor discovered the contagious hookworm parasite in the stool samples of several South Asian immigrants at Angel Island. Since a large percentage of South Asians carried this "Class A" (exclusion mandatory) disease, this virtually ended Indian immigration, which was already in decline at that station by the time the discovery was made public in late September. The US government closed a loophole to executive exclusion that had allowed the immigration of South Asians from Hawaii; but in 1912, South Asians immigrating from the Philippines, another American territory, began to arrive at San Francisco. This "back door" to the United States was somewhat more difficult to close, in that South Asians had passed medical inspection on arrival in the Philippines.

The relatively high rate of South Asian hookworm infection offered an ideal solution to the Philippines problem, even though many arrivals from the Philippines were not infected with the disease. Nevertheless, citing the case of one South Asian from Manila with hookworm, the IS, together with the War Department, which administered the territory's admissions, justified the passage of legislation forcing all migrants from the Philippines to pass reinspection on their arrival in the lower forty-eight states. By October 1913, South Asians from the Philippines were being rejected en masse for being LPC or for failing medical inspection, and transpacific steamship lines were refusing to sell tickets to the majority of South Asians attempting to book passage to the United States. In November, the Commissioner-General of Immigration, citing a dated study of fewer than six hundred residents of the Indian Subcontinent, reaffirmed the connection between South Asian immigrants and hookworm. The PHS's discovery of this parasite at Angel Island inspired Canadian officials to initiate unprecedented health screening of South Asian arrivals at BC ports in 1912 and 1913. After hearing rumours of the imminent arrival of South Asians in Vancouver, the Immigration Branch prepared a contingency plan to test for hookworm, although action on this plan was deferred before the arrival of the SS *Komagata Maru* shortly thereafter.

In 1912, interior minister Frank Oliver used incorrect Immigration Branch statistics about South Asian disease to defend his decision not to allow South Asian families to come to Canada, and there the matter rested for the next decade. Testimony collected in 1913 during a major BC provincial study of labour relations exemplified the enduring anti-Indian sentiment in most sectors of BC society, as did a series of popular reports published that year. Immigration authorities, roundly supported by almost all of the Dominion's federal MPs, justified the rejection of the *Komagata Maru*'s passengers in 1914 as a necessary measure to preserve the nation's health and genetic stocks. American observers watching the unfolding

Komagata Maru crisis in Vancouver's harbour between May and July 1914 surmised that its resolution could have serious consequences for South Asian immigration to the United States. The Commissioner-General of Immigration thus lobbied persistently for Indian exclusion legislation that would remove the need for executive restriction.

Congressional exclusionists, two of whom had introduced "Hindu exclusion" bills in late 1913, anxiously watched the results of the 1914 Hindu Immigration hearings in Washington, DC. Those hearings did not immediately bring about exclusion, even though testimony and debate during the hearings was slanted heavily towards exclusion and the idea that South Asian immigration was a public health menace. US labor secretary W.B. Wilson personally recommended the introduction of an anti-Hindu bill; however, South Asian immigration was linked, at least in the minds of Pacific coast exclusionists, to the politically delicate issue of Japanese immigration, and President Woodrow Wilson was reluctant to introduce any Asian immigration sanctions that would inflame tensions in Japan or disrupt Japanese–US relations. Even so, in late 1916 the House passed a version of the "Burnett Bill," which included the Indian Subcontinent within its Asian "Barred Zone" for immigrants. When the House and Senate passed the bill again over Wilson's veto, the Immigration Act of 1917 became law. The 1924 Asian Exclusion Act, part of the Johnson–Reed Act, would specifically exclude Indians by grouping them with other "non-white" races ineligible for citizenship, but by then, the 1917 legislation had already ended what little South Asian immigration had continued since the IS implemented executive restriction in 1910.

The link between Indian immigrants and disease and uncleanliness persisted in popular and official discourse well after legislative exclusion in both countries. In Canada, even after the murder of W.C. Hopkinson, the official tasked with South Asian surveillance in BC, federal MP for Vancouver H.H. Stevens and future Superintendent of Immigration F.C. Blair continued to oppose reopening immigration from India. After Canada agreed in 1919 to admit the families of resident South Asians, this small dispensation stirred up considerable controversy among politicians and residents of BC, who argued that any increase in the province's South Asian population would soon lead to greater allowances for that community. A key concession at issue was the franchise, as BC was the only province in which South Asians (along with other Asians) could not vote in municipal, provincial, and federal elections. In 1921, Canada's Conservative prime minister Arthur Meighen stated his hope that steps would be taken to enfranchise BC's South Asians, but his successor W.L.M. King, unwilling to inflame tensions in BC and among MPs from that province, decided not to pursue the matter himself. A Canadian speaking tour by Indian politician and rights activist V.S. Srinivasa Sastri did nothing to reverse this situation, and neither did opposition leader Meighen's investigation into the possibility of granting voting rights to members of Canada's small Indian expatriate population. Only in 1947, a quarter-century after Sastri's visit, did Canada extend the franchise to South Asians; immigration from India (and the newly independent nations of Pakistan and Ceylon [now Sri Lanka]) resumed a full five years after that.

The South Asian quest for voting rights in the United States met with similar resistance. While several individuals had become citizens in the first two decades of the century, in 1923 a major court decision revoked their new national status and decreed that South Asians could no longer become citizens. This influenced the admissibility of new and returning South Asians at US ports. California state reports published in the early 1920s affirmed the view that Indians would be undesirable citizens and inassimilable because of their health practices, general living standards, and morality. These reports also offered legitimacy to California's 1920 Alien Land Law, which reaffirmed 1913 legislation barring Asians from landownership, and the congressional enactment of the 1924 Johnson–Reed Immigration Act, which explicitly barred South Asians from immigrating.

Anti-Indian racism persisted in both countries after the period studied here. Canadian immigration records demonstrate that at least some officials with the Immigration Branch continued to view South Asians as undesirable. For example, after Canada allowed the wives and dependent children of resident members of the group to immigrate after 1919, one South Asian in Victoria requested that the government stretch its interpretation of "family member" and grant temporary entry to his half-brother. Although this prospective immigrant came with a very strong character reference from his former superiors in the Indian army, Percy Reid, the senior officer in charge of the Vancouver immigration office, rejected the application. Reid reasoned that "undoubtedly" the man would immediately apply for permanent residence once in Canada, and, with access to legal counsel, "there would be very little question but that they would succeed, and the practice would, no doubt, immediately become general, and would be a means of defeating the Immigration Act." Further exploration of these records is necessary to prove that these sentiments were understood and applied generally, but this case indicates that at least some Immigration Branch officials agreed with federal exclusion policy.[1]

Shortly before becoming Canada's assistant deputy immigration minister, in June 1922, Frederick C. Blair oversaw an "experiment" wherein agents at Victoria and Vancouver checked the Chinese and other Asian immigrants who continued to be admitted to Canada for hookworm. This bacteriological testing had been deferred after Jewalla Singh's inconclusive hookworm test in 1913, but since Asian immigrants were routinely detained for two to three weeks in the early 1920s, Blair's supervisor, D.A. Clark, suggested that they could be tested for hookworm and, if necessary, treated during this waiting period. The United States had continued to test most incoming Asian immigrants for the disease from 1910 onwards, and thus Clark proposed bilateral policy alignment on the matter, although the experiment would not apply to white immigrants, who were rarely detained for a significant amount of time on the coast. For example, an immigration agent at Vancouver, writing in the same month as Clark, reported that room shortages made it "inadvisable to keep *Europeans under detention unless absolutely necessary,*" as the station's detention quarters were "always occupied by Orientals."[2]

Interestingly, A.S. Munro, who was still the Department of Immigration and Colonization's medical inspector at Vancouver, privately informed Scott that Blair's proposal to examine the mostly Chinese arrivals for hookworm was unnecessary and would be a waste of departmental resources. He explained that hookworm and clonorchiasis (a similar parasitic infection) were "entirely different" from trachoma, a disease more commonly linked to Asians, and thus were not a "menace to the public health of Canada." Munro reasoned that "whether due to change in climatic conditions or not," Chinese treated in Vancouver hospitals for other conditions had never been found to have hookworm. Thus, "if the disease was present at the time of the entrance of the immigrant into Canada, the infection had disappeared after some months' or years' residence in the country." He added that Ellis Island's head physician, Dr. W.C. Billings, who in 1906 had examined some of the first South Asian arrivals to the US, now believed there was no danger of Chinese immigrants spreading the disease in the region.[3]

In April 1923, acting without departmental authorization, G.L. Milne, still medical inspector at Victoria, used a positive hookworm diagnosis to deport Lai Hung Sang, an otherwise healthy Chinese arrival. J.D. Page, the Department of Immigration and Colonization's head physician and chief of its Quarantine Division, later rebuked Milne for this decision, arguing that

> from the limited information so far available we are not persuaded that the disease of hookworm or liverflukes is so grave a menace to public health as you represent, and the question of whether or not it should be certified, and, if so, under what subjection of the Act, is still in abeyance. If, therefore, this man's general health was good and he was certified and deported purely as a result of the bacteriological findings for hookworm, it would appear that an injustice has been done.[4]

Yet just ten years earlier, the Immigration Branch had, under the minister's orders and with the initial support of Page's predecessor Peter H. Bryce, initiated hookworm testing on South Asian passengers on the SS *Sado Maru* and SS *Panama Maru*. The Branch planned, although it never implemented, the same test for South Asians on board the SS *Orterio* and another, unnamed vessel that had been expected to arrive in early 1914. The sole purpose of conducting these tests would have been to find and reject any Indians who carried the parasite. Since the interim decade had seen no new major studies on hookworm, and certainly no change in national policy regarding the disease, there seems to have been a remarkable inconsistency between the Dominion's treatment of South Asians in 1912–14 and that of other Asians (Chinese) ten years later. Page's admission that hookworm was not a serious public health threat, and his belief that it was a "major injustice" to reject a Chinese national for hookworm, demonstrate a significant discrepancy in the application of the Immigration Act, which, unlike US immigration legislation, had never named hookworm as an excludable disease. This intriguing inconsistency remains to be explored within the wider study of the comparative immigration, reception, and integration of Asian groups in BC in the early to mid-twentieth century.

Similarly, before legislative exclusion in the United States, IS officials had excluded South Asians by testing for hookworm, by informally persuading steamship companies not to sell tickets to Indian residents, and finally by imposing executive restriction measures at Vancouver, Seattle, Portland, and San Francisco. Beginning in 1910 and continuing until the official end of first-wave South Asian immigration in 1917, PHS officials tested South Asians for hookworm, a "Class A" contagious disease that excluded them under the Immigration Act. Yet since hookworm could be cured in under two weeks at Angel Island (as Surgeon General Rupert Blue explained in 1919), the PHS changed hookworm to a "Class B" disease in that year. The reclassification meant that all immigrants who were otherwise admissible would automatically be admitted if they first underwent and paid for treatment. Officials revised their policy as early as 1917, soon after the "Barred Zone" legislation officially barred Indian immigrants for the first time. While the timing of the PHS reclassification is certainly interesting, it may be a coincidence that it came so soon after South Asian legislative exclusion, especially since healthy South Asians arriving at Angel Island in the early years of that decade were generally rejected for being LPC and deported along with those South Asians who carried hookworm.[5]

While several decades separate us from these and the other events explored in this study, the challenges confronted by the first South Asian immigrants remain highly relevant to modern-day discourse on North American immigration. Most notably, the *Komagata Maru* debacle continues to command significant public attention as a defining moment in the twentieth-century South Asian experience in Canada. As we marked its centennial in 2014, recent years have seen its commemoration in a documentary film, a radio play, and a collaborative website. The incident has also repeatedly resurfaced in recent parliamentary debates. On August 3, 2008, soon after the House of Commons passed a Liberal motion for a government apology for the Dominion's actions at Vancouver in 1914, Conservative prime minister Stephen Harper apologized for Canada's handling of the affair.[6] While Harper had officially apologized in the House of Commons for Canada's treatment of Aboriginal children in residential schools and for the nation's imposition of a discriminatory "Head Tax" on Chinese immigrants in the nineteenth and early twentieth centuries, many South Asian Canadians felt cheated that Harper had chosen to apologize in Surrey, BC, and not in Parliament.

In May 2012, following along the lines of a 2010 Liberal motion on the matter, the New Democratic Party renewed the request for an in-House apology. In the ensuing debate, Jasbir Sandhu astutely observed that the *Komagata Maru* affair cannot be remembered simply as an isolated racist incident, because exclusion remained in effect for over four decades, until 1952.[7] Indeed, the incident and the legislation were deeply linked within a broader, long-term federal policy framework designed to exclude Indian arrivals. On May 28, 2012, after protracted debate, the motion was defeated by a vote of 147 to 118 in the Conservative-controlled House. I interviewed one MP who opposed the motion, who reported coming from a long family tradition of work in Canadian industry. His first family member in Canada was among a group of others who faced resentment, and who in some instances only escaped harassment by working longer hours and living at their workplaces. In his own political career decades later, he encountered some racism before being elected: voters in his riding sometimes assumed that he held radical beliefs or were surprised he spoke English. Besides the obvious propriety of following party policy, it seems likely that my informant's family and personal experience in overcoming socio-cultural obstacles to success had influenced the desire to leave the *Komagata Maru* affair in the past.[8]

Yet many Canadians continued to call for an official apology, and in the House of Commons on May 18, 2016, Prime Minister Justin Trudeau, whose Liberal party won the 2015 national election, formally apologized on behalf of Canada. In this speech, which for the Liberals had been eight years in the making, Trudeau declared that the nation's government in 1914 had been "without question responsible for the laws that prevented these passengers from immigrating peacefully and securely," and he stated that "for that, and for every regrettable consequence that followed, we are truly sorry." While the effect of these remarks was somewhat diminished by the delivery of the prime minister's other apology hours later, which addressed his personal actions during an unrelated altercation with opposition MPs that afternoon, many South Asian Canadians accepted Trudeau's remarks on the *Komagata Maru* debacle as an important milestone in the quest for furthering racial tolerance and equality and in the present day.[9]

The fact that debate on the apology issue continued for so long demonstrates that the *Komagata Maru* affair represents much more than the rejection of a few hundred South Asians over a century ago. For many, the affair remains a shared yet deeply personal reminder of the significant challenges that Indians faced in Canada. Ali Kazimi compares the event in 1914 with the 2010 arrival of the MV *Sun Sea,* which brought almost five hundred asylum-seeking Tamil migrants to the same city. Kazimi contends that the Canadian "moral panic" over that landing empowered the Conservatives to draft and pass Bill C-11 to amend the Immigration and Refugee Protection Act, which, since its amendment in 2011, targets human smugglers but also allows the imprisonment of some refugees, including minors, for months pending review of their claims.[10] Note also that the *Sun Sea* affair triggered a redirection of federal resources towards international surveillance and collaboration under a suite of policies ostensibly designed to curb human smuggling and refugee "queue jumping." While parliamentarians were debating the *Komagata Maru* apology in 2012, the *National Post* reported that the government had stopped a plan to help Sri Lankan migrants stranded in Togo come to Canada. Eighteen people were arrested in Ghana after a tip from Canadian intelligence officers, who had been "aggressively tracking suspected international migrant smugglers" to "prevent another influx of boat people arriving on Canada's shores."[11] Since public and official anxieties over the arrival of the *Komagata Maru* and *Sun Sea* passengers were similarly based on racial grounds, a comparison of these incidents offers scholars a promising field for future study.

Appendix
Key Individuals

Canada

Prime Ministers
John A. Macdonald, 1867–73
Wilfrid Laurier, 1896–1911
Robert Borden, 1911–20
Arthur Meighen, 1920–21; 1926
W.L. Mackenzie King, 1921–26; 1926–30; 1935–48
Justin Trudeau, 2015–

Ministers of the Interior (Responsible for Immigration)
Frank Oliver, 1905–11
Robert Rogers, 1911–12
William James Roche, 1912–17
H.H. Stevens (Acting), 1926

Superintendent of Immigration, Reporting to
Ministers of the Interior
W.D. Scott, 1902–19 (later Deputy Minister of Immigration and Coloniza-
   tion, 1919–24)

Immigration Branch Staff (Directly or Indirectly Reporting to
Superintendent)
E. Blake Robertson, Assistant Superintendent
Peter H. Bryce, Chief Medical Officer
A.S. Munro, Medical Inspector at Vancouver
G.L. Milne, Medical Inspector at Victoria
W.C. Hopkinson and Malcolm J. Reid, Immigration Inspectors at
   Vancouver
Thomas R. McInnes, Immigration agent (Ottawa)

F.C. Blair, Immigration agent (Ottawa) and later Director of Immigration (1936–43)

Others in Canada
Richard William Scott, Canada's Secretary of State in Ottawa
Frederick T. Underhill, Vancouver's Medical Officer of Health
Jewalla Singh, passenger on SS *Panama Maru*
Teja Singh, Vancouver resident
E.H. Lawson, physician on C.P.R. steamships
Agnes C. Laut, Toronto journalist

United States

Presidents
Theodore Roosevelt, 1901–9
William Howard Taft, 1909–13
Woodrow Wilson, 1913–21

US Congressmen (Except Secretaries of Labor)
Reps. Denver S. Church, John E. Raker and Julius Kahn (California)
Rep. Albert Johnson (Washington)
Sen. William P. Dillingham (Vermont)

Secretaries of (Commerce and) Labor (Responsible for the Immigration Service [IS], one of the two US agencies governing immigration)
Oscar S. Straus, 1906–9
Charles Nagel, 1909–13
W.B. Wilson, 1913–21 (Wilson was the first "Secretary of Labor" as this position was created in 1913)

Commissioners-General of Immigration (Reporting Directly to the Secretaries of Labor)
Frank P. Sargent, 1902–13
Daniel J. Keefe, 1909–13
Anthony Caminetti, 1913–21

Immigration Service (IS) Staff (Directly or Indirectly Reporting to the Commissioners-General)
William R. Wheeler and Benjamin S. Cable, Assistant Secretaries of Commerce and Labor in 1908–10 and 1910–13 respectively

John H. Clark, Immigration Commissioner in Montreal

Ellis DeBruler, Immigration Commissioner in Seattle

Hart Hyatt North, the first Commissioner of Angel Island Immigration Station

Surgeon General Rupert Blue (of the Public Health Service, the second US agency responsible for immigration), 1912–20

Public Health and Marine Hospital Service Staff (this agency was renamed the Public Health Service in 1912)

W.C. Billings, Medical Inspector at Vancouver (later Chief Medical Officer at Angel Island)

M.W. Glover, Assistant Surgeon at Angel Island

Others in the United States

A.E. Yoell, head of the Asiatic Exclusion League

Taraknath Das, IS translator at Vancouver

Bhagat Singh Thind, American Army veteran and appellant in naturalization case

India

V.S. Srinivasa Sastri, Indian politician and League of Nations delegate

Rudyard Kipling, writer

Colonel Falk Warren (Retired), Anglo-Indian Army veteran living in Vancouver

United Kingdom

Albert Grey (4th Earl Grey), Governor General of Canada

Edward Grey, Foreign Secretary

Lord Elgin (born Victor Bruce), Secretary of State for the Colonies

James Bryce, Ambassador to the United States

A. Carnegie Ross, Consul General in San Francisco

Notes

Introduction

1 *Blaine Journal*, September 13, 1907. The *Bellingham Herald* picked up the story on September 14, 1907; see Thoburn's Bellingham speech in this paper's edition of September 27, 1907.

2 This manuscript primarily employs the term "South Asian" as an inclusive means of designating a resident of the Indian Subcontinent, but also interchanges this term with "Indian" or "Indian immigrant" to reduce repetition. The original inhabitants of North America are referred to as Aboriginals. Some current-day scholars use "Asian Indian" to distinguish a South Asian individual from an Aboriginal person. During the period in question, the terms "Hindu," "Hindoo," "Sikh," and "East Indian" were used variously and in many cases interchangeably by Pacific coast populations and Indian immigrants alike. The male Sikh dress requirements (Kakkars), which are to be worn as well as the turban, are referred to as "the five K's" because of their Punjabi names: Kesh (uncut hair and beard), Kanga (comb), Kaccha (cotton underwear), Kirpan (small steel sword), and Kara (steel bracelet).

3 "First wave" refers to the first phase of South Asian immigration to North America (1899–1920s) before exclusion.

4 The 1908 Hayashi–Lemieux agreement with Japan limited the emigration of male Japanese labourers and domestic servants to four hundred individuals per year; however, this quota did not include the immediate families of resident Japanese. The quota was reduced to 150 per year in 1928.

5 I have borrowed the term "medical scapegoats" from J.B. Trauner, "The Chinese as Medical Scapegoats." The Book of Leviticus describes a scapegoat as the animal on which Aaron placed his hands and gave "all the evils, sins, and rebellions of the people of Israel." The goat was then driven away from the Israelites, "carry[ing] all their sins away with him into some uninhabited land." Old Testament, *Good News Bible*, Leviticus 16: 21–22.

6 See Howard Markel and Alexandra Stern, "Which Face? Whose Nation," 1316. See Higham, *Strangers in the Land*; see esp. 100–11. While Higham suggests that popular American opposition to immigrants during this period was motivated by an "undifferentiated ... xenophobia," and not a "dislike of particular races and classes," Schrag convincingly argues that after 1880, both "class rhetoric" and "popular literature" prove that immigrant nationality, race, religion, and class "were as important in the nation's declining enthusiasm for open borders as a general dislike of foreigners." See Schrag, *Not Fit For Our Society*, 47. Schrag cites Higham, "Origins of Immigration Restriction." See also Saxton, *The Indispensable Enemy*, 2, 274, 280.

7 Birn, "Six Seconds per Eyelid," 288–89; Fairchild, "The Rise and Fall"; Kraut, *Silent Travelers*, 3.

8 Jensen defines "executive restriction" as the set of informal practices employed by IS agents at Pacific coast ports to limit South Asian immigration without recourse to exclusionary legislation. Jensen, *Passage From India*, 113–14.

9 For example, in 1908 a South Asian living in Oregon wrote to the editor of his local newspaper in defence of the cleanliness and healthiness of his countrymen. See Letter to Editor by K. Kenchu Ram of Portland, *Morning Oregonian* (Portland), December 10, 1908, which is revisited in Chapter 3.

10 Ballantyne, *Between Colonialism and Diaspora*, 83.

11 See, for example, Johnston, *The Voyage of the Komagata Maru*; and Parnaby and Kealey, "The Origins of Political Policing."

12 Shah, *Stranger Intimacy*.

13 Barkan, *The Retreat of Scientific Racism*, 1–5.

14 For an example of the former, see Buchignani, Indra, and Srivastava, *Continuous Journey*: "the struggles of the first pioneers in British Columbia made it possible for those who have arrived more recently to enjoy this success." (233). For an example of the latter, see McClintock, *Imperial Leather*.

15 Panikkar, "In Defence of 'Old' History."

16 See Kant, *Critique of Teleological Judgment*; Foucault, *The Archeology of Knowledge*; and Hegel, *The Science of Logic*. The revised work was originally published in 1832. For a recent overview of both approaches, see Kreines, "The Logic of Life."

17 See McKeown, *Chinese Migrant Networks and Cultural Change*, 5–6; Ballantyne, *Between Colonialism and Diaspora*, 168; Fredrickson, "From Exceptionalism to Variability"; Elkins, *Slavery*.

18 Kenny, "Diaspora and Comparison," 135, 143; Kramer, "Imperial Histories," 1351.

19 Kenny, "Diaspora and Comparison," 143.

20 Lee, *At America's Gates*, 8, 11.

21 In 1991, Benedict Anderson convincingly argued that a nation is in fact an "imagined political community" that is "imagined as both inherently limited and sovereign." See Anderson, *Imagined Communities*, 6.

Chapter 1: "Leprosy and Plague Riot in Their Blood"

1 John A. Macdonald to Henry Sumner Maine, April 9, 1867, 7–8, formerly in the private collection of Alexander William Armour, The Nassau Club, Princeton, New Jersey, and sold by Heffel auctioneers in November 2006 to another collector. See *Ottawa Citizen*, November 17, 2006, and *Edmonton Journal*, November 25, 2006. Full text of the letter is at http://www.heffel.com/links/newsroom/Macdonald_Letter.pdf. The Book of 1 Kings describes Naboth's field as the vineyard owned by one Naboth of Jezreel during the ninth-century BC. According to this Biblical account, the Israelite King Ahab coveted the field, and when Naboth refused to sell it to him, Ahab, acting under instructions from his wife Jezebel, plotted to have Naboth killed so that the King could obtain the land. Although successful in his plan, Ahab was censured by the Prophet Elijah, who told him of God's angry reaction to Naboth's assassination. Old Testament, *Good News Bible*, 1 Kings 22:1–28.

2 In *Passage From India* (1988), one of the most complete works on the first-wave South Asian experience in North America to date, Joan Jensen erroneously states that 2,500 immigrants from India entered British Columbia in 1903. In fact, government sources indicate that only ten arrived that year, which predates the beginning of significant Indian immigration. See Jensen, *Passage From India*, 60; Library and Archives Canada [hereafter LAC], W.G. Parmalee to R.W. Scott, October 19, 1904, 1, RG 76 (Immigration), vol. 384, file 536999, pt. 1.

3 Forty-five people from India entered Canada in 1904, but immigration began in earnest in the 1905–6 season, when 387 arrived, followed by 2,124 in 1906–07 and 2,623 in 1907–08. See "Draft Minute on Asiatic Immigration," in LAC, Joseph Pope to Martin Burrell, January 22, 1912 (Table), 1, RG 25 (External Affairs) vol. 1118, file 66–1912.

4 Archdeacon, *Becoming American*, 137.

5 Biswas, *Colonial Displacements*, 26–27; Biswas cites Panikkar, *Culture, Ideology, Hegemony*, 22, 26–27; and Jensen, *Passage From India*, 7–8.

6 After New Zealand excluded Asians in 1881, South Africa's 1897 Immigration Restriction Act (also called the Natal Act) essentially stopped the immigration of all free (non-indentured) South Asians into that colony, while Australia barred new South Asian immigration with the 1901 "White Australia" policy.

7 1901 Census, Canada, CANSIM Table 075–0001.

8 LAC, Thomas Guigan to R.W. Scott, September 15, 1904, 1, RG 76, vol. 384, file 536999, pt. 1.

9 Nash, *Inescapable Ecologies*, 13, 14. Rhadika Mongia adds that the argument on the "cultural and climatic incompatibility of the Indians with the Canadian environment" generally evinced what Etienne Balibar terms "differential racism" at work in a system of "'racism without races' ... whose dominant theme is not biological heredity but the insurmountability of cultural differences." Mongia, "Race, Nationality, Mobility," 534; Balibar, "Is There a 'Neo-Racism?," in Balibar and Wallerstein, *Race, Nation, Class*, 21.

10 LAC, W.G. Parmalee to R.W. Scott, October 19, 1904, 1–2, RG 76, vol. 384, file 536999, pt. 1.

11 Roy, *A White Man's Province*, 47.

12 Ibid., 47; Goutor, *Guarding the Gates*, 36.

13 Ward, *White Canada Forever*, 100–8. In 1907, Vancouver's *Saturday Sunset* editor J.P. McConnell warned that while "a Chinese coolie is satisfied to remain one," it was "different with the Jap," who "sets up for himself" in Canada. *Saturday Sunset*, July 6, 1907.

14 Contagionism was the pre-germ theory association of infection with person-to-person contact.

15 Humphries, *The Last Plague*, 19, 26, 30–31.

16 Kelley and Trebilcock, *The Making of the Mosaic*, 84.

17 Ibid., 84; see also Curtis, "Social Investment in Medical Forms," 348, 360–65.

18 Humphries, *The Last Plague*, 45–46; Worboys, *Spreading Germs*, 234–277.

19 Razack, *Race, Space and the Law*, 53–54; Goldberg, *Racist Culture*, 187; Roediger, *Toward the Abolition of Whiteness*, 13.

20 Humphries, *The Last Plague*, 53–55; Sears, "Immigration Controls as Social Policy," 92–94; McKay, *Reasoning Otherwise*, 621–22. McKay cites Constance Backhouse, *Colour-Coded*, 15.

21 Feldberg, *Disease and Class*, 40; Humphries, *The Last Plague*, 53–55.

22 See Humphries, *The Last Plague*, 53–55; Roberts, *Whence They Came*, 70–71.

23 Humphries, *The Last Plague*, 46–47, 49.

24 Sears, "Immigration Controls as Social Policy," 92–97. Peter H. Bryce, Chief Medical Officer of the Immigration Branch, instructed medical inspectors at BC ports that, according to recent instructions, they were not to examine first-class passengers "unless some obvious case requires it." See LAC, P.H. Bryce to J.A.L. McAlpine, Medical Inspector, Vancouver, January 31, 1905, 1, RG 76, vol. 331, file 330483, pt. 1.

25 LAC, W.H. Bullock-Webster to B.C. Provincial Secretary, n.d., 1904, 1–4, and "Synopsis of Reports from Victoria and Vancouver," September 24–December 18, 1904," 1, both in LAC, RG 76, vol. 331, file 330483, pt. 1; LAC, H.W. Riggs to Frederick T. Underhill,

August 14, 1905, 1, RG 76, vol. 331, file 330483, pt. 4. See South Asian arrivals to Canada in 1905 in Canadian Government Original Data Passenger Lists, 1865–1935, Miscellaneous Publications, T-479-T-14939, tabulated on www.ancestry.ca; LAC, A.S. Munro to W.D. Scott, October 26, 1905, 1, RG 76, vol. 331, file 330483, pt. 5. At least one South Asian arriving in 1905 had trachoma: see LAC, J. Carroll to J.A.L. McAlpine, March 10, 1905, 1, RG 76, vol. 331, file 330483, pt. 2.

26   Government of Canada, "An Act Respecting Immigration and Immigrants," S.C., 1869, and Immigration Act, S.C., 1906; see also Kelley and Trebilcock, *The Making of the Mosaic,* 138.

27   Jensen, *Passage from India,* 60–61; Roy, *A White Man's Province,* 165.

28   Canadian Government Original Data Passenger Lists, 1865–1935, Miscellaneous Publications, T-479-T-14939, tabulated on www.ancestry.ca. Table 1 lists annual South Asian immigration to Canada statistics for the years 1904–21.

29   Indra, "South Asian Stereotypes," 168.

30   Ward, *White Canada Forever,* 7–8, 82.

31   For example, one physician testified in 1885 that Chinese immigrant "health is good for the reason that they are very cleanly." He added that they could not survive "in the hovels in which they dwell, were it otherwise." See "Testimony of Dr. McInnes," in Government of Canada, *Report of the Royal Commission on Chinese and Japanese Immigration* (Ottawa: King's Printer, 1885), 1005.

32   For example, a *Saturday Sunset* investigation undertaken by a reporter, two detectives, a local MP, and "several prominent labor men," found that the 9,000 residents who "infested" the city's Chinatown threatened population health. The neighbourhood's condition was not due to poverty but to a "taste ... inbred by generations of such methods of living." See "How Our Cooks Live In the Chinese Quarter" and "A Matter of Choice with the Chinks," both in *Saturday Sunset* (Vancouver), August 10, 1907, with the preceding quotes from the former. However, Roy points out that this resulted in a "paradox" whereby civic officials used the health code to elevate Asians to "'white standards'" in home hygiene, while relying on employment and franchise laws to maintain Asian segregation in the workplace and community. Roy, *A White Man's Province,* 30, 32–33, 36.

33   G.L. Milne to W.D. Scott, August 16, 1906, 1–2, and (Telegram) G.L. Milne to P.H. Bryce, n.d., both in RG 76, vol. 384, file 536999, pt. 1. An Immigration Branch staffer reported that he had given the documents to W.L. Mackenzie King, who was meeting with Laurier on the issue the next day; it seems likely that these reports made it to the prime minister. See LAC, L.M. Fortier to W.D. Scott, September 5, 1906, and A.S. Munro to W.D. Scott, August 16, 1906, 1–2, both in RG 76, vol. 384, file 536999, pt. 1.

34   LAC, A.S. Munro to W.D. Scott, August 16, 1906, 2–3, and (Telegram) A.S. Munro to W.D. Scott, October 15, 1906, both in RG 76, vol. 384, file 536999, pt. 1.

35   *Vancouver World,* October 8, 1906; *Ottawa Citizen,* September 20, 1906. This divide in opinion foreshadowed a significant (and largely unexplored) geographic disparity between public feeling in BC and Ontario on the issue.

36   These and the many other examples of labour agitation on the "Hindu" issue impugn Carlos Schwantes's argument that BC industrial unions were "subdued" compared to their counterparts in Washington State. See Schwantes, *Radical Heritage,* and a major counter-argument in Griffin, *Radical Roots.*

37   *Vancouver Province,* August 3 and 9, 1906; LAC, Victoria TLC, "Letter to the Working-men of British Columbia," August 6, 1906, 1, RG 76, vol. 384, file 536999, pt. 1; *Victoria Daily Times,* August 13, 1906; *Vancouver Province,* August 22, 1906.

38 LAC, (Telegram) Secretary, Amalgamated Society of Carpenters and Joiners, Vancouver Branch 1, to Minister of Emigration, n.d., 1, RG 76, vol. 384, file 536999, pt. 1.

39 LAC, (Copy) Medical Health Officer of Vancouver Health Department to Alderman Francis Williams, Chairman, Health Committee, August 22, 1906, 1, RG 76, vol. 384, file 536999, pt. 1; *Vancouver Province*, September 6, 1906.

40 *Vancouver World*, September 1 and 4, 1906.

41 Thorner and Frohn-Nielson, *A Country Nourished on Self-Doubt*, 73; *Vancouver World*, September 12, 1906; *Vancouver Province*, September 12 and 18, 1906; LAC, W.D. Scott Memorandum to Interior Department, November 2, 1906, 1, RG 76, vol. 384, file 536999, pt. 1.

42 LAC, Wilfrid Laurier to W. Zimmerman, September 24, 1906, 1, Manuscript Group (hereafter MG) 26-G C 838, vol. 427; LAC, (Telegram) Frederick Buscombe to Frank Oliver, September 4, 1906, 1, RG 76, vol. 384, file 536999, pt. 1; *Vancouver World*, September 6 and 7, 1906; LAC, "Resolution of Trades and Labour Congress of Canada, Victoria," September 17, 1906, 1, and Ed Stevenson, Saskatchewan Executive Committee, Trades and Labour Congress of Canada, Moose Jaw, to Secretary of State for the Colonies, London, November 19, 1906, 1, both in RG 76, vol. 384, file 536999, pt. 1. Government records dealing with medical inspections do not appear to indicate any incidence of venereal disease in South Asians. See, for example, LAC, RG 76, vol. 331, file 330483, pts. 1–5, and RG 36, vol. 306, file 28130, Victoria 1.

43 Medical rejections discussed in House of Commons Debate, 10th Canadian Parliament, 3rd Session, vol. 1, November 28, 1906, 234. For an overview of the evolution of the medical stipulations of the Immigration Act to 1906, see McLaren, "Stemming the Flood," 195.

44 Valverde, *Age of Light, Soap, and Water*, 111, 128.

45 Koshy, *Sexual Naturalization*, 11; McKay, *Reasoning Otherwise*, 621–22. McKay cites Backhouse, *Colour-Coded*, 15.

46 *Vancouver Province*, September 26, 1906; Public Archives of British Columbia [hereafter PABC], Death Certificate for Nara Singh, died September 24 at Vancouver, Registration No. 1906–09–122984. Hari Sharma of Simon Fraser University led one series of interviews in BC between 1984 and 1987, and Gurcharn S. Basran and B. Singh Bolaria led the second round of interviews in the province in 1985–86. See English transcript of Interview No. 22 by Gurcharn S. Basran and B. Singh Bolaria, July 5, 1985, 3, Indo-Canadian Oral History Collection, digitally archived by Simon Fraser University at http://digital.lib.sfu.ca/icohc-collection. See also Basran and Bolaria, *The Sikhs in Canada*.

47 A patient was admitted to the Vancouver General Hospital for tuberculosis in 1906; see LAC, "Individual Cases re East Indian Immigration to Canada," n.d., 1, RG 76, vol. 384, file 536999, pt. 4. Author's Interview 2 at Victoria, BC, June 30, 2010, 1. This informant is the uncle of informant 1, who is mentioned in relation to the same individual in Chapter 1.

48 *Victoria Daily Colonist*, September 19, 1906; *Vancouver Province*, September 20, 1906.

49 Glassberg, "The Design of Reform"; Valverde, *The Age of Light, Soap and Water*, 116; Humphries, *The Last Plague*, 36, 45–46. Humphries cites Worboys, *Spreading Germs*.

50 *Vancouver Province*, October 15, 1906; Ward, *White Canada Forever*, 65; LAC, Wilfrid Laurier to William Pringle, October 18, 1906, MG 26-G, vol. 429.

51 LAC, F. Grey, President, Victoria Trades and Labour Council, to W.D. Scott, October 15, 1906, 1, RG 76, vol. 384, file 536999, pt. 1.

52 Mary Wilson, Vancouver, letter to the *Vancouver News-Advertiser*, December 14, 1906.

53 LAC, F. Grey to W.D. Scott, October 15, 1906, 1, and Ed Stevenson, Saskatchewan Executive Committee, Trades and Labour Congress of Canada, Moose Jaw, to Secretary of State for the Colonies, London, November 19, 1906, 1, both in RG 76, vol. 384, file 536999, pt. 1; *Vancouver World*, October 16 and 23, 1906.

54 While the term "Anglo-Indian" can be used to designate individuals of mixed British and Indian ancestry, this book employs the term to mean individuals of U.K. ancestry living in India, especially during the period of the British Raj (1858–1947).

55 Col. Falk Warren to *Vancouver World*, October 20, 1906.

56 *Vancouver World*, October 16, 17, and 22, 1906. The CPR wharf incident ended by October 22, when only a small number of South Asians remained in the detention sheds awaiting work, along with the few being deported.

57 For news articles on the autumn 1906 labour shortage in BC, see, for example, "Scarcity of Labour and Its Remedy," *Vancouver World*, October 8, 1906; "Could Find Work for Some Hindus in Digging Potatoes," *Vancouver Province*, October 23, 1906; and "The Labour Famine in This Province," *Vancouver World*, October 26, 1906.

58 "Table: Oriental Immigration to Canada from 1 July 1904 to 1 December 1911," in LAC, "Draft Minute on Asiatic Immigration," prepared by Sir Joseph Pope, January 22, 1912, 5, RG 25, vol. 1118, file 66–1912; and (Table) "Census of Canada, 1901, Population of B.C. by Racial Origin, 1901–1941," in Roy, *A White Man's Province*, 171. According to the 1901 Canadian census, 14,885 Chinese and 4,957 Japanese lived in BC in that year; LAC, (Telegram) R. G. MacPherson to Frank Oliver, November 7, 1906, 1, (Telegram) Frank Oliver to R. G. MacPherson, November 9, 1906, 1, and Anonymous C.P.R. Representative to Frank Oliver, November 14, 1906, 1, all in RG 76, vol. 384, file 536999, pt. 1.

59 Although most men in the camps were healthy, a few succumbed to the effects of the long ocean voyage. Underhill learned that several Sikhs had requested the use of a plot of land for the religious practice of cremating their dead; this was eventually granted. Since, except for the small number of British Indian émigrés living in BC, most BC residents at this time saw South Asians as one homogenous Hindu group, reporting on Sikh burial rituals in Vancouver emphasized that "Hindoo" religious practices differed considerably from Christian custom. Jensen, *Passage from India*, 61; *Vancouver Province*, October 23 and November 10, 13, 15, 16, and 19, 1906; *Vancouver World*, November 6, 1906; Johnston, *Voyage of the Komagata Maru*, 13.

60 See English transcript of Interview 30, July 5 1985, 10, by Gurcharn S. Basran and B. Singh Bolaria, Indo-Canadian Oral History Collection, http://digital.lib.sfu.ca/icohc-collection.

61 On October 24, the *Vancouver World* declared that "our beturbaned cousins from India are becoming a cause of terror to [white] women," as South Asians travelling between homes were making "life unbearable" for housewives while their husbands were at work. *Vancouver World*, October 24 and 26, 1906; *Vancouver Province*, October 29, 1906.

62 *Vancouver Province*, November 15, 1906; *Vancouver World*, November 15, 1906. See also *Victoria Daily Times*, November 15, 1906. According to their marriage certificate, Harriett Hilda Mann married Alfred Laviolette in Victoria on January 4, 1906. See BC marriage certificate #1906–09–014505, PABC.

63 *Victoria Colonist*, November 16, 1906; *Vancouver News-Advertiser*, November 16, 1906.

64 *Vancouver Province*, November 16, 1906.

65 *Vancouver Province* (evening ed.), November 16, 1906.

66 In September 2012 the author submitted an "Access to Information" request for Harriett Laviolette's case file from the Vancouver police, but they replied that they do not retain records dating from before 1956.

67 Cohen, *Folk Devils and Moral Panics*, 1; LAC, "Resolution of Meeting of TLC of Canada, Victoria," September 17, 1906, 1, RG 76, vol. 384, file 536999, pt. 1.

68 Roy, *A White Man's Province*, 15. Roy quotes the following press accounts of the Kong incident: *Vancouver Province*, April 6, 1914; *Saturday Sunset* (Vancouver), April 11, 1914; *Prince Rupert Daily News*, April 8, 1914; *Nanaimo Herald*, April 7, 1914; *Vancouver News Advertiser*, April 7, 1914.

69 *Victoria Colonist*, 14 and 15 November, 1906. Also on November 15, the *Victoria Daily Times* reported that Dr. Milne had ordered the CPR to house the men until the men could find work, and that only twenty-five others had been rejected.

70 Jensen, *Passage From India*, 61; *Vancouver World*, November 17, 1906; Kelly, Rees, and Shutter, *Britain 1750–1900*, 18; Isaacs, *American Views of China and India*, 241; Luminet, *Black Holes*, 123.

71 Reitmanova, "Saving the Empire," 200–1; Humphries, *The Last Plague*, 46–47, 49.

72 Reitmanova, "Saving the Empire," 200–1. BC's population was 98,173 in 1891, 178,657 in 1901, and 392,080 in 1911. See these statistics in Roy, *A White Man's Province*, Appendix 1, 269.

73 *Vancouver Province* and *Vancouver World*, November 19, 1906; LAC, (Telegram) A.S. Munro to W.D. Scott, November 17, 1906, 1, and (Telegram) Frank Oliver to A.S. Munro, November 20, 1906, 1, both in Colonial Office fonds (hereafter CO) 42, vol. 908. Oliver also warned CPR officials that he would deport any of that company's former passengers who became indigent; see (Telegram) Frank Oliver to Thomas Shaughnessy, November 20, 1906, in ibid. See also *Vancouver News-Advertiser*, November 20, 1906.

74 *Vancouver Province* and *Vancouver News-Advertiser*, November 21, 1906. There may have been some discrepancy between the level of medical inspection at Vancouver and Victoria. While this is not evident in admissions records, after Dr. Milne passed a group of South Asians at his port, a *Province* reporter remarked that they had landed there to avoid "the eagle-eyed inspection of Dr. Monro [*sic*]" by landing at Victoria, where medical inspection was "not so rigid." The *Saturday Sunset* observed that Japanese migrants from Honolulu landed at Victoria because Milne was "much more lenient in his interpretation of the immigration act" than Vancouver officials. See *Vancouver Province*, October 16, 1906; and *Saturday Sunset* (Vancouver), August 17, 1907.

75 Buchignani, Indra, and Srivastava, *Continuous Journey*, 19; *Province*, November 26, 1906; PABC, Death Certificate for Easer Singh, died November 28 at New Westminster, 1906–09–08291; Cunha, *Pneumonia Essentials*, 4; Vancouver City Archives (hereafter VCA), *Annual Report of the Health Department of Vancouver for Year Ending 31 December 1906* (Vancouver: 1907), 4; LAC, "Copy of Resolution Passed by Vancouver City Council," November 26, 1906, 1, RG 76 vol. 384, file 536999, pt. 1.

76 Reitmanova, "'Disease Breeders Among Us,'" 73, 75, 77, 78, 95; Sears, "Immigration Controls as Social Policy," 92–97.

77 Reitmanova, "'Disease Breeders Among Us,'" 73, 75, 77, 78, 95; Bates, *Bargaining for Life*, 3; Kraut, *Silent Travelers*, 155–56; McQuaig, *The Weariness, the Fever and the Fret*, 4–6; Pernick, "Eugenics and Public Health," 1768.

78 Feldberg, *Disease and Class*, 181; The 1906 Certificates for Deaths in Vancouver and on Vancouver Island are as follows: Nara Singh, Registration No. 1906–09–122984; Hernam Singh, 1906–09–122085; Natta Singh, 1906–09–122092; Poomar Singh, 1906–09–08291; Sunder (Unknown First Name), 1906–09–051619; Easer Singh, 1906–09–082912; Brama Singh, 1906–09–082914. All certificates at PABC. See *Vancouver World*, November 6, 1906, and *Victoria Colonist*, November 1906. Vancouver's 1906 Health Department report shows that a total of forty-nine Vancouver residents of all "races" died of tuberculosis

in that year; we know that only two of these victims were South Asian. Divided into the 2,000 South Asians who remained in greater Vancouver, this number shows a tuberculosis mortality rate of approximately 0.15 percent. The city's tuberculosis death rate in 1906 was close to 1.1%. J.H. Elliot found that 199 in 100,000 Canadians died from the disease between 1900 and 1910. Page 6 of the Vancouver City Health Report indicates that 374 out of 41,000 whites in Vancouver died in 1906. Thus, the total death ratio percentages are 0.35 percent (South Asian) and 0.74 percent (white). See Elliot, "Present Status," 135; and VCA, *Vancouver City Health Report For Year Ending 31 December 1906* (Vancouver: 1907), 6.

79 *Vancouver Province*, December 12, 1906; LAC, E. Blake Robertson to W.D. Scott, December 27, 1906, 1–2, RG 76, vol. 384, file 536999, pt. 1; "No Need to Deport Hindoo: Assistant Superintendent of Immigration Makes Report," *Ottawa Free Press*, December 27, 1906.

80 *Vancouver Province*, November 27, 1906; LAC, A. McEvery (for Mayor) to Fred Buscombe, November 28, 1906, 1, RG 76, vol. 384, file 536999, pt. 1.

81 "*Canadian Annual Review of Public Affairs for 1906* (Toronto: Annual Review Publishing Company, 1907), 285, 295.

82 *Vancouver Province*, November 29, 1906; LAC, Dr. Robert McKechnie, Superintendent, Detention Hospital, to W.D. Scott, December 9, 1906, 2, RG 76, vol. 306. file 281230, Vancouver 1. Emphasis is McKechnie's.

83 A total of 2,351 Indians arrived in 1906, with 46 in December. See Canadian Government Original Data Passenger Lists, 1865–1935, Miscellaneous Publications, T-479-T-14939, tabulated on www.ancestry.ca. The death certificate of Arjan Singh shows he died May 22, 1907, of acute pulmonary tuberculosis at Vancouver, Reg., 1907–09–124947, PABC; *Vancouver Province*, November 28 and 30 and December 16, 1906; *World*, November 27, 1906.

84 *1st Session of 28th British Parliament, House of Commons Record*, vol. 16, December 12 and 13, 1906, 341 and 665, respectively. Though this estimated number of unemployed Indians was a large exaggeration, Frank Oliver himself had personally confirmed this number for use in the British House of Commons; see LAC, (Telegram) Frank Oliver to Dominion Office, London, December 11, 1906, RG 76, vol. 384, file 536999 1, pt. 1.

85 LAC, (Secret) Albert Grey to Colonial Secretary Victor Alexander Bruce (Earl of Elgin, hereafter Elgin), November 11, 1907, 1, RG 7 G10, vol. 13, January to December 1907; Stevens and Saywell, *Lord Minto's Canadian Papers*, xxiv. See also Hilliker, *Canada's Department of External Affairs*, esp. 7–9. Grey reported to Colonial Secretaries Alfred Lyttelton (1903–4), Lord Elgin (1905–8), Lord Crewe (1908–11), and Lewis Vernon Harcourt (1911–15). See Grey to Elgin, December 10, 1906, in CO 42, vol. 908, which enclosed Scott's autumn 1906 report. See also Hallett, "A Governor-General's Views."

86 LAC, "Draft Minute on Asiatic Immigration," January 22, 1912 (Table), RG 25, vol. 1118, file 66–1912. Six hundred had arrived between 1899 and 1905, with only twenty-one rejected among this group.

87 Geiger, *Subverting Exclusion*, 118–19; John H. Clark to F.P. Sargent, September 29, 1906, and B.R. Hunter, Vancouver, to John H. Clark, November 2, 1906, both in RG 85 E9 51403 23, US National Archives and Records Administration (hereafter NARA); NARA, L. Edwin Dudley to Robert Bacon, November 5, 1906, and A.K. Khan, Chico, California, to US Consul, Vancouver, received November 20, 1906, both in RG 85 E9 51388 005, pt. 2.

88 NARA, L. Edwin Dudley to Robert Bacon, November 22, 1906, RG 85 E9 51388 005, pt. 2.

89 NARA, "Memorandum Regarding Hindu Migration to the United States," January 23, 1914, 1, RG 85 E9 52903 110 C; Jensen, *Passage From India*, 10.

90 Roediger, *The Wages of Whiteness*, 12–14; see also Goutor, *Guarding the Gates*, 36. Much of the historiography on the 1882 Chinese Exclusion Act either defends or counters the "California thesis" of Asian exclusion, which was first posited by Mary Roberts Coolidge in 1909 and later developed by Elmer Clarence Sandmeyer in 1939. The California thesis holds that the "special circumstances" of California in the 1870s and 1880s, including the near-equal power of Californian and national Republican and Democratic parties, instigated and politicized the anti-Chinese movement and precipitated Asian exclusion in the United States. Alexander Saxton's classic study from 1971 defended the basic tenets of the California thesis, although Andrew Gyory countered in 1998 that labour unions were not a major force behind Chinese exclusion, as they focused on class, not race, in their efforts to counter imported labour. See Coolidge, *Chinese Exclusion*; Sandmeyer, *The Anti-Chinese Movement in California*; Saxton, *The Indispensable Enemy*, esp. 2, 274, 280; and Gyory, *Closing the Gate*. For a summary of both arguments, see Okihiro, *The Columbia Guide to Asian American History*, 74–76. See also Erika Lee, *At America's Gates*, 9–10.

91 Government attempts to control and quash the distribution and consumption of opium ultimately influenced the popular association between Chinese and narcotics. Another vice, Chinese female prostitution, came to signify "a sexualized danger with the power to subvert ... the domestic ideal," while the loose clothing and long hairstyle worn by male Chinese before China's 1911 Xinhai revolution disrupted American gender norms. Erika Lee, *At America's Gates*, 25–27.

92 Erika Lee, *At America's Gates*, 32; Daniels, *Asian America*, 109–10.

93 NARA, John H. Clark to Frank Sargent, December 24, 1906, 1–2, RG 85 E9 51403 23.

94 Fairchild, *Science at the Borders*, 135; NARA, John H. Clark to Frank Sargent, December 24, 1906, 1–2, RG 85 E9 51403 23.

95 C.W. Bennett to H.M. Durand, December 10, 1906, FO 371 160, 1, Public Records Office, United Kingdom.

96 Table 2 details US Asian immigration statistics for 1899–1921.

97 Birn, "Six Seconds Per Eyelid," 281–83; US Congress Act of March 3, 1891, 51 Cong. 2nd Sess., 26 Stat. 1084. The 1891 Act barred so-called idiots and the insane, along with paupers, criminals, political radicals, polygamists, and contract labourers. In 1903 the Act was amended to designate trachoma as a "Class A" (exclusion mandatory) condition; anarchists, prostitutes, and career beggars were later added to this list.

98 *Los Angeles Times*, December 4, 1906; Jensen, *Passage from India*, 15–16; NARA, "Bureau of Immigration Memorandum Regarding Hindu Migration to the United States," received January 23, 1914, 1, RG 85 E9 52903 110 C. Statistics of border crossings at Vancouver are in NARA, Inspector in Charge, Vancouver, to John H. Clark, February 21, 1907, 1, RG 85 E9 51403 23.

99 See Jensen's discussion on "executive restriction" and "LPC" in Jensen, *Passage from India*, 113–14; *Blaine Journal*, May 24, 1907. The *Journal* editor added that "there are none of them in Blaine, thank goodness."

Chapter 2: Riots, Plague, and the Advent of Executive Exclusion

Epigraph note: "Gifts of Famine: Invasion of Sikhs from the Punjaub [sic]," *International Woodworker* 17, 10 (October 1907): 4–5.

1 Laurier was addressing delegates of the national Trades and Labour Congress (TLC). See "Hindoos Not Diseased," *Toronto Daily Star*, January 10, 1907.

2　Roy, *A White Man's Province*, 164, 168; 108 South Asians arrived between January and March; Canadian Government Original Data Passenger Lists, 1865–1935, Miscellaneous Publications, T-479-T-14939, tabulated on www.ancestry.ca.

3　The patient was likely "Ameela" Singh, whom friends sent back to India in 1907. "Ameela" does not appear in passenger records, but six "Mela Singhs" arrived in 1906; see LAC, "Individual Cases regarding East Indian Immigration to Canada," n.d., 1, RG 76, vol. 384, file 536999, pt. 4. See also Canadian Government Original Passenger Lists; *Vancouver Province*, January 30 and February 15, 1907.

4　LAC, (Telegram) G.L. Milne to W.D. Scott, February 15, 1907, 1, and Frank Oliver to W.D. Scott, February 27, 1907, 1, both in RG 76, vol. 384, file 536999, pt. 1.

5　Mathieu, *North of the Colour Line*, 42. Mathieu cites the Scott quotation in Hill, *Alberta's Black Settlers*, 86. See also Erika Lee, *At America's Gates*, 22.

6　Omi and Winant, *Racial Formation in the United States*, 12–13.

7　LAC, W.D. Scott to G.U. Ryley, Grand Trunk Railway, Montreal, February 19, 1907, RG 76, vol. 384, file 536999, pt. 1; Williams and Nihal Singh, "Canada's New Immigrant," 385.

8　Williams and Nihal Singh, "Canada's New Immigrant," 388; Lockley, "The Hindu Invasion," 592, 595.

9　Arnold, "'An Ancient Race Outworn,'" 124–26, 131–33, 136, 140.

10　See 1907 death records for Albale Singh, 1907–09–124898; Mangal Singh, 1907–09–083437; Thaker Singh, 1907–09–020487; Arjan Singh, 1907–09–124912; Hira Singh 1907–09–124920; Bagga Singh, 1907–09–020499; Partap Singh, 1907–09–124943, and Fattch Singh, 1907–09–124947. All records at PABC. Also see Nayan Shah's treatment of the homophobia-motivated murder of Partap Singh, in Shah, *Stranger Intimacy*, 21, 30–34; "Winston Churchill, Response," *United Kingdom Parliamentary Debates, 2nd Session 28th Parliament*, vol. 1, February 18, 1907, 539. The 5 percent statistic is calculated by dividing the number of arrivals by the number rejected for medical reasons, using South Asian arrivals in 1906 (2,193) from E. Blake Robertson's above-mentioned report, housed in LAC, RG 76, vol. 384, file 536999. pt. 1.

11　LAC, George Halse, Acting Mayor, Col. Falk Warren, and A.S. Munro to Wilfrid Laurier, June 24, 1907, 1, RG 76, vol. 384, file 536999, pt. 1; *Vancouver World*, July 25 and August 14, 1907; *Vancouver Province*, August 14, 1907.

12　Kelley and Trebilcock, *The Making of the Mosaic*, 135–36.

13　Price, "'Orienting' the Empire,'" *BC Studies* 156 (Winter 2007–8): 53–57.

14　Biswas, "Colonial Displacements," 26–27. Biswas cites Panikkar, *Culture, Ideology, Hegemony*, 22, and Jensen, *Passage from India*, 7–8. By 1900, Bengal province had become a magnet for nationalism, as the middle class increasingly resented colonial measures designed to retain hegemony and profits in the hands of the governing white elite.

15　Gerald N. Hallberg's article remains the fullest historiographical account of the riot. See Hallberg, "Bellingham, Washington's Anti-Hindu Riot"; United States Government, *Reports of the Immigration Commission*, pt. 25, vol. 1, Senate Document, 633, 61st Cong., 2nd Sess. (Washington: US GPO, 1911), 331.

16　NARA, James Bryce to Alvey A. Adee (Acting Secretary of State), September 12, 1907, 1–2, RG 59, State Department Numerical and Minor Files 1906 to 1910, M862, reel 612.

17　*Bellingham Herald*, September 5 and 6, 1907.

18　A.W. Magnum, Bellingham, to "Mother," September 8, 1907, 1–2, Magnum Family Papers 483, folder 11, Wilson Library, University of North Carolina at Chapel Hill. Underline is Magnum's.

19 See Stout, *Chinese Immigration*; Kraut, *Silent Travelers*, 80–81. Kraut cites Stout's "Report on Chinese Immigration," in *First Biennial Report, State Board of Health in California* (Sacramento: California State Board of Health, 1870–71), 63.

20 Ross's ideas of biological determinism, which slightly pre-dated the American Eugenics movement, were by no means universally accepted in the nation's sociological circles. In 1907, W.I. Thomas compared the brain weight and academic performance of different racial groups in a phenotypically based argument very similar to that of the late sociologist J. Philippe Rushton of Western University (1943–2012). See Ross, "The Causes of Race Superiority," 82, 86–87; Rushton, *Race, Evolution, and Behavior*.

21 *Morning Olympian* (Olympia), August 12, 1910.

22 *San Francisco Call*, September 7 and 10, 1907; *Los Angeles Times*, September 9, 1907; *Bellingham Herald*, September 12, 1907; Jensen, *Passage from India*, 51; See *Blaine Journal*, May 24, 1907.

23 In a speech in Bellingham in late September, Thoburn declared that "the Hindu" and other Asians would soon "swarm this country" and that the nation "may as well try to sweep back the tides of the ocean as to try to keep them out." *Blaine Journal*, September 13, 1907; *Bellingham Herald*, September 14 and 27, 1914.

24 Shah, *Contagious Divides*, 150, 153–55.

25 Ibid., 120–23, 155. Shah quotes Todd, *Eradicating Plague from San Francisco*, 38.

26 Kraut, *Silent Travelers*, 90, 97, 104.

27 For press reports on plague in San Francisco, see *The Evening Statesman* (Walla Walla), August 29, 1907; *East Oregonian* (Pendleton), August 30, 1907; and *Los Angeles Herald*, August 31, 1907.

28 [Author unknown], "Gifts of Famine," *International Woodworker*, 4–5.

29 "Hindus are Undesirables" (Editorial), *Bellingham Herald*, December 30, 1909; Carter, "Oriental Sore of Northern India." Carter described clusters of parasites appearing on the skin of individuals living in certain villages in northern India. See Stiles's comments in *Spokane Spokesman-Review*, December 5, 1908.

30 Shah cautions that gaps between contemporary epidemiology and official, press, and popular etiological knowledge make it difficult to trace the "struggles between scientific bureaucracy and the socially marginalized races" during San Francisco's plague outbreaks. Shah, *Contagious Divides*, 123–24.

31 Barde, "Prelude to the Plague," 155–56, 160–61.

32 Klein, "Plague, Policy, and Popular Unrest," 724.

33 See Kraut, *Silent Travelers*.

34 *Vancouver World*, April 6, 1908; *Bellingham Herald*, April 7, 1908. According to Maynard Swanson, South Africa's "sanitation syndrome" of plague prevention in the late nineteenth and early twentieth centuries asserted that African and Asian urban settlement threatened public health. In the 1870s, Durban unsuccessfully strove to erect a *cordon sanitaire* between its white and South Asian populations, in order to contain what a local paper called Indian "breeding haunts and nursery grounds of disease, misery and discomfort." The city tried again in the 1890s to attain, in the mayor's words, "the isolation with better hopes of cure of this our social leprosy." Swanson argues that South Asians were a "special target" of sanitation efforts, because initially they were the most "obvious intrusive group," just as they were on their arrival in North America. Swanson, "The Sanitation Syndrome," 390–91."

35 Chang, *Pacific Connections*, 98.

36 *Vancouver World*, April 9, 1908; Kipling, *Letters to the Family*, 39–40, 62. In the full version of his diary entry, detailing his 1907 trip to the Pacific coast, he remarked it would take

only "the least little care and attention" to make the men excellent workers, although he felt that "some one ought to tell them not to bring their old men with them."

37 Hugh Johnston, *The Voyage of the Komagata Maru*, 11; author interview with informant 2, Victoria Khalsa Diwan Society, June 30, 2010, 1; author interview with informant 6 (Member of Parliament 3), House of Commons, April 12, 2010, 1. See also, for example, *Vancouver Province*, September 17, 1907.

38 Beiser, "The Health of Immigrants and Refugees," S31–S32; Reitmanova, "'Disease Breeders among Us,'" 74–75.

39 Taylor recalled a recent study on bubonic plague (likely a 1903 report on Hong Kong) that showed that plague originated in unclean areas of Chinese cities. Asking "Gwen" how she could "enjoy such persons as neighbors," Taylor made an imaginative leap in connecting Indian immigrants with plague in China. "Editorial – from a Woman's Point of View," *Vancouver World*, November 26, 1906. See also Simpson, *Report on the Causes*. Although Taylor also referred to a *Times* (London) article about plague in India, the editor neglected to mention that the article showed a nearly 75 percent decrease in plague mortality in India since Oct 1905; see *Times*, October 1, 1906.

40 Roy, *A White Man's Province*, 32–35. Roy cites Provincial Board of Heath, *Annual Report*, 1896, BCSP, 730 and 1898, 1177–78, 1144; and PABC, Secretary, Provincial Board of Health, to Attorney General, July 1900, GR 429, box 6.

41 "Regulations for Detection and Treatment of a Disease Known as Bubonic Plague," Approved 24 October 1907, *BC Sessional Papers 2nd Session 11th Parliament 1908* (Victoria: Wolfeden, 1908), G 19; *Vancouver World*, October 26 and 28, 1907; "Precautions against the bubonic plague," *Saturday Sunset* (Vancouver), November 2, 1907.

42 "Report of Inspector J. Hynes, N.D.," 1–2, City Records, Series 101, Health Inspectors ca. 1895–1911, VCA. This undated report very likely details work conducted in early November 1907, after the province's enactment of special measures to prevent plague in Asian dwellings.

43 *Vancouver World*, November 9, 1907; *Vancouver Province*, September 12 and 16, 1907.

44 Laurier declined Governor General Grey's request for federal help for the refugees from Bellingham, explaining that the government's attention was fully occupied with "the abominable outbreak against the Japs which has just disgraced Vancouver." LAC, Grey to Wilfrid Laurier, September 9, 1907, 1; LAC, Wilfrid Laurier to Grey, September 10, 1907, 1, MG 27 IIB2, vol. 2. In what Chris Lee has called an "institutional failure that must be urgently rectified," historians have traditionally downplayed the Vancouver riot, although since 2007 there has been a resurgence in scholarship on the subject. For example, see Chang, *Pacific Connections*, 89–117. See also Chris Lee, "The Lateness of Asian Canadian Studies," 2.

45 Taylor's editorial statements in *Vancouver World*, September 6 and 7, 1907. *Vancouver Province*, September 9, 1907; *Vancouver World*, September 9, 1907; Jensen, *Passage from India*, 66, 68. For the political consequences of the riot and the resulting 1908 Hayashi–Lemieux Agreement to limit Japanese emigration, see Price, *Orienting Canada*, 55–56.

46 LAC, Grey to Wilfrid Laurier, September 9, 1907, 1, and Wilfrid Laurier to Grey, September 10, 1907, 1, both in MG 27 IIB2, vol. 2. Price cites Chris Lee, "The Lateness of Asian Canadian Studies," 55–56.

47 LAC, (Secret) Grey to Elgin, November 11, 1907, 1, RG 7 G10, vol. 13, January to December 1907; LAC, (Telegram) Alexander Bethune to Wilfrid Laurier, 1, September 11, 1907, (Telegram) Wilfrid Laurier to Alexander Bethune, September 13, 1907, 1, (Telegram) Alexander Bethune to Wilfrid Laurier, September 13, 1907, 1, Taraknath

Das to Alexander Bethune, September 13, 1907, 1, all in MG 26-G C852, vol. 478; LAC, Grey to Wilfrid Laurier, September 13, 1907, 1, MG 27 IIB2, vol. 2; *Vancouver Province,* September 9 and 12, 1907; *Vancouver World,* September 9, 12, and 13, 1907; Jensen, *Passage from India,* 66.

48 Said, *Orientalism,* 12.

49 *Vancouver World,* September 17 and 18, 1907; Indra, "South Asian Stereotypes," 171–72; Said, *Orientalism,* 12.

50 Jensen, *Passage from India,* 113.

51 LAC, (Telegram) A.S. Munro to Frank Oliver, September 14, 1907, 1, and (Telegram) G. L. Milne to Frank Oliver, September 14, 1907, 1, both in RG 76, vol. 384, file 536999, pt. 1.

52 *Saturday Sunset* (Vancouver), September 21, 1907. Editor J.P. McConnell added that the *Monteagle's* South Asians had no formal aid (for locating housing, etc.) on arriving, as Munro's help was voluntary.

53 LAC, (Confidential) Wilfrid Laurier to Grey, September 16, 1907, 1, and Wilfrid Laurier to Grey, September 19, 1907, 1, both in MG 27 IIB2, vol. 2; LAC, Grey to Elgin, September 18, 1907, 1, MG 27 IIB2, vol. 14; Diary of W.L. Mackenzie King, September 19, 1907, 262, at www.collectionscanada.gc.ca/databases/king. The Vancouver press heralded Scott's visit, although with less enthusiasm than in 1906, when immediate Dominion intervention had been expected. See *Vancouver Province,* September 19, 1907, and *Vancouver World,* September 23 and 25, 1907.

54 *Vancouver World,* November 9, 1907. There is no record of bubonic plague in BC during this period; see Roy, *A White Man's Province,* 35. See also LAC, Grey to Elgin, November 11, 1907, 1, MG 27 IIB2, vol. 14; LAC, (Secret) (Telegram) Grey to Elgin, November 11, 1907, 1, RG 7 G10, vol. 13; LAC, Grey to Elgin, November 14, 1907, 2–3, MG 27 IIB2, vol. 14; and (Private and Confidential) Grey to Colonel Sir Claude Macdonald, British Embassy, Tokio [*sic*], October 1, 1907, 1, and Grey to John Morley, October 1, 1907, 2, both in 4th Earl Grey Papers, file GRE-B 210–7, Durham University Library.

55 See Mackenzie King's recollection of Laurier's views in Diary of W.L. Mackenzie King, September 28, 1907, 2104, at www.collectionscanada.gc.ca/databases/king; see also LAC, Wilfrid Laurier to Grey, October 1, 1907, 1, CO 42, vol. 913; LAC, Wilfrid Laurier Memorandum for W.W. Cory, October 1, 1907, 1, MG 26-G C-853, vol. 482; Jensen, *Passage from India,* 71–72; and LAC, (Very Confidential) Report of W.E.B. McInnes [pseudonym: real name was Thomas R. McInnes] to Frank Oliver, October 2, 1907, 7, 9, and 15, RG 25 G1, vol. 1138, file 1914 40 C.

56 LAC, "Report of W.E.B. McInnes," 9 and 15, RG 25 G1, vol. 1138, file 1914 40 C.

57 US officials at Vancouver reported to McInnes that from July 1 to 24, 82 of 84 men applying to the United States had passed examination, while from July 25 to August 24, 131 out of 154 passed, and from August 25 to September 24, 118 out of 133 passed; Jensen, *Passage from India,* 72; LAC, Grey to Laurier, November 16, 1907, 1, MG 27 IIB2, vol. 2.

58 LAC, (Telegram) W.W. Cory to Wilfrid Laurier, October 5, 1907, 1, [repeats Munro's telegram], and (Telegram) Wilfrid Laurier to W.W. Cory, October 5, 1907, 1, both in MG 26-G C-853, vol. 482; *Manitoba Free Press,* October 7, 1907; LAC, (Telegram) W.D. Scott to W.W. Cory, October 10, 1907, 1, RG 76, vol. 384, file 536999, pt. 1; *Vancouver World,* October 10, 1907.

59 "Statement of Taraknath Das of New York City," US Senate, Hearings on S.J. Res. 128, Before the Committee on Immigration, Providing for the Ratification and Confirmation of Naturalization of Certain Persons of the Hindu Race, 69th Cong., 2nd Sess.

(Washington: US GPO, 1926) Pt. 1, December 9, 1926, 22; LAC, MacDonnell, Henderson, and Jones to A.S. Munro, December 3, 1907, 1, RG 76, vol. 491, file 759510; LAC, "Individual Cases regarding East Indian Immigration to Canada," n.d., 1, RG 76, vol. 384, file 536999, pt. 4.

60 "English summary of Kartar Singh Ghag Interview by Hari Sharma, June 21, 1985, 1, Indo-Canadian Oral History Collection, http://digital.lib.sfu.ca/icohc-collection. Alan Sears points out that while British immigrants were not checked for trachoma, Europeans were, and a recession in 1907–8 caused an increase in inspections of both Britons and Americans at Canadian ports and entry points. Sears, "Immigration Controls as Social Policy," 98, 100.

61 Interview With Victoria informant 2, at Victoria, June 30, 2010, 1. This interviewee is the nephew of Victoria informant 3, who is mentioned in relation to the same individual in Chapter 1.

62 Singh, *Amrik Vich Hindustanee*, 42–45. Mr. Pooni of Vancouver orally translated this text for me from Gurumukhi. Two Kartar Singhs came on the *Tartar*, which carried 536 South Asians. This number is very close to Nawanchand's estimate.

63 *Vancouver World*, October 10, 1, 5 and 17, 1907; *Pittsburg Press*, August 31, 1901; *West Gippsland Gazette* (Australia), November 5, 1901. See also Fralick, *The Intravenous Infusion Method*.

64 LAC, Frank Oliver to Grey, October 27, 1907, 1–2, RG 76, vol. 384, file 536999, pt. 2. Scott's original report is missing, but it is quoted it in LAC, "Memorandum, W.D. Scott to W.W. Cory, 23 November 1911," 1, RG 76, vol. 384, file 536999, pt. 4.

65 LAC, Frank Oliver to Grey, October 27, 1907, 3–5, RG 76, vol. 384, file 536999, pt. 2.

66 *Vancouver World*, November 9, 1907; LAC, Grey to Elgin, November 11, 1907, 1, MG 27 IIB2, vol. 14; LAC, (Secret) (Telegram) Grey to Elgin, November 11, 1907, 1, RG 7 G10, vol. 13; LAC, Grey to Elgin, November 14, 1907, 2–3, MG 27 IIB2, vol. 14.

67 LAC, (Secret) Grey to Elgin, November 11, 1907, 1, RG 7 G10, vol. 13, January to December 1907; W.L. Mackenzie King, *Report of Royal Commission into the Methods by Which Oriental Labourers Have Been Induced to Come to Canada* (Ottawa: King's Printer, 1908), 11, 75, 76 80; *Vancouver World*, November 3, 1907; LAC, "Individual Cases regarding East Indian Immigration to Canada," n.d., 1, RG 76, vol. 384, file 536999, pt. 4. Witness 1's age and finances indicate that he was the man described in the *World*, November 3, 1907. See English transcript of Interview 32 by Gurcharn S. Basran and B. Singh Bolaria, July 10, 1985, 8, Indo-Canadian Oral History Collection, http://digital.lib.sfu.ca/icohc-collection.

68 Jensen, *Passage from India*, 75; See W. L. Mackenzie King's transshipment observation in *Report*, supra note 67, at 11, 75, 76 80.

69 Kelley and Trebilcock, *The Making of the Mosaic*, 147; Jensen, *Passage from India*, 60–61.

70 *Vancouver World*, December 3, 1907; LAC, P.H. Bryce to A.S. Munro, November 20, 1907, 1, RG 76, vol. 331, file 330483, pt. 5; see December 16 arrivals from the *Monteagle* in Canadian Government, Original Data Passenger Lists, 1865–1935, Miscellaneous Publications, T-479-T-14939, LAC, tabulated on www.ancestry.ca.

Chapter 3: "The Public Health Must Prevail"

Epigraph note: (Private Earl) Grey to John Morley, March 23, 1908, 2, 4th Earl Grey Papers, file GRE-B 210–7, Durham University Library.

1 "Government of Canada, Privy Council Orders 920 and 926, January 8, 1908." The money qualification only applied to South Asians; Chinese and Japanese were restricted

by separate legislation. Parnaby and Kealey explain that this "selective travel restriction" was "legally dubious, but politically sly." Jensen adds that the continuous journey order was "carefully worded to avoid express discrimination against British Indian subjects," which gave Laurier time to work out a diplomatic arrangement with India. Parnaby and Kealey, "The Origins of Political Policing," 224; Jensen, *Passage from India*, 75.

2 As Grey pointed out in a private letter to a colleague in November 1907, "Sir Wilfrid is genuinely alarmed ... [that more] Hindus [arriving] in B.C. either from across the Seas, or as refugees from oppression in the US, may precipitate another outbreak in Vancouver." LAC, Grey to Elgin, November 11, 1907, 1 and November 14 1907, 1, MG 27 IIB2 Grey, vol. 14; see also a second letter from the same date, LAC, (Secret) Grey to Elgin, November 11, 1907, 1, RG 7 G10, vol. 13, file January to December 1907.

3 LAC, Frank Oliver to Lord Strathcona, April 8, 1908, 1–2, RG 25, vol. 200, file 117–93 to 119–95; W.D. Scott, "The Immigration By Races" (1914), reprinted in Thorner and Frohn-Nielson, *A Country Nourished on Self-Doubt*, 83; LAC, H.H. Stevens to Mrs. M. Barber of the Anti-Asiatic League, February 7, 1923, 1, MG 27 III B 9, vol. 191, file Oriental Immigration 1923.

4 *Vancouver World*, February 12, 15, 25, and 27 and March 3 and 5, 1908; *Vancouver Province*, February 26 and March 3, 1908; LAC, Frank Oliver to L.M. Fortier, February 18, 1908, 1, and L.M. Fortier to G.L. Milne, February 18, 1908, 1, both in RG 76, vol. 474, file 729921, pt. 1; LAC, Frank Oliver to G.L. Milne, February 28, 1908, 1, RG 76, vol. 384, file 536999, pt. 2; LAC, Grey to Elgin, March 3, 1908, 1, MG 27 IIB2, vol. 14.

5 *Debates of the Canadian House of Commons, 10th Parliament, 4th Session*, vol. 3, March 24, 1908, 5490; LAC, (Personal) W.E.B. McInnes [pseudonym for Thomas R. McInnes] to Wilfrid Laurier, March 24, 1908, 1, MG 26-G C-860, vol. 511, 1–2; LAC, W.E.B. McInnes to Wilfrid Laurier, March 25, 1908, 1, CO 42, vol. 918; Jensen, *Passage from India*, 77–78; *United Kingdom Parliamentary Debates 3rd Session, 28th Parliament*, vol. 4, March 23, 1908, 1050; *United Kingdom Parliamentary Debate*, March 24, 1908, 1206, and March 25, 1908, 1404.

6 Durham University Library, (Private) Grey to John Morley, March 23, 1908, 2, 4th Earl Grey Papers, file GRE-B, 210–7. In the meantime, McInnes warned Oliver that steamship companies might soon begin selling through tickets from Calcutta to circumvent exclusion, a prediction shared by Vancouver's press. A noteworthy editorial cartoon portrayed Laurier as Canute, the eleventh-century English king who tried to stop the ocean's tide with his words. In the cartoon, "King Canute Laurier" held a stick with "Order in Council" written on it and asked a wave depicting the "Hindu Invasion" to "keep back." The caption read: "But the Cruel Waves Rolled On." LAC, (Confidential) W.E.B. McInnes to Frank Oliver, March 14, 1908, 2, CO 42, vol. 918; *Vancouver Province*, March 18, 1908.

7 *Vancouver World*, March 13 and 24, 1908; *Vancouver Province*, March 14 and 25, 1908; *Debates of the Canadian House of Commons, 10th Parliament, 4th Session*, vol. 3, April 8, 1908, 6431–36, 6441–44.

8 Paula Hastings affirms Stanley's interpretation of racism as a key "social configuration" within BC's "explicitly European (and largely British) masculinist project to establish dominance within the province." Hastings, "Review," 1.

9 This fact necessitates an expansion of Stanley's recent argument on the widespread and enduring nature of BC's anti-Chinese racism. Stanley borrows the term "texture of life" from Hannah Arendt's description of how Nazi Germany's anti-Semitism pervaded "day to day interactions and practices." Stanley, *Contesting White Supremacy*, 5–6. Stanley cites Arendt, "The Jew as Pariah."

10 While Kelley and Trebilcock incorrectly state that 2,623 South Asians arrived in Canada in 1908, in fact, only 354 came in that year, mostly in the gap between Orders. However, the authors astutely note that the continuous journey provision, in tandem with a renewed Asian requirement of $200, had an instant and profound effect on immigration from India. Kelley and Trebilcock, *The Making of the* Mosaic, 149; 47 came in January, 10 in February, 275 in March, and 5 in April. See Canadian Government, Original Data, Passenger Lists, 1865–1935, Miscellaneous Publications, T-479-T-14939, tabulated at www.ancestry.ca. Both Orders underwent court challenges in 1910 and 1914, but the government passed them again with slight revisions.

11 Dawson, *William Lyon Mackenzie King*, 157–60.

12 Some scholars have disputed Dawson's contention that King was Royally Commissioned to visit London because "an ostensible reason for the trip had to be found." Most recently, John Price asserts that Laurier sent King to London in March 1908 in order to influence British and Indian government policy on South Asian emigration. The broad scope of King's meetings on the issue and the breadth of his report suggest that Price's view is the correct one. Price, *Orienting Canada*, 23. King also failed to achieve Roosevelt's goal; as Price points out, a "hemispheric arrangement on exclusion proved elusive," because Britain felt that Japan would see through it and resent Anglo-American policy alignment on the matter. See also King Diary, March 3, 1908, at www.collection scanada.gc.ca/databases/king.

13 Government of Canada, *Report of Mackenzie King on His Mission to England in Connection with the Immigration of Asiatics Into Canada* (London: HMSO Office, 1908), 5. See LAC, Viceroy of India, Calcutta, to John Morley, London, January 22, 1908, 1, referenced in Government of India, Department of Commerce and Industry, Calcutta, to John Morley, March 11, 1909, 2, MG 26-J, vol. 12, file 11424 to 6.

14 *Vancouver World*, April 7 and 9, 1908; *Saturday Sunset* (Vancouver), April 11, 1908.

15 LAC, J. Obed Smith to W.D. Scott, June 29, 1908, 1, RG 76, vol. 384, file 536999, pt. 2; Lionel Curtis, Johannesburg, to Leopold Amery, July 20, 1908, 1–3, Leo Amery Papers, file AMEL 2/5/7, Churchill Archives Centre.

16 LAC, P.H. Bryce to W.D. Scott, June 17, 1908, 1, with enclosure "Detentions at Vancouver, April–May 1908," 1, W.D. Scott to P.H. Bryce, June 12, 1908, 1, and A.S. Munro to W.D. Scott, June 24, 1908, 3–4, all in RG 76, vol. 332, file Staff Hindus Monteagle.

17 *Vancouver Province*, August 22, 1908; Deportations listed in LAC, "Individual Cases regarding East Indian Immigration to Canada," n.d., 1, RG 76, vol. 384, file 536999, pt. 4.

18 Hawaiian Planters Association reply in the article "No Place for Hindus. Earth needs an annex, unless they stay at home," *Daily Capital Journal*, December 20, 1907; Jensen, *Passage from India*, 121–22.

19 Indeed, Jensen notes that Emma Goldman, a prominent anarchist member of the Industrial Workers of the World, addressed a South Asian audience before Swayne's arrival. Jensen, *Passage from India*, 122–23. For Swayne's estimate that three thousand South Asians remained in BC, see LAC, W.W. Cory to Wilfrid Laurier, November 6, 1908, 1, MG 26-G C-868, vol. 543.

20 Parnaby and Kealey, "The Origins of Political Policing," 225. As Hugh Johnston points out, Hopkinson began his Immigration Branch career in February 1909. See Johnston, *The Voyage of the Komagata Maru*, 35; also see Popplewell, *Intelligence and Imperial Defence*, 147–61. Hopkinson's records are housed in FO 115 1676, UK PRO, and in LAC, RG 24 C1, file 838. His Pacific coast surveillance reports comprise enough material for a full-length biographic monograph that remains to be written.

21 *Vancouver Province*, October 15 and November 14, 1908; *Ottawa Free Press*, October 20, 1908; *Vancouver World*, September 22 and December 7, 1908; LAC, W.W. Cory to Wilfrid

Laurier, November 6, 1908, 2, MG 26-G C-868, vol. 543; Durham University Library, Grey to Wilfrid Laurier, December 7, 1908, 1, 4th Earl Grey Papers, file GRE-B 173–5.

22 Canada, *The Indians in B.C.*; Durham University Library, (Telegram) Grey to the Earl of Crewe, December 8, 1908, 1, 4th Earl Grey Papers, file GRE-B 173–5; *Vancouver World*, December 10, 1908; LAC, T. Singh to J. Hill, December 24, 1908, 1, RG 76, vol. 384, file 536999, pt. 3; *Vancouver Province*, December 12, 1908.

23 LAC, J.H. MacGill to W.W. Cory, February 12, 1909, 1, and W.D. Scott to J.H. MacGill, March 23, 1909, 1, both in RG 76, vol. 384, file 536999, pt. 3. All BC–based immigration inspectors were already following this policy, however, as only two South Asians were landed at any BC port in the whole of 1909. See 1909 Arrivals in Canadian Government, Original Data, Passenger Lists, 1865–1935, Miscellaneous Publications, T-479-T-14939, tabulated at www.ancestry.ca. The memorandum "Asiatic Immigration: Its History and Present Position," August 28, 1929, 29, in LAC, RG 25, vol. 1549, file 1929 714, indicates that six South Asians arrived in 1909, but as mentioned above, only two appear to have arrived that year.

24 LAC, Grey to Elgin, December 8, 1908, 8–9, LAC, MG 27 IIB2 Grey, vol. 14.

25 Woodsworth, *Strangers within Our Gates*, 154–55. Agnes Foster Buchanan concurred that South Asians "lack[ed] physical endurance" because most followed a vegetarian diet, while F.G. Moorhead added that "physically they are unfit for the hard labor of opening a new country." See Buchanan, "The West and the Hindu Invasion," 312–13, Moorhead, "The Foreign Invasion of the Northwest."

26 Day, *Multiculturalism*, 144, 146. For immigration recruitment details from the period in question, and Canada's settlement of immigrants from the United Kingdom, Scandinavian countries, Italy, the rest of southern Europe, and eastern Europe, see Macdonald, *Canada*, esp. 117, 129, 148.

27 Day, *Multiculturalism*, 144, 146.

28 LAC, Wilfrid Laurier to Grey, November 17, 1908, 1, MG 27 IIB2 Grey, vol. 3; King Diary, December 3, 1908, 1, at www.collectionscanada.gc.ca/databases/king.

29 King Diary, December 3, 1908, 1, at ibid.

30 Jensen, *Passage from India*, 81.

31 LAC, Lords Minto, Kitchener et al., Government of India, to John Morley, 11 March 1909, 1, MG 26-J 1910, vol. 12. Most of the 350 South Asians who entered Canada in 1908 had arrived in the period of legislative limbo before the continuous journey provision was reinstated in April. LAC, Francis W. Giddens, "Statement on Chinese, Japanese and Hindoo Immigration," n.d., 1, RG 76, vol. 551, file 806018. For 1908 arrivals, see LAC, Canadian Government, Original Data, Passenger Lists, 1865–1935, Miscellaneous Publications T-479-T-14939, tabulated at www.ancestry.ca.

32 Kelley and Trebilcock, *The Making of the Mosaic*, 149. PC 920 and PC 926 were reissued May 9, 1910 under the revised Immigration Act. See LAC, W.D. Scott to Frank Oliver, February 4, 1911, 1, RG 76, vol. 384, file 53699, pt. 3; Avery, *Reluctant Host*, 52. See also Dawson, *William Lyon Mackenzie King*, 162–66.

33 Durham University Library, "Statement regarding Hindus in Canada," August 4, 1909, 1–2, 4th Earl Grey Papers, file GRE-B, 173–75; *Canadian Annual Review of Public Affairs for 1909* (Toronto: Annual Review Publishing Company, 1910), 39.

34 Buchignani, Indra, and Srivastava, *Continuous Journey*, 32; LAC, G.D. Kumar to India Office, enclosing "Petition of Public Meeting Swadesh Sevak Home, Fairview," April 24, 1910, 1, CO 42, vol. 943.

35 For Asian arrival statistics, see LAC, "Asiatic Immigration: Its History and Present Position," August 28, 1929, 7, 17, 28–29, RG 25, vol. 1549, file 1929, 714; see also LAC,

"Individual Cases regarding East Indian Immigration to Canada," n.d., 1, 4, RG 76, vol. 384, file 536999, pt. 4; and LAC, W.C. Hopkinson to W.W. Cory, January 11, 1911, 1, and W.C. Hopkinson to W.W. Cory, February 17, 1911, 1, both in RG 76, vol. 384, file 536999, pt. 3.

36 Hugh Johnston traces Hopkinson's reporting on the activities of Kumar and other South Asians on the Pacific coast throughout 1911. Peter Campbell further explores government monitoring of the relationships that developed in this period between BC Indian independence activists and the Socialist Party of Canada and the International Workers of the World. These accounts show that the Dominion and Imperial governments viewed some resident Indians as a political liability. See Johnston, "The Surveillance"; and Campbell, "East Meets Left." See also LAC, "Oaths of Allegiance and Office, Hopkinson, 15 February 1911," 1, RG 76, vol. 561, file 808722, pt. 1. This file's expense receipts offer information on Hopkinson's travel and other activities.

37 Jensen, *Passage from India*, 95, 102–3. For a discussion of the so-called American–Japanese War Scare of 1907, see Perras, *Stepping Stones to Nowhere*, 9; and Neu, *An Uncertain Friendship*, 87, 132.

38 Jensen, *Passage from India*, 113.

39 For Billings's comments, see NARA, John H. Clark to Frank Sargent, December, 24 1906, 1–2, RG 85 E9 51403 23. For South Asian rejections in 1907, see NARA, "Memorandum regarding Hindu migration to the United States," received January 23, 1914, 1, in RG 85 E9 52903 110 C. See Table 3 for South Asian immigrants rejections, admissions, and exits in the US between 1904 and 1914.

40 Fairchild, "The Rise and Fall," 338–39; Birn, "Six Seconds per Eyelid," 292, 308; Markel and Stern, "Which Face? Whose Nation?," 1316, 1319.

41 See Birn, "Six Seconds per Eyelid," 288–89, 295–96; and Yew, "Medical Inspection of Immigrants." Birn points out that the fact that both the eugenic and germ theories "coexisted" in medical screening theory and practice well into the twentieth century generally echoed the "ambiguity" between both schools in "American medicine as a whole in this period."

42 Birn, "Six Seconds per Eyelid," 288–89, 295–96; Fairchild, "The Rise and Fall," 338; Kraut, *Silent Travelers*, 3.

43 Fairchild, "The Rise and Fall," 338; Birn, "Six Seconds per Eyelid," 288–89, 295–96; Kraut, *Silent Travelers*, 3.

44 Daniels, *Asian America*, 109. Between 1892 and 1910, only 5,600 of the 80,000 Japanese rejected at US ports and border points were labelled "LPC." A further 2,500 were barred for failing medical inspection. Birn, "Six Seconds per Eyelid," 296, 300.

45 Daniels, *Asian America*, 109. For South Asian rejections in 1907, see NARA, "Memorandum regarding Hindu migration to the United States," received January 23, 1914, 1, RG 85 E9 52903 110 C. For 1908 statistics indicating that 1,710 South Asians were admitted, 438 excluded, and 124 departed in 1908, see "Table Showing Table Showing Arrivals, Deportations, and Departures of Hindus," in *Hindu Immigration Hearings*, House of Representatives, 63rd Cong., 2nd Sess. pt. 1, 68 (Washington: US GPO, 1914). These numbers do not include all border entries from Canada. "Rejection for disease" statistics found in United States Senate, *Reports of the Immigration Commission*, vol. 3, 326, Table 2. See Table 4 for reasons for South Asian rejections from the US Pacific coast, 1900–13.

46 Immigration Service, "Table Showing Arrivals, Deportations, and Departures of Hindus," *Hindu Immigration Hearings*, House of Representatives, 63rd Cong., 2nd Sess, pt. 1, 68 (Washington: US GPO, 1914). In 1908, 1,710 South Asians were admitted, 438 excluded, and 124 departed. NARA, J.H. Clark to F.P. Sargent, May 5, 1908, 1, and

F.H. Larned to Labor Secretary, September 25, 1908, 1, both in NARA, RG 85 E9 51388 005, pt. 2. Larned's letter contains Sargent's report.

47 NARA, John H. Clark to F.H. Larned, December 14, 1908, 1–2, RG 85 E9 51388 005, pt. 1; NARA, F.H. Larned, "Memorandums for the Assistant Secretary of Labor regarding 'Bhagwan' (Memorandum 1) and 'Gulsi Ram' (Memorandum 2)," March 6, 1909, both in RG 85 E9 52903 110.

48 NARA, A.S. Hollis, American Consul, Laurence Marquez, SE Africa, September 11, 1907, 1, RG 59, Numerical and Minor Files of the State Department, 1906 to 1910, M862, reel 612.

49 *San Francisco Call,* June 15, 1910; "Extract from Report of the Commissioner at Seattle," in *Annual Report of the Commissioner of Immigration, For Year Ending 30 June 1910* (Washington: US GPO, 1910), 148–49; Shah, *Stranger Intimacy,* 208. In fact, a total of twelve South Asians had been admitted at Seattle in the fiscal year ending March 1, 1910. See NARA, Daniel J. Keefe, Commissioner-General of Immigration, to Commissioner of Immigration, Seattle, March 12, 1910, 1, RG 85 E9 51391 21A.

50 See, for example, LAC Saskatchewan Executive Committee, Trades and Labour Congress of Canada, to Secretary of State for the Colonies, London, November 19, 1906, 1, RG 76, vol. 384, file 536999, pt. 1; Shah, *Stranger Intimacy,* 155–56, 206. Suspicions of "immorality" were largely unsupported by evidence. By 1910, one of the only press accounts to imply immoral behaviour was reported in January, when it emerged that a fifteen-year-old boy in Uplands, California, had been "captured" and "mistreated by several Hindus." Although this description implied pedophilic behaviour, and the incident had compelled local townspeople to drive out eight South Asian labourers, other reports indicated that the men had simply robbed and detained the boy, who was "not physically harmed by his captors." See *Medford Mail Tribune,* January 29, 1910; and *Los Angeles Times,* January 18, 1910.

51 Ettinger, "'We Sometimes Wonder,'" 162, 164, 170.

52 English summary of Imanat Ali Khan Interview by Hari Sharma, July 19, 1984, 1–2, Indo-Canadian Oral History Collection, http://digital.lib.sfu.ca/icohc-collection.

53 Chang, *Pacific Connections,* 89, 150. Chang describes the reaction to these arrivals as "anti-Asian racism defined [by] working-class politics and culture in the Pacific Northwest." Chang located the phrase "Republic and Dominion" in *Vancouver World,* August 26, 1907.

54 NARA, John Sargent to Commission General of Immigration, September 19, 1907, 1, in RG 85 E9 51630 44F; Chang, *Pacific Connections,* 151.

55 NARA, Frank P. Sargent, *Digest of, and Comment Upon, Report of Immigrant Inspector Marcus Braun,* September 1907, 1, 5, 6, 14, 21–24, 62, RG 85 E9 51630 44F. Braun specifically referred to racial feeling in California.

56 Chang, *Pacific Connections,* 151–52.

57 Dodd, "The Hindu in the Northwest," 1157–60.

58 *Reports of the Immigration Commission,* vol. 3, 325–326, Table 2; See NARA San Francisco Branch (SF), J.M. Crawford, Acting Commissioner, San Francisco, to Dr. W.C. Hobdy, March 4, 11, and 24 and 8 April, 1908, all in Public Health and Marine Hospital Services Records, vol. 1, box 27, "Letters Received from the Commissioner of Immigration (San Francisco) By the Medical Officer in Charge"; NARA, F.H. Larned, Memorandum for the Assistant Secretary of Labor, April 26, 1909, 1, RG 85 E9 52903 110.

59 Jensen, *Passage from India,* 99; Robertson, *The Passport in America,* 190.

60 In 1909, 331 were rejected; see NARA, "Memorandum Regarding Hindu Migration to the United States," January 23, 1914, 1, RG 85 E9 52903 110 C; Jensen, *Passage from India,* 96, 103, 113, also 95, 102–3.

61 Roger Daniels explains that "all of the available evidence indicates that the California politicians represented the prejudices of their constituents," particularly in their efforts to marginalize the state's growing Japanese community, which by 1910 had a population of close to 41,000, whereas there were about 38,000 Chinese. Daniels, *Asian America,* 137–38. The population estimates are from the 1910 US Census, tabulated at www.ancestry.ca, which lists 41,358 Japanese and 37,453 Chinese living in California in 1910. The Census lists 2,574 California residents born in India, but in fact twice that number lived in that US state.

62 Yoell, "The Hindoo Question in California," 12. Like Yoell, popular writer F.G. Moorhead observed that South Asians lived in housing that would have horrified whites, "even [those] from southern Europe." See Moorhead, "The Foreign Invasion of the Northwest, 9994."

63 Jensen, *Passage from India,* 16, 33; *Bellingham Herald,* October 11, 1907; *San Francisco Call,* November 15, 1907. See also *San Jose Evening News,* November 16, 1907; *San Francisco Chronicle,* December 5, 1907; Yoell, "Report of the Executive Board," in *Proceedings of the AEL, January 1910,* 5–7, 9–11.

64 F. Kenchu Ram, Letter to the Editor of the *Morning Oregonian* (Portland), December 19, 1908; Burnett, "Misunderstanding of Eastern and Western States, 257." In Stockton, California, some South Asians overcame what the *San Francisco Chronicle* called "a great prejudice against their nationality" by abandoning their turbans and impersonating "Negroes or Mexicans." *San Francisco Chronicle,* November 20, 1908.

65 Yoell, "Report of the Executive Board," in *Proceedings of the AEL, January 1910,* 5–7; *San Francisco Call,* January 23, 1910; Frank P. Sargent, *Annual Report of the Commissioner of Immigration (for 1902),* 42; Lee and Yung, *Angel Island,* 4.

66 David Hernández, "Undue Process," 74–75; Markel and Stern, "Which Face?," 1320, 1322. Markel and Stern add that class issues were "compounded by contemporary racial prejudices" in the examination of Asians travelling by first class. While this group circumvented Angel Island and instead received on-ship inspection, PHS workers generally neglected to perform the standard sterilization of equipment and handwashing used while inspecting white arrivals.

67 Lee and Yung, *Angel Island,* 150–51.

68 NARA, H.H. North to Commissioner General, July 30, 1910, 1, RG 85 E9 52961 10; *San Francisco Bulletin,* August 10, 1910; *San Francisco Chronicle,* February 1, 2, and 16 and August 30, 1910; "The Hindu Invasion," *Collier's Weekly,* March 26, 1910, 15; See "BSI SF, 4 February 1910, Re: Bant Singh," 1, "Findings of BSI, 2 February 1910," 1, "Findings of BSI, 3 February 1910," 1, and "Findings of BSI, 2 February 1910 re: Dulla Singh," 1, all in NARA, RG 85 E9 51308 24C, exhibit 12A. One of the nine men was debarred for scabies, while eleven more of the men were later rejected for having trachoma; see *San Francisco Call,* February 16, 1910.

69 Benjamin S. Cable, Memorandum for Daniel J. Keefe, April 25, 1910, 1, and Daniel J. Keefe to H.H. North, April 27, 1910, 1–6, both in NARA, RG 85 E9 52903 110.

70 Shah, *Stranger Intimacy,* 199–200.

71 Fairchild, *Science at the Borders,* 165–68. Fairchild cites Surgeon General Walter Wyman in "Minutes of Medical Conference to Discuss the Medical Examination of Immigrants, 8 February 1907," NARA, RG 85 51490/19. See also Markel and Stern, "What Face?," 1319.

72 Kraut, *Silent Travelers,* 65–66.

73 The AEL meeting was described in *San Francisco Call,* April 22, 1910.

74 NARA, Julius Kahn to Daniel J. Keefe, May 3, 1910, 1, RG 85 E9 52903 110. However, the climate argument, which was frequently used by Canadian opponents of South Asian labour, never gained much popularity in relatively warm and sunny California; when the fourth South Asian woman arrived in the state shortly after Kahn penned his letter, the *Chronicle* observed with alarm that the Indian community appeared to be putting down roots. *Evening Standard* (Ogden, Utah), August 27, 1910; *San Francisco Chronicle*, May 5 and 6, 1910.

75 NARA, Leon Ray Livingston, Hotel Colonia, Biggs, California, to Minister of the Interior, August 20, 1910, 1, RG 85 E9 52903 110; See also Livingston, *From Coast to Coast; San Francisco Call*, May 15 and August 14, 1910.

76 *San Francisco Chronicle*, June 9, 1910; "Health Officer W.J. McNutt, Report of the Board of Health on the Bacteriological Laboratory," *Annual Report of the Department of Public Health, San Francisco, 1910* (San Francisco: 1911), 276.

77 See Yoell's December 28, 1909, letter and the Senatorial replies in Yoell, "Report of the Executive Board," in *Proceedings of the AEL, Jan. 1910*, 5–7. See also See Yoell's memorandum at 9–11.

78 Fairchild, *Science at the Borders*, 133–34; Markel and Stern "Which Face?," 1320–21. Diplomats from China and Japan also avoided Angel Island.

79 Fairchild, *Science at the Borders*, 133–34.

80 Fairchild, *Science at the Borders*, 85; Shah, *Contagious Divides*, 195, 201; Daniels, "No Lamps Were Lit for Them," 5. Daniels questions "whether the intolerable conditions would have been allowed to go on for so long if the facility had held mostly Europeans."

81 *San Francisco Call*, June 18, 1910; Report of Dr. M.W. Glover, Inspection of Aliens at San Francisco, for Fiscal Year ending 30 June, 1910, 2, in NARA, RG 90, central file 1897 to 1923, box 785, file 16090; Lee and Yung, *Angel Island*, 152; *San Francisco Chronicle*, June 22, 1910.

82 *Medford Mail Tribune*, June 28, 1910; *San Francisco Call*, August 6 and 10, 1910.

83 Scheffauer, "The Tide of Turbans," 616. He added that between whites and "this dark, mystic race lies a pit almost as profound as that [which the white man] has dug between himself and the negro." See "Little Girl Tells Mayor How to Banish Hindus," *Los Angeles Herald*, October 3, 1907; *Los Angeles Herald*, September 26, 1907; *Bellingham Herald*, September 30, 1907; *San Francisco Chronicle*, August 27, 1910.

84 Snow, "The Civilization of White Men," 275.

85 *The White Man* (Organ of the Movement for Asiatic Exclusion, San Francisco), (Special Edition: The Hindu), August 1910, 2–3. Between the 1907 Bellingham Riot and his publication of "The White Man" in 1910, Fowler spent time in a psychiatric facility undergoing treatment for stress from his involvement in anti-Asian agitation; see *Morning Oregonian* (Portland), April 10, 1909.

86 NARA, (Personal) W.R. Wheeler to Charles P. Neill, August 11, 1910, 1–2, RG 85 E9 52903 110. Emphasis is Wheeler's.

87 William H. Michael, American Consul-General, Calcutta, to Assistant Secretary of State, August 11, 1910, 1–5, which contains a copy of Michael's August 10 telegram to the department, and see Benjamin S. Cable to Secretary of State, August 15, 1910, 1; all in NARA, RG 85 E9 52903 110; *San Francisco Chronicle*, August 12 and 13, 1910.

88 *Evening Bulletin Honolulu*, August 20, 1910; *San Francisco Chronicle*, August 23 and September 10, 1910; *The Englishman (Calcutta)*, August 28, 1910; *San Francisco Call*, September 5, 1910.

89 *San Francisco Call*, September 11, 1910; *San Francisco Chronicle*, September 11, 1910.

Chapter 4: Amoebic and Social Parasites, 1910–13

Epigraph notes: Vallejo Trades and Labor Council to A. Caminetti, 13 September 1913, RG 85 E9 52903 110 A, NARA; E.H. Lawson, MD, Highland, Alberta, Letter to the *Victoria Daily Colonist,* 25 September 1913.

1 NARA, M.W. Glover, (Passed Assistant Surgeon, Medical Division, San Francisco,) to Surgeon General, October 1, 1910, 1, RG 90, central file 1897–1923, box 785, file 16090; *San Francisco Chronicle,* September 23 and 29, 1910.

2 Shah, *Contagious Divides,* 191.

3 Shah, *Stranger Intimacy,* 200–2; *Contagious Divides,* 180.

4 *Evening Standard Ogden* (Utah), September 20, 1910; *San Francisco Bulletin,* September 29 and 30, 1910.

5 M.W. Glover to Surgeon General, October 1, 1910, 1, and Surgeon General to M.W. Glover, October 19, 1910, 1, both in NARA, RG 90, central file 1897 to 1923, box 785, file 16090.

6 Shah, *Contagious Divides,* 191–192.

7 Fairchild, *Science at the Borders,* 14, 15–16, 289. Foucault, *Discipline and Punish,* 25–26, 138. See McCarthy, "The Critique of Impure Reason." See also Allen, "The Entanglement of Power and Validity." In three similarly invasive studies beginning in 1912, leading eugenics advocate H.H. Goddard employed experimental intelligence techniques at Ellis Island. Goddard's and Glover's tests were different, yet both demonstrated and reinforced the utter subjectivity of immigrant detainees to medical examiners. See Kraut, *Silent Travelers,* 73–74.

8 Shah, *Contagious Divides,* 191–92; Tomes, "American Attitudes," 39; Nash, *Inescapable Ecologies,* 123.

9 Fairchild, "The Rise and Fall," 342–45.

10 Shah, *Contagious Divides,* 191–92.

11 Ettling, *The Germ of Laziness,* 2–5.

12 *Virginia Gazette* (Williamsburg), November 11, 1909; NARA, Glover to Commissioner of Immigration, San Francisco, October 14, 1910, 1–3, RG 90, central file 1897 to 1923, box 785, file 16090. In a follow-up letter of the same day, Glover clarified that he had only tested seventy-five passengers for hookworm.

13 Shah, *Contagious Divides,* 190–91; NARA, "Report of M.W. Glover, Medical Inspection of Immigrants, San Francisco, for Year ending 30 June 1911," 1, RG 90, central file 1897 to 1923, box 785, file 16090.

14 Shah, *Stranger Intimacy,* 202; NARA, "Transcript Notes and Translations Made Incident to the Visit to Angel Island Immigration Station on June 6, 1911, of Committee Representing the Down Town Association," 4–9, RG 85 E9 52961 file 240 Tour of Angel Island 1911; NARA, Daniel J. Keefe, Commissioner General, [Approved by Benjamin S. Cable, Assistant Secretary of Labor,] to Commissioner of Immigration, Angel Island, August 23, 1912, 1, RG 90, central file 1897 to 1923, box 785, file 16090.

15 Lee and Yung, *Angel Island,* 152; See hospital statistics in NARA, H. Edsell to Washington, December 10, 1910, 1, RG 85 E9 52903 110 A; *San Francisco Chronicle,* October 11 and 28, 1910, *Deseret Evening News* (Ohio), October 28, 1910; NARA, Charles Earl, Acting Secretary, to Secretary of State, October 20, 1910, 1, RG 85 E9 52903 110.

16 Jensen, *Passage from India,* 158–59; Report from El Paso (15 October) is included in NARA, Charles Earl, Acting Secretary, to Secretary of State, October 20, 1910, RG 85 E9 52903 110; *Tombstone Epitaph* (Arizona), October 9, 1910; NARA, J.W. Tappan, El

Paso, Texas, to Surgeon General, April 14, 1911, 1, RG 85 E9 51931 14B, Vancouver; See Kraut, *Silent Travelers*, 65.

17 *San Francisco Chronicle*, September 23 and 29, 1910.

18 Shah, *Stranger Intimacy*, 200. The quotation is Shah's.

19 *Proceedings of the Asiatic Exclusion League October 1910*, 62–63; *Los Angeles Times*, November 25, 1910.

20 *San Francisco Chronicle*, October 14, 1910.

21 *San Francisco Chronicle*, December 8, 1910; *Washington Post*, September 30, 1910; NARA, H. Edsell to Washington, DC, December 10, 1910, 1, RG 85 E9 52903 110 A. According to "East Indians Admitted Year ending 31 Dec 1910," 106, the numbers of South Asians admitted in 1910 were as follows: January (95), February (377), March (47), April (169), May (231) June (183), July (65), August (189), September (45), October (1), November (1), December (2), total: 1405.

22 Jensen, *Passage from India*, 116; NARA, H.H. North to Daniel J. Keefe, September 14, 1910, 1, RG 85 E9 52903 110; Hester, *Deportation*, 287; *San Francisco Examiner*, September 22, 1910; NARA, Samuel Bond, SF, to Charles Nagel, September 27, 1910, 1, and A.E. Yoell to Daniel J. Keefe, September 28, 1910, 1, both in RG 85 E9 52903 110.

23 Jensen, *Passage from India*, 142–49; *Evening Bulletin* (Honolulu), December 5, 1910.

24 English summaries of Hari Sharma's interviews with Imanat Ali Khan, July 19, 1984, 1, and Kehar Singh Kailey, December 5, 1984, 1, Indo-Canadian Oral History Collection, http://digital.lib.sfu.ca/icohc-collection; Hester, *Deportation*, 287; Shah, *Stranger Intimacy*, 203; NARA, Ellis DeBruler to Commissioner General of Immigration, March 27 and November 22, 1912, 1, RG 85 53173 40.

25 Acting Secretary of Labor to the Secretary of War, July 13, 1912, 1, Robert Shaw Oliver, Assistant Secretary of War, to Secretary of Commerce and Labor, July 17, 1912, 1, and Ellis DeBruler to Daniel J. Keefe, November 22, 1912, 1, all in NARA, RG 85 53173 40. The SS *Minnesota* brought forty-seven South Asians from Manila on August 30, 1912, and forty-nine on November 29, 1912; Ellis DeBruler to Daniel J. Keefe, December 4, 1912, 1, and March 21, 1913, 1, both in ibid.; "Report of Commissioner of Immigration, Seattle, in Charge District 16, Comprising Washington State," in US Government, *Annual Report of the Commissioner of Immigration, For Year Ending June 30, 1913* (Washington: US GPO, 1913), 224.

26 Commissioner General of Immigration, Memorandum for W.B. Wilson, April 7, 1913, 1–2, and Wilson to Lindley M. Garrison, April 7, 1913, 1–2, both in NARA, RG 85 53173 40; Jensen, *Passage from India*, 148–49; Shah, *Stranger Intimacy*, 203–5.

27 NARA, W.B. Wilson to Lindley M. Garrison, May 22, 1913, RG 85 53173 40; see also Glover, "Hookworm among Oriental Immigrants." The affidavit of Ottam Singh, who arrived at Angel Island in September 1913, indicates that Dr. W.N. Lemmon of the Pacific Mail Service examined him for both hookworm and trachoma in July 1913, while the Pacific Mail medical clearance form in the case file of Natha Singh, who sailed from Manila to San Francisco on September 13, 1913, certifies that he was microscopically tested for hookworm also. See NARA SF, "Affidavit of Ottam Singh," Angel Island, October 25, 1913, 1, RG 85 AICF file 12924/4–4 (Case File of Ottam Singh). See also NARA SF, "Pacific Mail Form 4 for Natha Singh," September 11, 1913, 1, RG 85 AICF, file 12973/8–3 (Case File of Natha Singh).

28 (Telegram) Bissell, SF, to Immigration DC, May 24, 1913, 1, Dept. Labor Memo, May 16, 1913, 1, and Warrant Arrest of Alien, Dept. of Labor, to Samuel Backus, Angel Island, May 27, 1913, 1, all in NARA, RG 85 53173 40. Wilson allowed the four healthy men to leave custody under bond during their appeal.

29 *New York Times,* June 20, 1913; Jensen, *Passage from India,* 147–8.

30 "Editorial: Leprosy and Safeguards," *Washington Post,* June 21, 1913; Moran, *Colonizing Leprosy,* 18–19; Shah, *Contagious Divides,* 97–101.

31 See US Government, *Reports of the Immigration Commission,* pt. 25, 326 (Table 2), which shows rejection reasons; NARA, H.H. Stevenson, City Passenger Agent, Milwaukee and Puget Sound Railway Co., New Westminster BC, to Commissioner of Emigration, Washington, DC, July 4, 1913, 1, RG 85 E9 53173 40A; "Editorial: There's No Law to Bar a 100 Million," *Seattle Star,* June 26, 1913. Capitalization in original.

32 Public Records Office, United Kingdom, (Telegram) S. Singh, President, Sikh Temple, Victoria, to British Embassy, July 2, 1913, 1, FO 115 1731; (Telegram) Bhag Singh to Secretary of Commerce and Labor, July 3, 1913, 1, and Anthony Caminetti to San Francisco Immigration Branch, July 3, 1913, 1, both in NARA, RG 85 E9 53173 40A. See also *San Francisco Chronicle,* August 14, 1913. See also Vallejo Trades and Labor Council to Anthony Caminetti, September 13, 1913, 1, and Geo. A. Dean, Recording Secretary, Central Labor Council of San Joaquin Valley to Immigration Service, September 10, 1913, 1, both in NARA, RG 85 E9 52903 110 A.

33 Anthony Caminetti, "US Immigration Service Circular, No. 30, Distribution of Hookworm Inspection, November 1 1913," 1, reprinted in House Committee on Immigration and Naturalization, *Hearings Relative to the Restriction of Immigration of Hindu Laborers (Part 1),* 63 Cong., 2 Sess. (1914), 63. The circular quoted from the Rockefeller Sanitary Commission's *Hookworm Infection in Foreign Countries* (Washington: 1911), 59.

34 See NARA, "List of Certificates for Hookworm at the Port of San Francisco, June 30 to Oct 30 1913," RG 85 54261 184, which indicates that only nine in twenty-seven South Asians inspected in September and October had the disease. See also *Democratic Banner* (Ohio), November 21, 1913; Anthony Caminetti, "Circular No. 30, Distribution of Hookworm Inspection, 1 November 1913," 1, reprinted in House Committee on Immigration and Naturalization, *Hearings Relative to the Restriction of Immigration of Hindu Laborers (Part 1),* 63 Cong., 2 Sess. (1914), 63; Samuel Backus to Anthony Caminetti, "Regarding Dhian Singh," November 28, 1913, 1, and Samuel Backus to Anthony Caminetti, regarding Sucha Singh, November 28, 1914, 1, both in NARA, RG 85 E9 53667 through 69.

35 NARA, F.H. Larned to Acting Secretary of Immigration, December 3, 1913, Enclosing "Memorandum of General Facts and Circumstances Requiring Consideration," 1–5, RG 85 E9 53627 58 A and B; NARA SF, Report of W.H. Chadney to Commissioner of Immigration, Angel Island, "Re Investigation of Hindus," October 8, 1913, 1–3, RG 85, AICF file 12924/4–3 (Case File of Nika Singh). For Chadney acting as Chair in BSI hearings, see, for example, NARA SF, "BSI Ruling in the Case of Arjan Singh, 15 October 1913," RG 85, AICF file 12973–8-5 (Case File of Arjan Singh).

36 Luibheid, *Entry Denied,* 7–8.

37 NARA, "Memorandum of General Facts and Circumstances Requiring Consideration," 6, RG 85 E9 53627 58 A and B.

38 Argen Singh's case mentioned in "Memorandum of General Facts," 6, ibid.; NARA SF, "Amended Petition for a Writ of Habeas Corpus, District Court of United States Northern District of California," n.d., 2–3, RG 85, AICF file 12973–014–03, box 736 (Case File of Bram Singh), and Immigration Service, "Brief for Alien Battan Singh, Arrived at Angel Island on the SS *Persia* 12 October 1913," 1, both in RG 85, AICF file 12973–8-6.

39 NARA SF, "Hearing in the Case of Ottam Singh, Angel Island, 24 September 1913," 1, 5–6, RG 85, AICF file 12924/4–4 (Case File of Ottam Singh).

40 Ibid; Webber, *Communicable Disease Epidemiology and Control,* 112.

41 "Copy of Letter from F.H. Larned to Commission of Immigration, Angel Island," November 18, 1913, 1, and Samuel Backus to Inspector in Charge, Angel Island, "Regarding Ottam Singh," October 14, 1913, 1, both in NARA SF, RG 85, AICF file 12924/4–4 (Case File of Ottam Singh). According to the latter document, Ottam Singh was released from custody on October 14, earlier than the other hookworm sufferers (Sarwan and Bir Singh), after paying a $500 bond. See "Affidavit of Ottam Singh," October 15, 1913, 1, Commissioner of Immigration to Medical Examiner of Aliens, Angel Island, February 3, 1914, 1, and W.C. Billings, "Medical Certificate of Release," February 10, 1914, all in ibid. See also NARA SF, F.H. Larned, "Memorandum General Facts and Circumstances Requiring Consideration," 4, RG 85 E9 53627 58 A and B; and NARA SF, "Memorandum re: Joala Singh," September 22, 1913, 1, in RG 85, AICF file 12924/4–11 (Case File of Joala Singh). Ottam Singh's case file indicates that he was eventually granted permission to undergo PHS treatment for the disease in February 1914. See Shah, *Stranger Intimacy*, 202; LAC, P.H. Bryce to G.L. Milne, December 28, 1911, 1, RG 76, vol. 584, file 820636.

42 See Sproule-Jones, "Crusading for the Forgotten."

43 In 1910, interior minister Frank Oliver created what would become the most important Immigration Branch file pertaining to the early-twentieth-century public health aspects of South Asian immigration in Canada. Titled "Prevalence of Hook Worm Among Hindus Applying for Admission to the US and Among the Negroes (Blacks) of the US," the file's focus shifted soon afterwards to the Canadian situation. The dossier is a gold mine on the public health aspects of South Asian immigration after 1911. See LAC, RG 76, vol. 584, file 820636; *Victoria Times*, October 17, 1910; LAC, Frank Oliver to W.D. Scott, October 18, 1910, 1, RG 76, vol. 584, file 820636.

44 LAC, G.L. Milne to P.H. Bryce, November 14, 1911, and P.H. Bryce to GL Milne, December 28, 1911, 1–2, RG 76, vol. 584, file 820636. See Cuban conference summary in G. T. Swarts, "The Havana Meeting," 895–96.

45 LAC, W.C. Hopkinson to W.W. Cory, April 15, 1912, 1, and W.W. Cory to W.D. Scott, April 16, 1912, 1, RG 76, vol. 384, file 536999, pt. 5. See Jensen and Johnston for a detailed discussion of Hopkinson's key role in South Asian immigration inspection and community surveillance before his 1914 murder.

46 LAC, W.D. Scott telegrams to G.L. Milne and Malcolm J. Reid, April 17, 1912, 1, RG 76, vol. 384, file 536999, pt. 5; LAC, G.L. Milne to W.D. Scott, April 20, 1912, both 1, RG 76, vol. 584, file 820636; Malcolm J. Reid to W.D. Scott, April 18, 1912, 1, and Malcolm J. Reid to W.D. Scott, April 27, 1912, 1, all in RG 76, vol. 384, file 536999, pt. 5.

47 LAC, P.H. Bryce Memorandum to W.D. Scott, May 14, 1912, 1, J.H. Chapman to P.H. Bryce, May 23, 1912, 1, P.H. Bryce to J.H. Chapman, May 28, 1912, 1, Bryce Memorandum to W.D. Scott, May 28, 1912, 1; W.D. Scott to J.H. Chapman, May 30, 1912, 1, all in RG 76, vol. 584, file 820636.

48 LAC, P.H. Bryce to W.D. Scott, May 14, 1912, 1, P.H. Bryce to J.H. Chapman, May 28, 1912, 1, P.H. Bryce to W.D. Scott, May 28, 1912, 1, W.D. Scott to J.H. Chapman, May 30, 1912, 1, all in RG 76, vol. 584, file 820636. Hopkinson was hired as Immigrant Inspector in 1909 with an annual salary of $1,200. See LAC, W.W. Cory to W.D. Scott, February 26, 1912, 1, RG 76, vol. 561, file 808722, pt. 1; and Johnston, "The Surveillance," 16.

49 Nayan Shah, *Stranger Intimacy*, 200–2; and *Contagious Divides*, 180, 196; Fairchild, *Science at the Borders*, 39, 181–82.

50 Stern, *Eugenic Nation*, 46–47; Beiser, "The Health of Immigrants and Refugees," S30–31.

51 Census data in LAC, F.C. Blair to Sir Joseph Pope, July 25, 1922, 1, RG 25 G1, vol. 1300, file 1011 FPi.

52 W.D. Scott Memorandum, September 30, 1913, 1–2, and (Confidential) W.C. Hopkinson to W.W. Cory, August 1, 1913, 1, both in LAC, RG 76, vol. 385, file 536999, pt. 6; *Ottawa Free Press*, October 8, 1913. The South Asians were admitted on July 30; see arrivals for that vessel on www.ancestry.ca.

53 Johnston, *The Voyage of the Komagata Maru*, 48.

54 Johnston, Ibid., 45–48; LAC, G.L. Milne to W.D. Scott, November 26, 1913, 1, RG 76, vol. 385, file 536999, pt. 8; *Vancouver Province*, October 23, 1913; *Vancouver News-Advertiser*, October 24, 1913; W.C. Hopkinson, October 25, 1913, 6, and G.L. Milne to W.D. Scott, 1, October 27, 1913, both in LAC, RG 76, vol. 385, file 536999, pt. 6.

55 LAC, W.D. Scott to W.W. Cory, October 28, 1913, 1, in RG 76, vol. 385, file 536999, pt. 6. Ministerial permission granted in W.D. Scott to G.L. Milne, November 8, 1913, 1, in ibid; LAC, W.P. Walker, Victoria, to G.L. Milne, November 18, 1913, 1, RG 76, vol. 584, file 820636. This was almost certainly the thirty-five-year-old "Jowalla Singh" described in the department's passenger manifest – see "Jowalla Singh," ex. SS *Panama Maru*, arrived October 17, 1913, in Canadian Passenger Index, www.ancestry.ca. See W.H. Schultz, "Remedies for Animal Parasites." See also *New York Times*, October 7, 1911. Schultz, a US government pharmacologist, was credited in 1911 with being the first to widely publicize the effectiveness of thymol, a natural derivative of the herb thyme, in treating hookworm.

56 *Victoria Colonist*, November 28, 1913. See PC 2642, December 8, 1913.

57 LAC, G.L. Milne to W.D. Scott, December 12, 1913, 1–2, RG 76, vol. 584, file 820636.

58 LAC, Anthony Caminetti, "Circular No. 30, Distribution of Hookworm Inspection, 1 November 1913," forwarded by G.L. Milne to W.D. Scott, December 26, 1913, RG 76, vol. 584, file 820636. Scott had already requested copies of the circular in W.D. Scott to J.H. Clark, December 19, 1913, 1, ibid; see also LAC, W.D. Scott to G.L. Milne, January 7, 1914, 1, and W.D. Scott to Malcolm R. Reid, January 7, 1914, 1, both in ibid.

59 *Toronto Mail and Empire, Toronto News*, and *Gazette* (Montreal), November 11, 1913, and *Gazette* (Montreal), December 4, 1913. By December, Stevens had unaccountably switched his focus to lung fluke.

60 E.H. Lawson, MD, Highland, Alberta, Letter to *Victoria Daily Colonist*, September 25, 1913. Bernard Harris shows that other physicians in this period also attempted to disprove Social Darwinist conceptions that certain immigrant groups, particularly Jews, were especially prone to disease. See Harris, "Pro-Alienism," 195–96.

61 LAC, David Ross to Robert Borden, July 28, 1914, 1–3, MG 26 H (Borden Papers) 1 (a), vol. 40.

62 P.H. Bryce to W.D. Scott, January 26, 1914, 1, W.D. Scott Memorandum for W.W. Cory, February 2, 1914, 1, and W.D. Scott Memorandum for W.W. Cory, February 19, 1914, 1, all in LAC, RG 76, vol. 584, file 820636. Hopkinson's report and Cory's January 28 memorandum are described in LAC, W.D. Scott Memorandum to W.W. Cory, February 10, 1914, in ibid. For a detailed discussion of this correspondence and the government's hookworm testing operations, see author, "Komagata Maru Revisited."

63 W.D. Scott to W.W. Cory, February 10, 1914, 1–2, W.D. Scott to G.L. Milne, February 10, 1914, and W.D. Scott to British Consulate General, Yokohama, February 26, 1914, all in LAC, RG 76, vol. 385, file 536999, pt. 8; W.D. Scott to Malcolm J. Reid, March 2, 1914, and H.E. Young, Provincial Secretary and Acting Secretary of BC Board of Health, to W.J. Roche, February 21, 1914, both in LAC, RG 76, vol. 584, file 820636; LAC, W.D. Scott to C.J. Davidson, Act. British Consulate General, Yokohama, February 26, 1914, RG 76, vol. 385, file 536999, pt. 8.

64 LAC, P.H. Bryce Memo to W.J. Roche, March 25, 1914, 1–4, RG 76, vol. 584, file 820636.

65 John Ettling, *The Germ of Laziness*, 2–5.
66 LAC, P.H. Bryce Memo to W.J. Roche, March 25, 1914, 1–4, RG 76, vol. 584, file 820636.
67 See LAC, (RUSH) M.J. Reid to W.D. Scott, March 31, 1914, 1–2, and W.D. Scott to W.W. Cory, April 1, 1914, 1, in ibid. While vessels arrived with varying numbers of passengers aboard, 400 would be a mid-sized number. The above-mentioned salary example for immigration inspector W.C. Hopkinson indicates that he was hired in 1909 at an annual salary of $1,200, although this had climbed to $1,800 by early 1912. See LAC, W.W. Cory to W.D. Scott, February 26, 1912, 1, RG 76, vol. 561, file 808722 pt. 1, and Hugh Johnston, "The Surveillance," 16.
68 LAC, (RUSH) M.J. Reid to W.D. Scott, March 31, 1914, 1–2, RG 76 Vol. 584 File 820636.
69 PC 1914–897 of March 31, 1914, renewed PC 1913–2642 of December 1913. See Kelley and Trebilcock, *The Making of the Mosaic*, 150; LAC, W.D. Scott to W.W. Cory, April 1, 1914, and W.D. Scott to M.J. Reid, 14 April 1914, both in RG 76 Vol. 584 File 820636. For the legislative history of PC 897–1914 (formerly 1913–2642), see Ryder, "Racism and the Constitution," 670.

Chapter 5: South Asians, Public Health, and Eugenic Theory
Epigraph notes: PABC, Testimony of James McVety of the BC Federation of Labour, March 10, 1913, 266–69, box 1, file 8, GR 0684; Denver S. Church, "Hindu Immigration Hearings," 63rd Congress, 2nd Session, February 19, 1914, pt. 2, 76 and 85.
1 Victoria Friends of the Hindus, "Summary of the Hindu Question"; English transcript of Phanga Singh Gill interview by Gurcharn Basran and B. Singh Bolaria, July 12, 1985, 5, Indo-Canadian Oral History Collection, http://digital.lib.sfu.ca/icohc-collection; Friends of Moral Reform to Grey, June 6, 1911, enclosing "Memoir Regarding Hindus in Canada," n.d., LAC, RG 76, vol. 384, file 536999, pt. 4.
2 LAC, (Confidential) G.L. Milne to W.D. Scott, July 8, 1911, 1, RG 76, vol. 384, file 536999, pt. 4. Milne was referring to the *Times of London* editorial, "The Problems of Hindu Immigration into Canada," July 8, 1911.
3 Ward, *White Canada Forever*, 81; Transcript of Norman King Interview by Gurcharn S. Basran and B. Singh Bolaria, January 1, 1985, Indo-Canadian Oral History Collection, http://digital.lib.sfu.ca/icohc-collection; PABC, (Sound Recording) "Ellen King Interview," August 6, 1965, Imbert Orchard/CBC fonds, TO815:0001.
4 Ward, *White Canada Forever*, 82.
5 W.D. Scott to W.W. Cory, October 11 1911, 1, and November 14, 1911, 1, both in LAC, RG 76, vol. 384, file 536999, pt. 4; Thorner and Frohn-Nielson, *A Country Nourished on Self-Doubt*, 73. Scott later reversed his ruling and allowed South Asians to use the certificates to re-enter Canada when transpacific travel resumed after the First World War.
6 "Individual Cases regarding East Indian Immigration to Canada," n.d., 6, and W.C. Hopkinson to W.W. Cory, August 4, 1911, 1, both in LAC, RG 76, vol. 384, file 536999, pt. 4; Magocsi, *Encyclopedia of Canada's Peoples*, 1152.
7 Abella and Troper, *None Is Too Many*, 280–85; LAC, W.D. Scott to H.E. Hume (for Interior Minister), December 21, 1912, 1, RG 76, vol. 384, file 536999, pt. 5.
8 Previous official Immigration Branch visits to BC were: W.C. Scott (twice in 1906), E. Blake Robertson (1906), Thomas R. McInnes (1906), and W.L. Mackenzie King (1908); *Ottawa Free Press*, January 8, 1912.
9 F.C. Blair, "Private Memorandum regarding Hindu Immigration, Particularly With Reference to the Present Agitation for the Admission of Wives of Hindus Now Resident in Canada," January 26, 1912, 1 and 3, in VCA, ADD MSS No. 69 (H.H. Stevens Papers), vol. 1 file 1, pp. 1–36d, location 509D7.

10   VCA, Robert Marrion to Frederick T. Underhill, Vancouver Medical Health Officer, January 9, 1912, 1–2, published in *Vancouver Health Report for 1912*, PDS 11; *Vancouver Province*, January 29, 1912.

11   F.C. Blair, "Private Memorandum regarding Hindu Immigration," 4–5, 6–7 and 9–10, *supra* note 9.

12   Buchignani, Indra, and Srivastava, *Continuous Journey*, 41.

13   *Vancouver Sun*, February 16, 1912; *Vancouver Province*, January 27, 1912.

14   *Victoria Daily Times*, January 9, 1912; *Vancouver Province*, January 26, 1912.

15   Stevens, "The Oriental Problem," 8–9. This document is briefly cited in Roy, *A White Man's Province*, 231.

16   *Toronto World*, February 17, 1912; LAC, H.H. Stevens, "Address to Women's Canadian Club, Toronto, Regarding Hindu Immigration," February 17, 1912, 7, 8, 15–16, MG 27 III B 9, vol. 165, File Immigration Oriental Hindu Question December 1911 to February 1911. Italics are Stevens's. In the provincial legislature in February 1912, Richard McBride similarly declared that South Asians could not assimilate and that in Canada's "complete change of environment" the men had proven to be poor workers. "Address of Premier Richard McBride to BC Legislative Assembly, Regarding Oriental Immigration," February 14, 1912.

17   Nayan Shah, *Stranger Intimacy*, 215.

18   LAC, H.H. Stevens to W.A. Holman, Attorney General, Sydney, Australia, February 21, 1912, 1–2, MG 27 III B 9, vol. 165, File Immigration Oriental Hindu Question December 1911 to February 1912.

19   Dua, "Racializing Imperial Canada," 71, 78, 81.

20   Dua, 71, 78 and 81; Goutor, *Guarding the Gates*, 72.

21   Avery, *Reluctant Host*, 53.

22   *Debates of the Canadian House of Commons 12th Parliament 1st Session*, vol. 2, February 27, 1912, 3930–32. See also *Debates of the Canadian House of Commons 14th Parliament 2nd Session*, vol. 1, February 21, 1923, 497, 507–10. See *Vancouver Province*, February 28, 1912.

23   See for example, Roy, *A White Man's Province*, 30. However, this book offers an authoritative, well-researched and well-argued discussion of the Chinese and Japanese situations in BC during this period.

24   John Beckwith quoted in *Toronto Daily Star*, November 15, 1912; "Fair Play" and "Kumar Singh" letters in *Victoria Daily Times*, September 6, 1912; "Hindus Are Touchy: Mayor of Victoria Being Sued for Remark He Made," *Ottawa Citizen*, September 13, 1912.

25   McLaren, *Our Own Master Race*, 27, 47. He emphasizes the importance of anti-Semitism and anti-radicalism in the spread of Canadian eugenic theory, and quotes Conn, "Immigration," 119, 129. See also Furedi, *The Silent War*, 71–72.

26   See PABC, file GR 0684 (BC Royal Commission on Labour, 1912–14). After a major coal strike in the province, Commission Chairman H.G. Parson and his associates spent much of 1913 travelling the province and compiling testimonials. Several scholars have mined this documentation, which offers invaluable insight into labour conditions in the immediate prewar period, but none have explored the nineteen testimonials addressing South Asians. *The Report of the Royal Commission on Labour* (Victoria: W. Cullin, 1914) was submitted to BC's legislature in early 1914. See Hinde, *When Coal Was King*, 4; Roy, *A White Man's Province*, 252.

27   Testimony of J.A. Gill, President of the Kamloops Board of Trade, January 22, 1913, 210, 219, box 1, file 3; testimony of Frederick S. Stevens, Manager of Okanagan Saw Mills Company, Enderby, April 28, 1913, 298, box 2, file 3; testimony of Charles D. Rodgers, Owner of Canyon City Lumber Company, Creston, n.d., 161, box 2, file 10; testimony of R.H. Alexander, Manager of Hastings Mill, Vancouver, October 23, 1913,

344, box 3, file 3; testimony of William Lyle Maczes, President of the Chilliwack Board of Trade, Chilliwack, March 4, 1913, 26, box 1, file 7; unknown mill owner, unknown location and date, 305–6, box 2, file 12. All of the foregoing are in PABC, GR 0684. Descriptive information for the latter interview has been lost or misfiled: the finding aid for GR 0684 states that "it should be noted that most of the files were received in a state of disarray."

28 See testimony of James McVety of the BC Federation of Labour, March 10, 1913, 266–69, box 1, file 8, PABC, GR 0684. See also McKay, *Reasoning Otherwise*, 366; McKay quotes McVety, "Suggests Violence" and adds that, despite his anti-Indian stance, McVety's later *BC Federationist* editorial during the 1914 *Komagata Maru* incident was somewhat sympathetic to the vessel's passengers.

29 Shah, *Stranger Intimacy*, 28.

30 Testimony of William Hutchinson, Accountant for Brayden and Johnson Mills, Salmon Arm, January 23, 1913, 257, box 1, file 3; testimony of C.F. Burkhart, representing the Journeyman Barbers Association, unknown location, January 20, 1913, 108, box 1, file 2, both in PABC GR 0684; also, Molina, *Fit to Be Citizens?*, 201. Molina explains that Santa Ana officials used this case to justify the destruction of that city's Chinatown.

31 Testimony of Mr. Staples, unknown first name, occupation and location unknown, October 24, 1913, box 3, file 4, 416–17; testimony of Kenneth Duncan, Mayor of Duncan, October 24, 1913, 488, box 3, file 4, both in PABC, GR 0684.

32 "Once a Household Name, E.H. Lukin Johnston Is All but Forgotten Today," *Cowichan Valley Citizen*, April 1, 2011; testimony of Lukin Johnston, Editor of the *Cowichan Leader*, Duncan, October 24, 1913, 487, box 3, file 4, PABC, GR 0684; E. Johnston, "The Case of the Oriental in B.C.," 315. Johnston achieved a modest level of provincial fame later in life, both for editing the *Vancouver Province* and for being lost at sea in 1933, shortly after privately interviewing Adolf Hitler.

33 Gosnell, "B.C. and British Int'l Relations," 11.

34 "The Hindu's Pastime," *New Westminster News*, 6 January 6, 1914; *Vancouver Sun*, December 15, 1913; VAC, H.H. Davies to H.H. Stevens, December 19, 1913, 1, ADD MSS No. 69, vol. 1, file 1, 1 to 136d, location 509D7.

35 G.D. Kumar, "The Hindu Grievance," editorial in *Vancouver Sun*, March 17, 1913. Kumar's editorial was published in the *Vancouver Province*, April 15, 1913. See also, (Personal) Malcolm J. Reid to H.H. Stevens, April 16, 1913, and (Personal) H.H. Stevens to Malcolm J. Reid, April 22, 1913, both in VAC, ADD MSS No. 69, vol. 1, file 1, 1 to 136d, location 509D7; and VCA, (Personal) Malcolm J. Reid to H.H. Stevens, April 30, 1913, ADD MSS No. 69, vol. 1, file 6, location 509-D-7 349–521.

36 Hugh Johnston, *The Voyage of the Komagata Maru*, 39. For this author's review of the book's third edition, see author, "Review of Hugh Johnston," 2015. LAC, W.C. Hopkinson to W.W. Cory, August 1, 1913, 1, RG 76, vol. 385, file 536999, pt. 6; LAC, W.D. Scott to Malcolm J. Reid, November 27, 1915, 1, RG 76, vol. 385, file 536999, pt. 9. The 1911 census recorded 2,342 South Asians in Canada (2,292 in BC). Data at www.ancestry.ca.

37 *Debates of the Senate of Canada, 1912–1913, 2nd Sess., 12th Parliament,* June 2, 1913, 930, 932–33.

38 H.H. Stevens remarks in *Vancouver Daily News Advertiser*, July 11, 1913; Chang, *Pacific Connections*, 98.

39 J.M.G. Davis comments in article "Canada Should Exclude Hindus," *Vancouver Province* [date unknown- April–May 1912?,] this clipping in LAC, MG 27 III B 9, vol. 171, file Hindu Immigration Incident, January 1, 1912–May 1914; W.J. Ottley remarks in *Vancouver World*, July 25, 1913, and *Vancouver Sun*, July 28, 1913.

40 King, *Orientalism and Religion*, 113–14. See, for example, Das, "Gender Studies."

41 Avery, *Reluctant Host*, 54; see, for example, *Vancouver Sun*, August 1 and 12, 1913; VCA, H.H. Stevens to William James Roche, August 8, 1913, 1, and William James Roche to H.H. Stevens, September 4, 1913, 1, ADD MSS No, 69, vol. 1, file 1, 1 to 136d, location 509D; PC 2218, 2448, August 25, 1913, 1. See also PC 2218, August 25, 1913, 1–2.

42 NARA, Malcolm J. Reid to Anthony Caminetti, December 17, 1913, 2, RG 85 E9 52903 110 C. Reid explained that Chinese were exempt from the order as their admission was governed by other legislation.

43 LAC, T.W. Holderness, India Office, Whitehall, to Under Secretary of State for the Colonial Office, December 9, 1913, RG 25, series a3a, vol. 1129, file 1913 66; Broad, *An Appeal for Fair Play*, 1. See Hugh Johnston's discussion of Broad in Johnston, *Jewels of the Qila*, 42. See also Laut, *Am I My Brother's Keeper?*

44 Leier in Laut, *Am I My Brother's Keeper?*, iii, v–vi. Quotations are Leier's.

45 Laut, *Am I My Brother's Keeper?*, 43, 44, 48, 52, 55–57, 62, 63. All italics are Laut's.

46 *Saturday Sunset (Vancouver)*, November 8, 1913; "The Hindu's Pastime" (Editorial), *New Westminster News*, January 6, 1914.

47 PC, 23, January 7, 1914, replaced PC 920, May 9, 1910. PC 24, January 7, 1914, replaced PC 926, May 9, 1910. In 1930, Prime Minister R.B. Bennett introduced an Order in Council barring "any immigrant of any Asiatic race," which included South Asians. See Kelley and Trebilcock, *The Making of the Mosaic*, 325; and PC 1930–2215.

48 Diary of W.L.M. King, January 14, 1914, 2420, 14, 8; R.L. Borden to Duke of Connaught, January 19, 1914, 1, and E. Blake Robertson, "Re: Wives and Children," January 5, 1914, 1, both in LAC, RG 25 G1, vol. 1138, file 1914 40 C. William Roche hand-wrote "I heartily concur with the above memo's views."

49 PC 1914–897, March 31, 1914, renewed PC 1913–2642, December 8, 1913, which was a temporary measure requiring renewal to stay in force. See Kelley and Trebilcock, *The Making of the Mosaic*, 150.

50 See Hugh Johnston, *The Voyage of the Komagata Maru;* Ward, *White Canada Forever*, 92–93; McKay, *Reasoning Otherwise*, 613–16; and Kazimi, *Undesirables*, 8.

51 H.B. Hetherington, Canadian Immigration Branch official stationed at Ellis Island, New York, appears to have reminded the branch that the method could be still be useful on the vessel's arrival. See LAC, W.D. Scott Memorandum to W.W. Cory, April 29, 1914, RG 76, vol. 601, file 879545, pt. 1. I would like to thank Reader 1 for alerting me to the location of this document.

52 Malcolm J. Reid's telegram re: 15 percent rejection for eye diseases quoted in W.D. Scott's 'Memorandum for Mr. Mitchell,' May 26, 1914, 1, in RG 76, vol. 601, file 879545, pt. 2, LAC; Malcolm J. Reid to W.D. Scott (Night Lettergram), May 25, 1914, 1; W.D. Scott to Malcolm J. Reid, May 26, 1914, 1; Munro's detailed examinations described in Malcolm J. Reid to W.D. Scott, May 31, 1914, 1–2, all in RG 76, vol. 601, file 879545, pt. 1, LAC.

53 Scott's statement that "the medical and civil examinations [were] in progress" as late as June 6 in LAC, W.D. Scott "Memorandum to Mr. Mitchell," June 6, 1914, 1–2, RG 76, vol. 601, file 879545. pt. 2; see Scott granting permission for tropical specialist in LAC, W.D. Scott to Malcolm J. Reid, May 26, 1914, 1, RG 76, vol. 601, file 879545. pt. 1, LAC; Reid's statement that ninety men had ultimately been rejected for medical reasons is in Malcolm J. Reid's May 28 telegram to W.D. Scott, 1.

54 LAC, Anonymous, Vancouver, to Robert Borden, June 2, 1914, 1, MG 26 H 1(a), vol. 40.

55 English transcript of Bishan Singh Aujla interview by Gurcharn S. Basran and B. Singh Bolaria, July 26, 1985, 8, Indo-Canadian Oral History Project, http://digital.lib.sfu.ca/icohc-collection.

56 LAC, J. Farmer to Robert Borden, Enclosing "Meeting Minutes of Council of North Vancouver, 16 July 1914," 1, MG 26 H 1(a), Vol. 40.

57 LAC, "Minutes of a Public Meeting, Dominion Hall, 23 June 1914," 1, MG 26 H 1(a), vol. 40; *Vancouver Sun*, June 24, 1914; Jensen, *Passage from India*, 133. Jensen cites NARA, John H. Clark to Anthony Caminetti, June 30, 1914, RG 85, file 52903. See also McKay, *Reasoning Otherwise*, 605; McKay cites *Vancouver Sun*, June 23, 1914. See also LAC, Dr. Malcolm T. MacEachearn, Vancouver Hospital, to H.H. Stevens, June 23, 1914, 1, MG 26 H 1(a), vol. 40.

58 LAC, C.H.N. Lester, Westmount, Quebec, to Robert Borden, June 15, 1914, 1, MG 26 H 1(a), vol. 40; *Vancouver Province*, July 8 and 22, 1914.

59 House of Commons, 12th Parliament, 3rd Session, vol. 5, May 26, 1914, 4214; May 27, 1914, 4295; May 30, 1914, 4533; June 1, 1914, 4562, 4565.

60 Said, *Orientalism*, 2–3.

61 *House of Commons*, 12th Parliament, 3rd Session, vol. 5, June 1, 1914, 4565; June 6, 1914, 4954–55; Johnston, *Voyage of the Komagata Maru*, 44. Seventy-seven of the eighty-eight men identified as having medical issues may have had trachoma, although this percentage is not clearly demonstrated in the archival record; *House of Commons*, 12th Parliament, 3rd Session, vol. 5, June 8, 1914, 5026; Johnston, *The Voyage of the Komagata Maru*, 36–37; *Vancouver News-Advertiser*, May 22, 1914; Nayan Shah, *Contagious Divides*, 61–63; Buchignani, Indra and Srivastava, *Continuous Journey*, 44; *Vancouver Sun*, June 1, 1914; Johnston in *The Voyage*, 80, points out that Singh suffered from asthma; PABC, "Death Certificate for Santa Singh," died Vancouver, June 5, 1914, 1, Registration, 1914–09–139730.

62 *Vancouver Sun*, June 1, 1914; *Vancouver Province*, May 23 and June 2, 1914.

63 For a complete list of the prescription medications and "medical comforts," see Dr. Raghunath Singh's 14 June, 1914, prescription request list for the SS *Komagata Maru*, 1–2, in LAC, RG 76, vol. 601, file 879545, pt. 2. The list includes Epsom salts but not the other ingredients (thymol, chenopodium, or male fern) required to treat hookworm at that time.

64 *Vancouver Province*, May 23 and June 2, 1914; *Vancouver Sun*, July 7 and 17, 1914. The Shore Committee, comprising several South Asians in Vancouver, raised money for some of Gurdit Singh's expenses. Indo-Canadian Oral History Collection participant no. 22 recalled that her husband had told her that he had contributed to this fund. See English transcript of Interview 22 by Gurcharn S. Basran and B. Singh Bolaria, July 5, 1985, 8, http://digital.lib.sfu.ca/icohc-collection.

65 See "Re Munshi Singh (July 6 1914, 1914), 20 BCR. 243 (BC Court of Appeal)," and Canada, *Commission to Investigate Hindu Claims*.

66 LAC, Robert Borden to C.J. Doherty, Minister of Justice, July 22, 1914, 1, MG 26 H 1(a), vol. 40. Borden referred to a *Halifax Chronicle* article of July 13, 1914.

67 PC 1914–23 ordered that immigrants arrive in Canada by "continuous journey" from their country of birth and/or nationality, and PC 1914–24 ordered that Asian immigrants, except those whose entry was governed by other legislation (Chinese and Japanese nationals), have $200 in their possession on arrival. These January 1914 Orders replaced PC 920 and 926 of 1910, which were updated versions of the original Orders 920 and 926 of January 1908. See Singh, "The Gadar Party," 41.

68   United States, *Annual Report of the Commissioner* ... Appendix III: Report of the United States Commission of Immigration for Canada, District, 1, 200–1; NARA, Anthony Caminetti Memorandum for W.B. Wilson, June 13, 1914, 1–2, RG 85 E9 52903 110 D; Wilson's statement is typewritten in red on page 2. See also NARA, W.B. Wilson to John L. Burnett, July 3, 1914, 1, RG 85 E9 52903 110 D.

69   Tichenor, *Dividing Lines*, 128–31. Tichenor adds that the commission's intensive research demonstrated how the ascendance of "social-scientific expertise" became "an institutionalized feature of the American policymaking process" and shaped that nation's government structures.

70   Haller, *Eugenics*, 153; see also Palumbo-Liu, *Asian/American*, 23; and Hing, *Defining America*, 46.

71   See, for example, Chiswick, "Jewish Immigrant Wages"; and Pula, "American Immigration Policy"; United States, *Reports of the Immigration Commission*, Pt. 3, 323, 331, 334, 337, and vol. 2, *Agriculture*, 110.

72   Employer opinion on the productivity of South Asian workers varied widely, especially among California farmers. One beet farmer asserted that the South Asian worker was "generally complained of on account of his uncleanliness," but his high productivity made this irrelevant. Another California employer attempted to overcome local prejudice against his South Asian orange pickers by calling them "Turks" and segregating them in housing miles away from other people. United States, *Reports of the Immigration Commission*, Pt. 3, 341, 344, 346, 349; see also 28 and 97.

73   US Government, Abstracts of Reports in *Reports of the Immigration Commission*, 47, 677, 681–82, 691.

74   A. Carnegie Ross, San Francisco, to James Bryce, March 13 and 14, 1912, 1–2, both in FO 115 1676, Public Records Office, United Kingdom.

75   A. Carnegie Ross to James Bryce, 14 March 1912, 1–2, and James Bryce to Edward Grey, 25 March 1912, both in FO 115 1676, Public Records Office, United Kingdom.

76   "Table 3: Alien Applicants for Admission to U.S. and Percent Debarred By Nationality, July 1, 1910–June 30, 1932," in Lee and Yung, *Angel Island*, 330–31. The Chinese rejection rate was 4.41 percent, the Japanese rejection rate was 1.30 percent, and the Korean rate was 4.54 percent. The general rejection rate at the station was 2.78 percent.

77   See NARA, "Transcript Notes and Translations Made Incident to the Visit to Angel Island," 4–9, RG 90, central file 1897 to 1923, box 785, file 16090.

78   *San Francisco Chronicle*, October 29, 1913; United States, *Restriction of Immigration Hearings*, 3–9.

79   United States, *Restriction of Immigration Hearings* ... Pt. 2, December 11 and 12, 1913, 125–26, 147, 174.

80   Schrag, *Not Fit For Our Society*, 77–78; Palumbo-Liu, *Asian/American*, 26–27.

81   Proceedings and Debates, 63rd US Cong., 3rd Sess. (House of Rep.), vol. 51, Pt. 3, January 31, 1914, 2679–81.

82   Palumbo-Liu, *Asian/American*, 27; Higham, *Strangers in the Land*, 166; Leong, *The China Mystique*, 7–11. Leong cites Hunt, *Ideology and Foreign Policy*, 16.

83   *Morning Oregonian* (Portland), December 9, 1913; *Los Angeles Times*, December 10, 1913; NARA, Daniel J. Keefe, The Oriental Hotel, Kobe, Japan, to Warner A. Parker, January 26, 1914, 1 RG 85 E9 52903 110 D.

84   Jensen, *Passage from India*, 153–54.

85   In 1910, 1,782 South Asians were admitted, and 411 were debarred; in 1911, 517 were admitted and 862 were debarred; in 1912, 165 were admitted and 104 debarred; in 1913, 188 were admitted and 236 were debarred. See NARA, Immigration Service,

Washington, DC. "Memorandum regarding Hindu migration to the United States," received January 23, 1914, RG 85 E9 52903 110 C; Jensen, *Passage from India,* 158.
86 Jensen, *Passage from India,* 150.
87 Jensen, *Passage from India,* 153–54.
88 NARA, W.B. Wilson to Speaker of the House of Representatives, January 20, 1914, 1–3, 9, RG 85 E9 52903 110 C. The Church and Humphrey bills were HR 9044 and 6440, respectively.
89 "Statement of Dr. Sudhindra Bose," in *Hindu Immigration Hearings of the Committee on Immigration and Naturalization,* House of Representatives, 63rd Cong., 2nd Sess., Pt. 1, February 13, 1914, 7, 15, 29; ibid., "Statement of Mrs. R.F. Patterson," 7, 24, 26, 27, 29, 30, 31, 35.
90 Ibid., "Statement of Anthony Caminetti," 36, 37, 44–46, 48, 49, 51. See also *Washington Herald,* February 14, 1914; *Los Angeles Times,* February 16, 1914; *San Francisco Chronicle,* February 16, 1914. See also *New York Times,* February 17, 1914.
91 *Hindu Immigration Hearings, supra* note 89, Pt. 2, February 19, 1914, 85, 86, 97; Pt. 1, 53. See also Charles Nesbitt, "The Health Menace of Alien Races," 1–4. See also Ring's discussion of Nesbitt in *The Problem South,* 89. Raker introduced the Nesbitt article in the first hearing, but it is included in the second hearing record.
92 Arnold, "An Ancient Race Outworn," 123, 125, 126, 127, 128–29, 133.
93 *Hindu Immigration Hearings, supra* note 89, Pt. 2, 69, 70, 76–80, 85.
94 *Hindu Immigration Hearings, supra* note 89, Pt. 4, April 16, 1914, 129, 130, 132, 137–38, 145–46; Pt. 5, April 30, 1914, 153, 156, 163, 170, 177; Jensen, *Passage from India,* 159; NARA, Anthony Caminetti Memorandum for W.B. Wilson, June 13, 1914, 1–2, RG 85 E9 52903 110 D; United States, *Annual Report ... (Year Ending 30 June 1914),* 2, 10. Wilson's statement is typewritten in red on page 2; NARA, W.B. Wilson to John L. Burnett, July 3, 1914, 1, RG 85 E9 52903 110 D.
95 NARA, Pearson Robbins, Inspector in Charge, Vancouver, to John H. Clark, February 21, 1910, 1, RG 85 E9 51391 21 21A. John H. Clark to Anthony Caminetti, May 27, 1914, 3, and W.B. Wilson to John L. Burnett, July 3, 1914, 3, both in NARA, RG 85 E9 52903 110 D. NARA, O.C. Gould, Consular Assistant, Curling, Bay of Islands, Newfoundland, to Secretary of State, December 16, 1914, 1, RG 85 E9 53854 133. *Los Angeles Times,* October 1 and 3, 1915.
96 Jensen, *Passage from India,* 159; *Los Angeles Times,* November 8, 1915; "Report of the Commissioner of Immigration, San Francisco," in United States, *Annual Report ... (Year Ending 30 June 1915),* 37; see Caminetti's prediction on page xvi.
97 *Debates of the 63rd United States Congress, 3rd Sess.,* February 4, 1915, 3053.
98 Inspector Edward T. Ross, "Sanitary Report, 397 regarding Camp, 7, Lower Jones Tract," submitted to California State Board of Health, Bureau of Administration, Sacramento, January 3, 1916, 4; Ross to Dr. W.A. Sawyer, "Regarding camps in delta region owned or control by George Shima, (Camps 6–9, Shima Tract and Bacon Island)," January 5, 1917, 1, 2, 6; Ross, "Report on camps owned or controlled by the California Delta Farms Company, Stockton, (Camp 3. Cohn Tract)," January 6, 1917, 1; Ross, "Camps in Stockton owned or controlled by the Staten Island Land Co, SF, (Camp 21, Staten Island), January 6, 1917, 1. All of the foregoing in R384-007-1-24, Public Health Dept. Records 1876–1974, California State Archives.
99 J.C. Misrow, "East Indian Immigration on the Pacific Coast,", 11, 22, 24, 26, 30.
100 Assistant to the Secretary of the California State Board of Health, to Carson C. Cook, General Manager, Ridge Land and Navigation Company, Stockton, January 27, 1917, 1, R384–007–1-24 Public Health Dept. Records 1876–1974, California State Archives.

101   Siu, "'The Sojourner,'" 34. See also Atal's discussion of Siu in "Outsiders as Insiders," 136–38.
102   La Brack, *The Sikhs of Northern California*, 20–21.
103   Shah, *Stranger Intimacy*, 101–3. See also Archdeacon, *Becoming American*.
104   Jensen, *Passage from India*, 159; Stern, *Eugenic Nation*, 46–47; Walter W. Baker, Portland, Letter to the Editor, *San Jose Evening News*, May 31, 1917.
105   Stern, *Eugenic Nation*, 28–31, 46–47.
106   Pernick, "Eugenics and Public Health," 1768–70. By the 1910s, American scientists supported August Weismann's anti-Lamarckian belief that the hereditary "germ plasm" (later known as "genes") could not be corrupted by environmental factors, but many thought that disease could affect the health of future children.
107   *United States Congressional Record*, 64th Cong., 1st Sess. vol. 53, Pt. 5, March 2, 1916, 4864; Jensen, *Passage from India*, 142–43.
108   "Appendix to Congressional Record: Extension of Remarks of Hon. Denver S. Church to the House of Representatives," *United States Congressional Record*, 64th Cong., 1st Sess. vol. 53, Pt. 5, April 14, 1916, 724.
109   Jensen, *Passage from India*, 141–42.

Chapter 6: Franchise Denied

Epigraph note: LAC, Charles Herbert Dickie to Arthur Meighen, September 25, 1922, MG 26I, vol. 98.

1   See esp. VCA, F.C. Blair, "Private Memo re: Hindu Immigration," January 26, 1912, 1, 3, ADD MSS No. 69, vol. 1, file 1, 1 to 136d, location 509D7; and House of Commons, 12th Parl., 1st Sess., vol. 2, February 27, 1912. See also W.D. Scott, "The Immigration by Races," 1914, in *Canada and Its Provinces*, vol. 7 (Toronto: Glasgow, 1914), ed. A. Short and A. Doughty, reprinted in Thorner and Frohn-Nielson, *A Country Nourished on Self-Doubt*, 73–93.
2   VCA, H.H. Stevens to L.A. Davis, October 14, 1915, 1–2, ADD MSS 69, vol. 1, file 5, location 509-D-7 349–521.
3   Razack, *Race, Space and the Law*, 53–54. Razack adds that if a mixed-race person could "*pass* as white," he or she could "disrupt Euro-Canadian dominance" by attaining white rights of franchise and citizenship.
4   McKay, *Reasoning Otherwise*, 621–22.
5   Hugh Johnston, "The Surveillance," 26–27.
6   Parnaby and Kealey, "The Origins of Political Policing,", 234–35.
7   LAC, W.W. Cory to Joseph Pope, December 4, 1914, 1, RG 25, vol. 1139, file 1914–40-C; LAC, (Confidential) E.J. Chambers, Chief Press Censor, to G.D. Perry, GNW Telegraph Company, January 19, 1916, 1, RG 6 E, vol. 524, file 150-D-1 P 1; Hugh Johnston, "The Surveillance," 23–24.
8   LAC, H.C. Clogstoun to Dr. Roche, November 1915, 1, G 25 G1, vol. 1300, file 1011 FPi. See also Harry L. Good, Immigration Inspector, to H.C. Clogstoun, August 14, 1915, 1–2, included as an Appendix to Clogstoun's November 1915 report on the *Komagata Maru* incident, which was published as Canada, *Commission to Investigate Hindu Claims*.
9   Buchignani, Indra, and Srivastava, *Continuous Journey*, 75; English transcript of Interview 51 by Gurcharn S. Basran and B. Singh Bolaria, January 1, 1985, 8, Indo-Canadian Oral History Collection, http://digital.lib.sfu.ca/icohc-collection; *Toronto Weekly Star*, October 17, 1922; E.H. Lawson, MD, Letter to the Editor of the *Victoria Daily Colonist*, September 25, 1913.

10 As the resident South Asian population dwindled down to less than 1,200 in 1917, Scott observed with satisfaction that the "the East Indian difficulty in BC is largely solving itself." W.D. Scott to Joseph Pope, January 7, 1916, 1, and Joseph Pope Memorandum for Robert Borden, n.d., both in LAC, RG 25, series A3a, vol. 1185, file 1916 897. See also LAC, W.D. Scott to Malcolm J. Reid, November 27, 1915, 1, RG 76, vol. 385, file 536999, pt. 9; and W.D. Scott Memo to William Roche, April 20, 1917, 1, W.D. Scott to Robert Campbell, July 26, 1917, 1, and William Roche to Governor General, (Council), November 27, 1917, 1, all in RG 76, vol. 385, file 536999, pt. 10. LAC, E. Blake Robertson Memorandum to W.W. Cory for Robert Borden, received May 6, 1918, 1, and W.D. Scott Memorandum to Hon. Mr. Crerar, October 21, 1918, 1–2, both in LAC, RG 76, vol. 385, file 536999, pt. 11; PC 641, March 26, 1919; *The Critic* (Vancouver), April 19, 1919.

11 See Flick's opposition to the 1938 Japanese interment in Harrington and Stevenson, *Islands in the Salish Sea,* 70; Charles Flick, Lt.-Col. Commanding, 3 Special Battalion, 1 Special Brigade, Karachi, April 24, 1919, Letter to the Editor of *Vancouver Sun,* June 22, 1919; LAC, Malcolm J. Reid to W.W. Cory, June 23, 1919, 1, RG 76, vol. 386, file 536999, pt. 12.

12 Most social and sexual interactions in Vancouver between homosexual men were restricted to Chinatown, Gastown, and the business district, because these neighbourhoods were "separated spatially and socially from working-class and middle-class white families." Shah, *Stranger Intimacy,* 57–58, 62, 131–32.

13 These lists do not explain why some were held longer than the usual short period for observation, but they do indicate that only one South Asian was rejected in these years; he failed the continuous journey provision because he was neither a dependent nor a returning immigrant. LAC, "Record of Persons Detained or Rejected at Victoria, 15 February 1921," 3, RG 76, vol. 306, file 281230, Vancouver 4; LAC, "Record ... 12 June 1921" and "Record ... Vancouver, July 7 1921," RG 76, vol. 306, file 281230, Vancouver 5; LAC, "Record ... Victoria, February 1922," "Record ... Victoria, 22 May 1922," and "Record ... Victoria ... 17 June 1922," all in LAC, RG 76, vol. 306, file 281230, Victoria 7. See also Canadian Government, Original Data Passenger Lists, 1865–1935, Miscellaneous Publications, T-479-T-14939, tabulated on www.ancestry.ca, which show that forty-five South Asians arrived in 1920 and seventy-one arrived in 1921. See also English summary of Kartar Singh Ghag interview by Hari Sharma, June 21, 1984, 1, and English transcript of Ratan Kaur Thauli interview by Hari Sharma, May 14, 1987, 1, both in Indo-Canadian Oral History Collection, http://digital.lib.sfu.ca/icohc-collection.

14 VCA, Arthur G. Price, Medical Health Officer, "1919 Report of Victoria Sanitary Inspector, Office of Board of Health, to Mayor," January 1920, 3. The City of Vancouver's annual "Health Reports" for 1910–24 are housed in VCA, PDS 11. See "1922 Report of the Medical Health Officer (Abridged)," in *Vancouver City Annual Report* (Vancouver: 1923), 81. The "Oriental" death rate was 21.327/1000, while the white death rate was 10.526/1000. See also "1923 Report of the Medical Health Officer (Abridged)," *Vancouver City Annual Report* (Vancouver: 1924), 83.

15 Between 1910, the first year for which these data are available, and 1924, an average of five South Asians died each year, along with 59 Japanese, 80 Chinese, and 479 whites (classified as Canadians). The city's Health Report statistics for these years show an average annual white mortality rate of 0.46 per thousand, while Asians died at an average rate of 1.56 per thousand. The city lumped Asians together in its population statistics for "Asiatics," so it is difficult to use these data to ascertain mortality rates for different groups. We only know that a combined 9,648 Chinese, Japanese, and South Asians

lived in Vancouver in these years, compared to 103,609 whites. However, the 1911 census indicated that a very large majority of BC's approximately 2,342 South Asians lived in areas covered in the Health Report. With the following exceptions, all mortality numbers are on page 14 of the *Vancouver City Annual Reports* (except 1911 [pg. 19], 1912 [pg. 33], and 1914 [pg. 16]). See individuals with the first and/or last name Singh, and self-identified "Hindus" and "Sikhs" in "Vancouver City," "New Westminster," and "Richmond" subdistricts, tabulated in the 1911 Canadian Census, at www.ancestry. ca. The government's total 1911 census tally of South Asians is detailed in LAC, F.C. Blair to Dr. McLaurin, April 21, 1943, 1, RG 76, vol. 387, file 536999, pt. 17.

16 *Conference of Prime Ministers and Representatives of UK, the Dominions and India, June, July and Aug 1921* (London: King's Printer's, 1921). The 1921 census data that show that 1,016 South Asians remained in Canada in 1921 are in LAC, F.C. Blair to Dr. McLaurin, April 21, 1943, 1, RG 76, vol. 387, file 536999, pt. 17; see Buchignani, Indra, and Srivastava, *Continuous Journey*, 81; see also LAC, W.L.M. King to Joseph Pope, July 22 and 28, 1922, 1, RG 25 G1, vol. 1300, file 1011, Sastri.

17 Joseph Pope, Empress Hotel, Victoria, to Maurice Pope, August 16, 1922, 2, accession 20030022–001 (Maurice Arthur Pope Collection), box 4, file 28, Military History Research Centre, Canadian War Museum.

18 LAC, Joseph Pope to W.L.M. King, August 13, 1922, 1, and Joseph Pope to John Oliver, August 13, 1922, 1, RG 25 G1, vol. 1300, file 1011, Sastri. Sastri's statements are contained in LAC, A. Ireland, "Memorandum Regarding Status of East Indians in B.C.," October 23, 1946, 2, RG 25, series G2, vol. 3706, file 555040, pt. 2. The latter file was declassified and opened April 15, 2010, on the author's Access to Information Request to LAC.

19 LAC, A. Ireland, "Memorandum Regarding Status of East Indians in BC," October 23, 1946, 2–3, RG 25, series G2, vol. 3706, file 555040, pt. 2. Looking back at the debate, A. Ireland's 1946 memo correctly recalled that "no support was forthcoming for the Indian cause from any party."

20 Graham, *Arthur Meighen*, 186. Graham and others have overlooked the relationship between the two men, and the key correspondence between Meighen and his federal MPs from BC after Sastri's visit. See LAC, V.S. Srinivasa Sastri to Arthur Meighen, September 22, 1922, 1, MG 26I, vol. 98. Meighen's letter to BC Conservative Members of Parliament is copied in VCA, (Private and Confidential) Arthur Meighen to H.H. Stevens, September 6, 1922, 1–2, ADD MSS 69, vol. 1, file 5, location 509-D-7 349–521.

21 VCA, H.H. Stevens to Arthur Meighen, September 20, 1922, 1–2, ADD MSS 69, vol. 1, file 5, location 509-D-7 349–521.

22 See VCA, Leon Ladner, "National Liberal Conservative Association of Vancouver South, Government Candidate, Memorial to Fellow Citizens," November 31, 1921, 1, AM641, Leon Johnson Ladner fonds, box 2, file Asiatic Exclusion Chinese; and LAC, Leon Ladner to Arthur Meighen, September 19, 1922, 1–3, MG 26I, vol. 98.

23 (Personal) Leon Ladner to Arthur Meighen, October 2, 1922, 1; (Private and Confidential) William Garland McQuarrie to Arthur Meighen, September 30, 1922; (Personal) Leon Ladner to Arthur Meighen, October 2, 1922, 1; and Leon Ladner to Arthur Meighen, November 1, 1922, 1, all in LAC, MG 26I, vol. 98.

24 LAC, Charles Herbert Dickie to Arthur Meighen, September 25, 1922, 1, MG 26I, vol. 98.

25 Meighen to V.S. Srinivasa Sastri, October 9, 1922, 1, and Arthur Meighen to Leon Ladner, October 9, 1922, 1, both in LAC, MG 26I, vol. 98.

26 Diary of W.L.M. King, March 23, 1923; *Debates of the Canadian House of Commons*, 14th Parliament, 2nd Session (1923), vol. 1, February 21, 1923, 497, 507, 510–11; *Debates* ...

vol. 5, June 19, 1923, 4077, and June 29, 1923, 4645, 4647. For more on Jacobs's role in Montreal's Jewish community, see Figler, *Sam Jacobs*.

27 Supra note 26, *Debates*, vol. 5, 4660–62, 4667; LAC, A. Ireland, "Memorandum Regarding Status of East Indians in B.C.," October 23, 1946, 2–3, RG 25, series G2, vol. 3706, file 555040, pt. 2; See *Debates of the Canadian House of Commons*, 18th Parliament, 1st Session, vol. 1, February 20, 1936, 373.

28 (Confidential) F.C. Blair to Joseph Pope, July 21, 1922, 5, and F.C. Blair to Joseph Pope, July 25, 1922, 1, both in LAC, RG 25 G1, vol. 1300, file 1011; LAC, F.C. Blair to M. Cowie, Punjab, January 3, 1924, 1, RG 76, vol. 387, file 536999, RO pt. 3; LAC, F.C. Blair to Dr. McLaurin, Ontario, April 21, 1943, 1, RG 76, vol. 387, file 536999, pt. 17.

29 Ignatiev, *How the Irish Became White*, Roediger, *The Wages of Whiteness*, 13–14. As Tony Ballantyne reminds us, the Aryan image had become an especially "crucial element within the culture of empire" by the twentieth century, as it offered both "a powerful lens for analyzing the pre-colonial past of colonized societies" and a way to interpret the "imperial present." See Ballantyne, *Orientalism and Race*, 3–4.

30 Arnold, "'An Ancient Race Outworn,'" 123, 125, 126, 127, 128–29, 133.

31 See Jensen, *Passage from India*, 256, Okihiro, *The Columbia Guide*, 21; and Hess, "The Hindu in America," 66–67.

32 The author wishes to thank Dr. Barrington Walker for his input in this area.

33 Hernan Shah, "Race, Nation and Citizenship," 257–58. Hess similarly concluded that "shortly after the passage of the Immigration Act, any public sympathy for the alien Indian was destroyed by the well-publicized uncovering of the Hindu conspiracy." See Hess, "The 'Hindu' in America," 65.

34 NARA, Mrs. I. Malone, New York City, to Department, n.d. (received by F. Nixon, Acting Commissioner General of Immigration, October 16, 1922), 1, RG 85 E9 53854 133B.

35 "United States v. Bhagat Singh Thind, *U.S. Senate*, 261 US 204 [1923]. Sutherland added that while European immigrants blended quickly into American society, "the children born in this country of Hindu parents would retain indefinitely the clear evidence of their ancestry."

36 R.L.H. Jr., "Aliens: Naturalization: Who is a White Person?," 353.

37 "Interview with Inder Singh (Hindu), El Centro, California," May 31, 1924, by William C. Smith, Southern California, Major Documents file 28–237, Survey of Race Relations, Hoover Institution, Stanford University Library.

38 "Section 13, An Act to Limit the Migration of Aliens into the United States," approved May 26, 1924, 68 Cong., 1 Sess., Ch. 185, 190, *The Statutes at Large of the United States of America*, December 1923–March 1925, vol. XLII, pt. 1, (Washington: US GPO, 1925), 153–69. Markel and Stern point out that, like the 1921 Immigration Act that first established national immigration quotas, the Johnson–Reed legislation was "based on a mixture of nativist thought, arguments about the potentially devastating eco effects of open immigration and sensational eugenic 'evidence' of the effects of immigrants on the national 'germ plasm.'" See Markel and Stern, "Which Face?," 1320.

39 NARA Pacific Branch, Minutes of a BSI at Angel Island, August 1, 1925, Joginder Singh of SS *Tenyo Maru* (d.o.b. June 26, 1925), 1–2, RG 85, file 24291–4-2, Immigrant Arrival Case (IACF) Passenger Files.

40 Hernan Shah, "Race, Nation and Citizenship," 260. In late 1923 the US Supreme Court ruled that California's alien land law, first passed in 1913 and repassed in a revised form in 1920, did not violate the 14th Amendment of the US Constitution. See Jensen, *Passage from India*, 265.

41 See statements of "Taraknath Das" and "V.R. Kokatnur." See also "Raymond G. Crist, Commission of Naturalization, to Secretary of Labor (Through Chief Clerk), 26 Oct

1926," in US Senate, *Hearings on S.J. Res. 128, Before the Committee on Immigration, Providing for the Ratification and Confirmation of Naturalization of Certain Persons of the Hindu Race*, 69th Cong., 2nd Sess., Pt. 1, December 9, 1926 (Washington, US GPO, 1926), 5, 22, 30; see also Jensen, *Passage from India*, 264, and Nayan Shah, *Stranger Intimacy*, 248–50. Crist called attention to the criminal record and "anarchism" of Taraknath Das, the chief South Asian proponent of the Reed bill.

42   V.S. McClatchy to Hiram Johnson, 30 November 1926, 1, in *Hearings on S.J. Res. 128*, I, 20; see also Okihiro, *Cane Fires*, 66. See also V.S. McClatchy to Hiram Johnson, December 2, 1926, in *Hearings on S.J. Res. 128*, pt. 2, December 15, 1926, 43.

43   Hess, "The Hindu in America," 70; see also Jensen, *Passage from India*, 264. Hess explains that in 1927 and 1928, Senators Copeland and Cellar attempted to introduce legislation recognizing South Asians as "white persons," but these attempts were tabled; see Hess, "The Hindu in America," 70–71.

44   "Excerpts from the report of Mr. Fieldbrave, a worker among East Indians on the Pacific Coast, 1924," 2–3, file 28–245, Excerpts Fieldbrave Report, Major Documents, and "Hindus in Los Angeles," by Willard A. Schurr, n.d., 22, file 29–273 Hindus Los Angeles, Major Documents, all in Survey of Race Relations, Stanford University Library. See also Theodore Fieldbrave, "Work Among the Hindus," *The Baptist* (Chicago), January 24, 1925, and "East Indians in the United States," *Missionary Review of the World* 57 (1934): 291–93.

45   Mitchell, *The Lie of the Land*, 44–45; Street, *Beasts of the Field*, 577.

46   California, "Report on Fresno, Pt. II," 4 and 9; "Report on Fresno Pt. III, The Chinese," 9–10, and "Report on Fresno Pt. IV, East Indians," 1–2, all in Commission of Immigration and Housing [California], *Report on Fresno's Immigration Problem* (Sacramento: California State Printing Office, 1918).

47   See "Amendments to the Constitution, and Proposed Statutes, to Be Submitted to the California Electors at the General Election on 2 November 1920," http://library. uchastings.edu/ballot_pdf/1920g.pdf; California State Board of Control, *California and the Oriental: Japanese, Chinese, and Hindus* (19 June 1920), republished under the same title (New York: Arno Press, 1978); see, for example, Roger Daniels, *The Politics of Prejudice: The Anti-Japanese Movement in California and the Struggle for Japanese Exclusion* (Berkeley, California: University of California Press, 1962), 123.

48   California, State Board of Control, *California and the Oriental*, 7, 10–11, 45, and 101.

49   California, State Board of Control, *California and the Oriental*, 110–111. See the following four complaint files regarding unsanitary conditions at South Asian–run camps: "Labor Camp Report regarding Camp of Lashman Singh," December 2, 1922, 1, container 80, file 67; "Labor Camp Report regarding Camp of Chanon Singh," November 21, 1922, 1, container 80, file 64; "Labor Camp Report regarding Camp of Bishan Singh," February 6, 1922, 1, container 80, file 62; "Labor Camp Report regarding Babu Singh," October 4, 1922, 1, container 80, file 61; all of the foregoing in BANC, MSS CA 194, at Bancroft Library, University of California–Berkeley. See California, State Board of Control, *California and the Oriental*, 109–10.

50   English transcript of Interview 46 by Gurcharn S. Basran and B. Singh Bolaria, January 1, 1985, 5, Indo-Canadian Oral History Collection, http://digital.lib.sfu.ca/ icohc-collection.

Conclusion

1   Percy Reid, Division Commander, Vancouver, to S.N. Reid, Immigration Agent, May 31, 1924, 1. This letter is contained in a later (1968) file of a Victoria resident asking

for his wife's entry to Canada. Under the "Access to Information" terms I agreed to, I cannot identify the immigrant's name; LAC Burnaby Branch, RG 76 1984–85/279 GAD VFRC#FAD83–27, box 1, file 2222H.

2 Blair uses the term "experiment" in F.C. Blair Memorandum to J.E. Featherstone, April 5, 1923, 1, see also D.A. Clark, Assistant Deputy Minister, Department of Health, to F.C. Blair, June 21, 1922, 1, both in LAC, RG 76, vol. 584, file 820636; LAC, A.L. Joliffe to Department Secretary, June 23, 1922, 1, RG 76, vol. 306, file 281230, Van 5. Underscore in original.

3 LAC, A.S. Munro Memorandum to W.D. Scott "Regarding Medical Examination of Chinese Immigrants at Port of Vancouver," October 5, 1922, 1,, RG 76, vol. 584, file 820636.

4 J.D. Page to Milne, April 5, 1923, 3, in LAC, RG 76, vol. 584, file 820636.

5 NARA, Rupert Blue to Commissioner General of Immigration, March 14, 1919, 2–3, RG 85 54261 184; See Kraut, *Silent Travelers*, Appendix II, 275–76. Deirdre Maloney incorrectly states that this policy was first implemented in 1925; see Maloney, *National Insecurities*, 114–15.

6 See Kazimi "Continuous Journey," and Varughese, "Entry Denied." See also "Komagata Maru," a Simon Fraser University and Citizenship and Immigration Canada website, at http://komagatamarujourney.ca; Ruby Dhalla's motion in *Debates of the Canadian House of Commons*, 40th Parliament, 3rd Session, Entry 49, May 26, 2010.

7 *Debates of the Canadian House of Commons*, 41st Parliament, 1st Session, vol. 146, 127, May 18, 2012, 1005. As stated above, limited immigration from India resumed only in 1952, over forty years after legislative exclusion was first introduced in 1908.

8 The record of the motion's defeat on May 28, 2012, is in *Debates supra* note 7, 128. This Member of Parliament has requested anonymity; interview conducted April 12, 2010, on Parliament Hill. The interview took place before the 2012 motion for an in-House apology.

9 *Debates of the Canadian House of Commons*, 42nd Parliament, 1st Session, vol. 58, May 18, 2016, 1515. This apology occurred four years to the day of Jasbir Sandhu's remarks. For an example of a South Asian Canadian's reaction to Trudeau's remarks, see *Toronto Star*, 20 May 2016.

10 Bill C-11, which became law as a 2011 amendment to Canada's 2002 Immigration and Refugee Protection Act, was codified as S.C.2011, c. 8; Kazimi, *Undesirables*, 11.

11 *National Post*, 25 May 2012.

Bibliography

Archives and Newspapers

Archives

Bancroft Library, University of California at Berkeley
AAS ARC 2000/62 – Angel Island Oral History Project
BANC MSS CB 581 – Governor Hiram Johnson Papers
BANC MSS CA 194 – California Industrial Relations Commission of Immigration and
  Housing

British Columbia Archives, Victoria
E/D/D843 – Richard Low Drury Accession
GR 429 – Attorney General Records
GR 0684 – BC Royal Commission on Labour Records
GR 0441 – British Columbia Premier's Records
GR 1195 – British Columbia Legislative Assembly Records
GR 2856 – Alberni County, British Columbia, County Court Records
Imbert Orchard / Canadian Broadcasting Corporation Accession
M.S. Bryant Accession
Records of Municipal Death Certificates

California State Archives, Sacramento
R384–007–1-24 – Public Health Department Records
F3743–26 – California Industrial Relations Commission of Immigration and
  Housing

Churchill Archives Centre, Cambridge, UK
AMEL 2/5/7 – Leopold Amery Papers

Durham University Library, UK
4th Earl Grey Papers

Hoover Institution, Stanford University
Survey of Race Relations Records

Library and Archives Canada, Ottawa
CO 42 – Colonial Office Fonds
MG 26-G – Wilfrid Laurier Papers
MG 26-J – W.L. Mackenzie King Papers

MG 26 H 1a – Robert Borden Papers
MG 27 IIB2 – Governor General Grey Papers
MG 27 III B 9 – H.H. Stevens Papers
MG 26I – Arthur Meighen Papers
MG26-J13 – Diaries of William Lyon Mackenzie King
RG 2 – Privy Council Office
RG 6 – Secretary of State
RG 7 – Governor General's Office
RG 13 – Department of Justice
RG 18 – Royal Canadian Mounted Police
RG 24 – Department of National Defence
RG 25 – Department of External Affairs
RG 29 – Department of Health and Welfare
RG 76 – Department of Immigration

Library and Archives Canada, Burnaby (Pacific Regional Office)
RG 76 Accession 86–87/244 – Vancouver, Immigration Case Files, Canada Immigration
   Centre
RG 76 1984–85/279 GAD VFRC#FAD83–27 – Victoria, Lookout, Hindu and Chinese
   Case Files

Military History Research Centre, Canadian War Museum, Ottawa
Accession 20030022–001 – Maurice Arthur Pope Collection

National Archives and Records Administration, College Park, Maryland
RG 59 – State Department
RG 90 – Public Health Service

National Archives and Records Administration, Washington, D.C.
RG 85 – Immigration and Naturalization Service

National Archives and Records Administration, San Bruno (California Branch)
RG 85 – Records of the Immigration Service, Alien Passenger Arrival Files
RG 90 – Records of the Public Health and Marine Hospital Service, Angel Island, San
   Francisco

Public Records Office, London, UK
FO 115 – Foreign Office Embassy and Consulates, US Correspondence
FO 371 – Foreign Office Embassy and Consulates, US General Correspondence
   (Political)

Simon Fraser University Archives, Vancouver
CA SFU F145 – Indo-Canadian Oral History Collection

University of California at Davis, Pacific Regional Humanities Center
Angel Island Oral History Project

University of North Carolina at Chapel Hill, Wilson Library
MG 483 – Magnum Family Papers

Vancouver City Archives
ADD MSS 69 – H.H. Stevens Papers
AM641 – Leon Johnson Ladner Papers
Series 101 – Health Inspectors' Reports
Series 483 – Files of the City Clerk
Series 605 – Vancouver Medical Health Officer Annual Reports
Series 616 – Annual Reports of the Chief Constable

Victoria City Archives
Reports of Victoria Sanitary Inspector to Mayor

Newspapers
Bellingham Herald (Washington)
Bisbee Daily Review (Arizona)
Blaine Journal (Washington)
Cowichan Valley Citizen (British Columbia)
Critic (Vancouver)
Democratic Banner (Ohio)
Deseret Evening News (Salt Lake City, Utah)
Evening Bulletin Honolulu
Gazette (Montreal)
Halifax Chronicle
Los Angeles Times
Manitoba Free Press
Marysville Appeal (California)
Medford Mail Tribune (Oregon)
Morning Oregonian (Portland)
National Post
New York Times
New Westminster News
Ogden Evening Standard (Utah)
Ottawa Citizen
Ottawa Free Press
Prince Rupert Daily News
Sacramento Record-Union
San Francisco Bulletin
San Francisco Call
San Francisco Chronicle
San Francisco Examiner
San Jose Evening News
Saturday Sunset (Vancouver)
Seattle Star
Spokane Spokesman-Review
Tacoma Times (Washington)
Times of London
Tombstone Epitaph (Tombstone, Arizona)
Toronto Star
Toronto Mail and Empire
Vancouver Province

Vancouver Sun
Vancouver World
Victoria Daily Times
Victoria Colonist
Virginia Gazette (Williamsburg)
Washington Herald
Washington Post

Legislative Debates

Legislative Debates and Hearings

Canada
Debates of the House of Commons. 10th Parliament.
3rd Session, vol. 1, November 28, 1906, 234
4th Session, vol. 1, December 4, 1907, 177, and December 16, 1907, 692; vol. 3,
    March 24, 1908, 5490, and April 8, 1908, 6431–36 and 6441–44
– . 12th Parliament
1st Session, vol. 2, February 27, 1912, 3930–32
3rd Session vol. 5, May 26, 1914, 4214, May 27, 1914, 4295, May 30, 1914, 4533, June 11,
    1914, 4562 and 4565, June 1, 1914, 4565, and June 6, 1914, 4954–55
– . 14th Parliament
2nd Session, vol. 1, February 21, 1923, 497, and 507–11, vol. 5, June 19, 1923, 4077,
    and June 29, 1923, 4645, 4647, 4660–62, and 4667
3rd Session, vol. 1, March 14, 1924, 355
– . 18th Parliament
1st Session, vol. 1, February 20, 1936, 373
– . 40th Parliament
3rd Session, May 26, 2010, entry 49
– . 41st Parliament
1st Session, vol. 146, May 18, 2012, 1005
– . 42nd Parliament
1st Session, vol. 58, May 18, 2016, 1515
Debates of the Senate of Canada., 12th Parliament.
2nd Session, June 2, 1913, 930, and 932–33

United Kingdom
Debates of the British House of Commons. 28th Parliament.
1st Session, vol. 16, December 12, 1906, 341, and December 13, 1906, 665
2nd Session, vol. 1, February 18, 1907, 539
3rd Session, vol. 4, March 23, 1908, 1050, March 24, 1908, 1206, and March 25, 1908,
    1404

United States
Proceedings and Debates of the United States Congress. 60th Congress.
1st Session, vol. 42, Pt. 8, May 27, 1908, 205
– . 63rd Congress
3rd Session, vol. 51, Pt. 3, January 31, 1914, 2679–81, and February 4, 1915, 3053
– . 64th Congress.
1st Session, vol. 53, Pt. 5, March 2, 1916, and April 14, 1916, 724 (Appendix)

United States Congressional Committee on Immigration and Naturalization. *Hindu Immigration Hearings.* 63rd Congress, 2nd Session Pt. 1, February 13, 1914, Pt. 2. February 19, 1914, Pt. 4, April 16, 1914, and Pt. 5, April 30, 1914. Washington: Government Printing, 1914.
– . *Restriction of Immigration Hearings.* 63rd Congress, 2nd Session, Pt. 1, December 6 and 7, 1913, and Pt. 2, December 11 and December 12, 1913. Washington: Government Printing, 1913.

Interviews
Conducted under General Research Ethics Board Clearance (granted May 2010)

Ottawa (3)
Informant 1, Ottawa Gurdwara, March 21, 2010
Informant 1, second interview, April 3, 2010.
Narinder Singh, March 21, 2010.

Parliament Hill (4)
Interview with Hon. Member of Parliament Sukh Dhaliwal, May 5, 2010
Interview with Member of Parliament 2, April 12, 2010
Interview with Member of Parliament 3, March 24, 2010
Interview with Member of Parliament 4, March 30, 2010

Stockton (1)
Interview with Stockton informant 1, August 7, 2011

Vancouver (2)
Interview with Secretary Ross St Gurdwara Joginder Singh Sunner, July 8, 2010, General Secretary Gurdwara Sahib Khalsa Diwan Society, 8000 Ross St., Vancouver
Interview with Vancouver informant 2, July 8, 2010.

Victoria (3)
Interview with Victoria informant 1, July 9, 2010
Interview with Victoria informant 2, June 30, 2010
Interview with Victoria informant 3, June 30, 2010

Unpublished Works
Biswas, Paromita. "Colonial Displacements: Nationalist Longing and Identity among Early Indian Intellectuals in the US." PhD Diss., University of California at Los Angeles, 2008.
Hester, Torrie. "Deportation: Origins of a National and International Power. PhD Dissertation, University of Oregon, 2008.
La Brack, Bruce. "The Sikhs of Northern California: A Sociohistorical Study." PhD diss., Syracuse University, 1980.
Misrow, J.C. "East Indian Immigration on the Pacific Coast." MA thesis, Stanford University, 1915.
Reitmanova, Sylvia. "'Disease Breeders Among Us': Canadian Press Coverage of Immigrant Tuberculosis: A Critical Discourse Analysis." PhD diss. Faculty of Medicine, Memorial University, September 2010.

Published Works
Abella, Irving M., and Harold Troper. *None Is Too Many: Canada and the Jews of Europe, 1933–1948.* 3rd ed. Toronto: Lester Publishing, 1991.

Allen, Amy. "The Entanglement of Power and Validity: Foucault and Critical Theory." In *Foucault and Philosophy*, ed. Timothy O'Leary and Christopher Falzon, 78–98. Oxford: Wiley Blackwell, 2010. http://dx.doi.org/10.1002/9781444320091.ch4.

Anderson, Benedict. *Imagined Communities: Reflections on the Origin and Spread of Nationalism.* 3rd ed. London: Verso, 2006.

Anderson, Warwick. *Colonial Pathologies: American Tropical Medicine, Race, and Hygiene in the Philippines.* Durham: Duke University Press, 2006. http://dx.doi.org/10.1215/9780822388081.

Archdeacon, Thomas J. *Becoming American: An Ethnic History.* New York: Free Press, 1983.

Arendt, Hannah. "The Jew as Pariah: A Hidden Tradition." *Jewish Social Studies* 6, 2 (April 1944): 99–122.

Arnold, David. "'An Ancient Race Outworn': Malaria and Race in Colonial India, 1860–1930." In *Race, Science and Medicine, 1700–1960*, ed. Walter Ernst and Bernard Harris, 123–45. London: Routledge, 1999.

Atal, Yogesh. "Outsiders as Insiders: The Phenomenon of Sanwich Culture: Prefatorial to a Possible Theory." In *The Indian Diaspora: Dynamics of Migration*, ed. Naranyana Jayaran, 204–18. New Delhi: Indian Sociological Society, 2004.

Avery, Donald. *Reluctant Host: Canada's Response to Immigrant Workers, 1896–1994.* Toronto: McClelland and Stewart, 1995.

Backhouse, Constance. *Colour-Coded: A Legal History of Racism in Canada, 1900–1950.* Toronto: Osgoode Society/University of Toronto Press, 1999.

Balibar, Etienne, and Immanuel Wallerstein. *Race, Nation, Class.* London: Verso, 1993.

Ballantyne, Tony. *Between Colonialism and Diaspora: Sikh Cultural Formations in an Imperial World.* Durham: Duke University Press, 2006. http://dx.doi.org/10.1215/9780822388111.

—. *Orientalism and Race: Aryanism in the British Empire.* London: Palgrave Macmillan, 2006.

Banton, Michael. *The Idea of Race.* London: Tavistock, 1977.

Barde, Robert. "Prelude to the Plague: Public Health and Politics at America's Pacific Gateway, 1899." *Journal of the History of Medicine and Allied Sciences* 58, 2 (April 2003): 153–86. http://dx.doi.org/10.1093/jhmas/58.2.153.

Barkan, Elizar. *The Retreat of Scientific Racism: Changing Concepts of Race in Britain and the United States between the World Wars.* Cambridge: Cambridge University Press, 1992.

Basran, Gurcharn, and B. Singh Bolaria. *The Sikhs in Canada: Migration, Race, Class, and Gender.* New Delhi: Oxford University Press, 2003.

Bates, Barbara. *Bargaining for Life: A Social History of TB, 1876–1938.* Philadelphia: University of Pennsylvania Press, 1994.

Beiser, Morton. "The Health of Immigrants and Refugees in Canada." *Canadian Journal of Public Health* 96, Supp. 2 (March–April 2005): S30–44.

Birn, Anne-Emanuelle. "Six Seconds Per Eyelid: The Medical Inspection of Immigrants at Ellis Island, 1892–1914." *Dynamis Acta Hisp. Med. Sci. Hist. Illus.* 17 (1997): 281–316.

Broad, Isabella Ross. *An Appeal for Fair Play for the Sikhs in Canada.* Victoria: 1913.

Buchanan, Agnes Foster. "The West and the Hindu Invasion." *Illustrated Overland Monthly* 51 (April 1908): 308–13.

Buchignani, Norman, Doreen M. Indra, and R. Srivastava. *Continuous Journey: A Social History of South Asians in Canada.* Toronto: McClelland and Stewart, 1985.

Burnett, A.G. "Misunderstanding of Eastern and Western States regarding Oriental Immigration." *Annals of the American Academy of Political and Social Science* 34, 2 (September 1909): 37–41. http://dx.doi.org/10.1177/000271620903400205.

California. State Board of Control. *California and the Oriental: Japanese, Chinese, and Hindus.* Sacramento: California State Printing Office, 1922.

——. Commission of Immigration and Housing. *Report on Fresno's Immigration Problem.* Sacramento: California State Printing Office, 1918.

——. State Assembly Chief Clerk. "Amendments to the Constitution, and Proposed Statutes, To Be Submitted to the California Electors at the General Election on November 2, 1920." Sacramento, California.

Campbell, Peter. "East Meets Left: South Asian Militants and the Socialist Party of Canada in B.C., 1904–1914." *International Journal of Canadian Studies* 35 (1999): 35–66.

Canada [Government of]. *Commission to Investigate Hindu Claims Following Refusal of Immigration Officials to Allow Over 300 Hindus Aboard the SS Komagata Maru to Land at Vancouver.* Vancouver: Government Printing Office, 1914.

——. Censuses of 1901, 1911, and 1921. Ottawa, ON.

——. *The Indians in British Columbia: A Report Regarding the Proposal to Provide Work in British Honduras for the Indigent Among Them.* Ottawa: King's Printer, 1908.

——. Order in Council 1908–2227. "Hindoo delegation to visit Honduras." Introduced October 2, 1908. Ottawa, ON.

——. Order in Council 920. "That Immigrants Arrive in Canada by Continuous Journey." Introduced January 8, 1908, updated in 1910, and again in January 1914 as P.C. 1914–23. Ottawa, ON.

——. Order in Council 926. "That Asiatic Immigrants Show $200 Upon Arrival." Introduced January 8, 1908, updated in 1910, and again in January 1914 as P. C. 1914–24. Ottawa, ON.

——. Original Data Passenger Lists. 1865–1935. Miscellaneous Publications T-479-T-14939, tabulated on www.ancestry.ca.

——. *Report of Mackenzie King Report by W.L. Mackenzie King on his Mission to England to Confer with the British Authorities on the Subject of Immigration to Canada from the Orient and Immigration from India in Particular.* London: HMSO, 1908.

——. *Report of the Royal Commission on Chinese and Japanese and Immigration.* Ottawa: King's Printer, 1885.

——. *Report of the Royal Commission to Inquire into the Methods by which Oriental Labourers have been Induced to Come to Canada.* Ottawa: King's Printer, 1908.

——. *Reports of the Royal Commission on Chinese Immigration.* Ottawa: King's Printer, 1885 and 1902.

——. *Report of the Select Committee on Chinese Labour and Immigration.* Ottawa: House of Commons, Journals, 1879.

——. *Report on the Need for the Suppression of the Opium Traffic in Canada.* Ottawa: King's Printer, 1908.

——. *Amended "Immigration and Refugee Protection Act.* S.C.2011, c. 8.

[Author Unknown]. *Canadian Annual Review of Public Affairs for 1906.* Toronto: Annual Review Publishers, 1907.

[Author Unknown]. *Canadian Annual Review of Public Affairs for 1909.* Toronto: Annual Review Publishers, 1910.

Carter, R. Markham. "Oriental Sore of Northern India a Protozoal Infection: A Preliminary Communication on the Etiology of the Disease and the Extra-Corporeal Cycle of the Parasite." *British Medical Journal* 2541, 2, (September 11, 1909): 647–50. http://dx.doi.org/10.1136/bmj.2.2541.647.

Chang, Kornel. *Pacific Connections: The Making of the U.S.–Canadian Borderlands.* Berkeley: University of California Press, 2012.

Chiswick, B.R. "Jewish Immigrant Wages in America in 1909: An Analysis of the Dillingham Commission Data." *Explorations in Economic History* 29, 3 (July 1992): 274–89. http://dx.doi.org/10.1016/0014-4983(92)90039-Y.

Cohen, Stanley. *Folk Devils and Moral Panics.* 3rd ed. New York: Routledge, 2002. Conn, J.R. "Immigration." *Queen's Quarterly* 8 (1900): 119, 129.

Coolidge, Mary Roberts. *Chinese Exclusion.* New York: Henry Holt, 1909.

Cunha, Burke E. *Pneumonia Essentials.* 3rd ed. Sudbury: Jones and Bartlett, 2010.

Curtis, Bruce. "Social Investment in Medical Forms: The 1866 Cholera Scare and Beyond." *Canadian Historical Review* 81, 3 (2000): 359–61.

Daniels, Roger. *Asian America: Chinese and Japanese in the United States since 1850.* Seattle: University of Washington Press, 1988.

—. "No Lamps Were Lit for Them: Angel Island and the Historiography of Asian American Immigration." *Journal of American Ethnic History* 17, 1 (Fall 1997): 3–18.

Das, Veena. "Gender Studies, Cross-Cultural Comparison, and the Colonial Organization of Knowledge." *Berkshire Review* 21 (1986): 24–54.

Dawson, R. MacGregor. *William Lyon Mackenzie King: A Political Biography, 1874–1923.* Toronto: University of Toronto Press, 1958.

Day, Richard J.F. *Multiculturalism and the History of Canadian Diversity.* Toronto: University of Toronto Press, 2000.

Dodd, Werter D. "The Hindu in the Northwest." *World Today* 13 (November 1907): 1157–60.

Dua, Enakshi. "Racializing Imperial Canada: Indian Women and the Making of Ethnic Communities." In *Sisters or Strangers? Immigrant, Ethnic, and Racialized Women in Canadian History,* ed. Marlene Epp, Franca Iacovetta, and Frances Swyripa, 71–85. Toronto: University of Toronto Press, 2004.

Elkins, Stanley M. *Slavery: A Problem in American Institutional and Intellectual Life.* Chicago: University of Chicago Press, 1959.

Elliot, J.H. "Present Status of Anti-tuberculosis Work in Canada, *Transactions of the Sixth Annual Conference on Tuberculosis,* vol. 4, Pt. 1. Philadelphia: Wm. F. Fell, 1908.

Ettinger, Patrick. "'We Sometimes Wonder What They Will Spring on Us Next': Immigrants and Border Enforcement in the American West, 1882–1930." *Western Historical Quarterly* 37, 2 (Summer 2006): 159–81. http://dx.doi.org/10.2307/2544 3330.

Ettling, John. *The Germ of Laziness: Rockefeller, Philanthropy, and Public Health in the New South.* 2nd ed. Cambridge, MA: Harvard University Press, 2000.

Fairchild, Amy L. "Policies of Inclusion: Immigrants, Disease, Dependency, and American Immigration Policy at the Dawn and Dusk of the Twentieth Century." *American Journal of Public Health* 94, 4 (April 2004): 528–39. http://dx.doi.org/10.2105/AJPH.94.4.528.

—. "The Rise and Fall of the Medical Gaze: The Political Economy of Immigrant Medical Inspection in Modern America." *Science in Context* 19, 3 (September 2006): 337–56. http://dx.doi.org/10.1017/S0269889706000962.

—. *Science at the Borders: Immigrant Medical Inspection and the Shaping of the Modern Industrial Labor Force.* Baltimore: Johns Hopkins University Press, 2003.

Feldberg, Georgina. *Disease and Class: Tuberculosis and the Shaping of Modern North American Society.* New Brunswick: Rutgers University Press, 1995.

Figler, Bernard. *Sam Jacobs: Member of Parliament.* Montreal: Harpell, 1970.

Fieldbrave, Theodore. "East Indians in the United States," *Missionary Review of the World* 57 (1934): 291–93.

—. "Work Among the Hindus," *The Baptist* (Chicago), January 24, 1925, 438 (1 pg).

"The Filth of Asia." *The White Man* (organ of the Movement for Asiatic Exclusion, San Francisco, Special Edition: "The Hindu") 1, 2. (August 1910): 6–8.

Foucault, Michel. *The Archeology of Knowledge.* New York: Pantheon, 1972.

——. *Discipline and Punish: The Birth of the Prison.* New York: Vintage Books, 1979.

Fralick, Wilfred G. *The Intravenous Infusion Method of Treatment for Tuberculosis.* Chicago: Windermere, 1902.

Fredrickson, George M. "Fredrickson, "From Exceptionalism to Variability: Recent Developments in Cross-National Comparative History." *Journal of American History* 82, 2 (September 1995): 587–604. http://dx.doi.org/10.2307/2082188.

Furedi, Frank. *The Silent War: Imperialism and the Changing Perception of Race.* New Brunswick: Rutgers University Press, 1998.

Geiger, Andrea. *Subverting Exclusion: Transpacific Encounters with Race, Caste, and Borders, 1885–1928.* New Haven: Yale University Press, 2011.

[Author Unknown]. "Gifts of Famine: Invasion of Sikhs from the Punjaub." *International Woodworker* 17, 10 (October 1907): 4–5.

Glassberg, David. "The Design of Reform: The Public Bath Movement in America." In *Sickness and Health in America: Readings in The History of Medicine and Public Health.* 3rd ed., ed. Judith W. Leavitt and Ronald L. Numbers, 485–94. Madison: University of Wisconsin Press, 1997.

Glover, M.W. "Hookworm among Oriental Immigrants." *Journal of the American Medical Association* 58, 24 (June 15, 1912): 1837–40. http://dx.doi.org/10.1001/jama.1912.04260060186003.

Goldberg, David. *Racist Culture: Philosophy and the Politics of Meaning.* Oxford: Blackwell, 1993.

Good News Bible, 1986 Edition.

Gosnell, E.R. "British Columbia and British International Relations." *Annals of the American Academy of Political and Social Science* 45, 1 (January 1913): 1–19. http://dx.doi.org/10.1177/000271621304500101.

Government of British Columbia. Court of Appeal "Regarding Munshi Singh." (July 6, 1914), 20 B.C.R. 243.

——. "Regulations for Detection and Treatment of a Disease Known as Bubonic Plague." Approved October 24, 1907, *B.C. Sessional Papers 2nd Session 11th Parliament 1908.* Victoria: Wolfeden, 1908, G 19.

Goutor, David. *Guarding the Gates: The Canadian Labour Movement and Immigration, 1872–1934.* Vancouver: UBC Press, 2008.

Graham, Roger. *Arthur Meighen: A Biography.* Vancouver: Clarke, Irwin, 1965.

Griffin, Harold. *Radical Roots: The Shaping of British Columbia.* Vancouver: Commonwealth Fund, 1999.

Gyory, Andrew. *Closing the Gate: Race, Politics, and the Chinese Exclusion Act.* Chapel Hill: University of North Carolina Press, 1998.

Hallberg, Gerald N. "Bellingham, Washington's Anti-Hindu Riot." *Journal of the West* 12 (January 1973): 163–71.

Haller, Mark. *Eugenics: Hereditarian Attitudes in American Thought.* New Brunswick: Rutgers University Press, 1963.

Hallett, Mary. "A Governor-General's Views on Oriental Immigration to British Columbia, 1904–1911." *BC Studies* 14 (Summer 1972): 51–72.

Harrington, Sheila, and Judi Stevenson. *Islands in the Salish Sea: A Community Atlas.* Surrey: Land Trust Alliance of BC, 2005.

Harris, Bernard. "Pro-Alienism, Anti-Alienism and the Medical Profession in Late-Victorian and Edwardian Britain." In *Race, Science, and Medicine, 1700–1960*, ed. Waltraud Ernst and Bernard Harris, 189–217. London: Routledge, 1999.

Hastings, Paula. "Review of *Contesting White Supremacy.*" *Journal of Colonialism and Colonial History* 13, 1 (Spring 2012): 1–2.

Hegel, Georg Wilhelm Friedrich. *The Science of Logic.* Cambridge: Cambridge University Press, 2010.

Hernández, David Manuel. "Undue Process: Racial Genealogies of Immigrant Detention." In *Constructing Borders/Crossing Boundaries: Race, Ethnicity, and Immigration*, ed. Caroline B. Brettell, 59–86. London: Lexington Books, 2007.

Hernández, Tanya. "The Construction of Race and Class Buffers in the Structure of Immigration Controls and Laws." *Oregon Law Review* 76, 3 (Fall 1997): 731–65.

Hess, G.R. "The Hindu in America: Immigration and Naturalization Policies and India, 1917–1946," *Pacific Historical Review* 38, 1 (February 1969): 59–79.

Higham, John. "Origins of Immigration Restriction, 1882–1897: A Social Analysis." *Mississippi Valley Historical Review* 39, 1 (June 1952): 77–88. http://dx.doi.org/10.2307/1902845.

——. *Strangers in the Land: Patterns of American Nativism 1860–1925.* 3rd ed. New York: Atheneum, 1985.

Hill, Judith S. *Alberta's Black Settlers: A Study of Canadian Immigration Policy and Practice.* Calgary: University of Alberta Press, 1981.

Hilliker, John F. *Canada's Department of External Affairs*, vol. 1. Ottawa: Institute of Public Administration, 1990.

Hinde, John. *When Coal Was King: Ladysmith and the Coal-Mining Industry on Vancouver Island.* Vancouver: UBC Press, 2003.

"The Hindu Invasion." *Collier's Weekly*, March 26, 1910, 15.

Hing, Bill Ong. *Defining America through Immigration Policy.* Philadelphia: Temple University Press, 2004.

Humphries, Mark Osborne. *The Last Plague: Spanish Influenza and the Politics of Public Health in Canada.* Toronto: University of Toronto Press, 2013.

Hunt, Michael. *Ideology and Foreign Policy.* New Haven: Yale University Press, 1988.

Ignatiev, Noel. *How the Irish Became White.* London: Routledge, 1996.

Indra, Doreen M. "South Asian Stereotypes in the Vancouver Press." *Ethnic and Racial Studies* 2, 2 (January 1979): 166–89. http://dx.doi.org/10.1080/01419870.1979.9993261.

Isaacs, Harold Robert. *American Views of China and India.* 2nd ed. Westport: Greenwood Press, 1973.

Jensen, Joan. *Passage from India: Asian Indian Immigrants in North America.* New Haven: Yale University Press, 1988.

Johnston, E. Lukin. "The Case of the Oriental in BC." *Canadian Magazine* 57 (August 1929): 315.

——. *Jewels of the Qila: The Remarkable Story of an Indo-Canadian Family.* Vancouver: UBC Press, 2011.

——. "The Surveillance of Indian Nationalists in North America, 1909–1918." *BC Studies* 78 (1988): 3–27.

——. *The Voyage of the Komagata Maru: The Sikh Challenge to Canada's Colour Bar.* 3rd ed. Vancouver: UBC Press, 2014.

Kant, Immanuel. *Critique of Teleological Judgment.* New York: Clarendon Press, 1928.

Kazimi, Ali. *Undesirables: White Canada and the Komagata Maru: An Illustrated History.* Toronto: Douglas and McIntyre, 2012.

Kelley, Ninette, and Michael Trebilcock. *The Making of the Mosaic: A History of Canadian Immigration Policy.* Toronto: University of Toronto Press, 1998.

Kelly, Nigel. R. Rees, and J. Shutter. *Britain 1750–1900.* Oxford: Heinemann, 1998.

Kenny, Kevin. "Diaspora and Comparison: The Global Irish as a Case Study." *Journal of American History* 90, 1 (June 2003): 134–62. http://dx.doi.org/10.2307/3659794.

King, Richard. *Orientalism and Religion: Post-Colonial Theory, India, and the 'Mystic East.* New York: Routledge, 1999.

Kipling, Rudyard. *Letters to the Family: Notes on a Recent Trip to Canada.* Toronto: Macmillan, 1908.

Klein, Ira. "Plague, Policy, and Popular Unrest in British India." *Modern Asian Studies* 22, 4 (1988): 723–55. http://dx.doi.org/10.1017/S0026749X00015729.

Koshy, Susan. *Sexual Naturalization: Asian Americans and Miscegenation.* Stanford: Stanford University Press, 2004.

Kramer, Paul. "Imperial Histories of the United States in the World." *American Historical Review* 116, 5 (2011): 1348–91. http://dx.doi.org/10.1086/ahr.116.5.1348.

Kraut, Alan. *Silent Travelers: Germs, Genes, and the "Immigrant Menace."* Baltimore: Johns Hopkins University Press, 1995.

Kreines, James. "The Logic of Life: Hegel's Philosophical Defense of Teleological Explanation of Living Beings." In *The Cambridge Companion to Hegel and Nineteenth-Century Philosophy,* ed. Frederick C. Beiser, 344–77. New York: Cambridge University Press, 2008. http://dx.doi.org/10.1017/CCOL9780521831673.014.

La Brack, Bruce. "Immigration Law and the Revitalization Process: The Case of the California Sikhs." *Population Review* 25 (1982): 59–66.

——. *The Sikhs of Northern California, 1904–1975.* New York: AMS Press, 1988.

Laut, Agnes C. *Am I My Brother's Keeper? A Study of BC's Labour and Oriental Problems.* Toronto: Saturday Night Publishing, 1913. (Reprinted in Mark Leier, ed., *Am I My Brother's Keeper?* Vancouver: Subway Books, 2003)

Lee, Chris. "The Lateness of Asian Canadian Studies." *Amerasia Journal* 33, 2 (2007) 1–17.

Lee, Erika. *At America's Gates: Chinese Immigration during the Exclusion Era, 1882–1943.* Chapel Hill: University of North Carolina Press, 2003. Lee, Erika, and Judy Yung. *Angel Island: Immigrant Gateway to America.* Oxford: Oxford University Press, 2011.

Leong, Karen. *The China Mystique: Pearl S. Buck, Anna May Wong, Mayling Soong, and the Transformation of American Orientalism.* Berkeley: University of California Press, 2005.

Livingston, Leon Ray. *From Coast to Coast with Jack London.* Erie: A-1 Publishing Company, 1917.

Lockley, Frederick. "The Hindu Invasion: A New Immigration Problem." *Pacific Monthly* 17 (May 1907): 587.

Luibheid, Eithne. *Entry Denied: Controlling Sexuality at the Border.* Minneapolis: University of Minnesota Press, 2002.

Luminet, Jean-Pierre. *Black Holes.* Cambridge: Cambridge University Press, 1999.

Macdonald, Norman. *Canada: Immigration and Colonization, 1841–1903.* London: Aberdeen University Press, 1966.

Magocsi, P.R., ed. *Encyclopedia of Canada's Peoples.* Toronto: University of Toronto Press, 1999.

Maloney, Deirdre. *National Insecurities: Immigrants and US Deportation Policy Since 1882.* Chapel Hill: University of North Carolina Press, 2012.

Markel, Howard, and Alexandra M. Stern. "Which Face? Whose Nation? Immigration, Public Health, and the Construction of Disease at America's Ports and Borders, 1891–1928." *American Behavioral Scientist* 42, 9 (June–July 1999): 1314–31. http://dx.doi.org/10.1177/00027649921954921.

Mathieu, Sarah-Jane. *North of the Colour Line: Migration and Black Resistance in Canada, 1870–1955.* Durham: University of North Carolina Press, 2010.

McClintock, Anne. *Imperial Leather: Race, Gender, and Sexuality in the Colonial Contest.* New York: Routledge, 1995.

McInnes, T. *Oriental Occupation of British Columbia.* Vancouver: Sun Publishing Company Limited, 1927.

McKay, Ian. *Reasoning Otherwise: Leftists and the People's Enlightenment in Canada, 1890–1920.* Toronto: Between the Lines, 2008.

McKeown, Adam. *Chinese Migrant Networks and Cultural Change: Peru, Chicago, Hawaii, 1900–1936.* Chicago: University of Chicago Press, 2001.

McLaren, Angus. *Our Own Master Race: Eugenics in Canada, 1885–1945.* Toronto: McClelland and Stewart, 1990.

——. "Stemming the Flood of Defective Immigration." In *The History of Immigration and Racism in Canada: Essential Readings*, ed. Barrington Walker, 173–204. Toronto: Canadian Scholars' Press, 2008.

McQuaig, Katherine. *The Weariness, the Fever, and the Fret: The Campaign against Tuberculosis in Canada, 1900–1950.* Kingston and Montreal: McGill–Queen's University Press, 1999.

McVety, James. "Suggests Violence in Case Asiatics Are Landed." *British Columbia Federationist* (June 5, 1914).

Mongia, Radhika. "Race, Nationality, Mobility: A History of the Passport." *Public Culture* 11, 3 (Fall 1999): 527–55. http://dx.doi.org/10.1215/08992363-11-3-527.

Mitchell, Don. *The Lie of the Land: Migrant Workers and the California Landscape.* Minneapolis: University of Minnesota Press, 1996.

Molina, Natalia. *Fit to Be Citizens? Public Health and Race in LA, 1879–1939.* Berkeley: University of California Press, 2006.

Moorhead, F.G. "The Foreign Invasion of the Northwest." *The World's Work* (Marc. 1908): 9994–97.

Moran, Michelle. *Colonizing Leprosy: Imperialism and the Politics of Public Health in the United States.* Durham: University of North Carolina Press, 2007.

Nash, Linda. *Inescapable Ecologies: A History of Environment, Disease, and Knowledge.* Berkeley: University of California Press, 2006.

Nesbitt, Charles T. "The Health Menace of Alien Races." *The World's Work* (November 1913): 1–4.

Neu, Charles E. *An Uncertain Friendship: Theodore Roosevelt and Japan, 1906–1909.* Cambridge, MA: Harvard University Press, 1967. http://dx.doi.org/10.4159/harvard.9780674182950.

Okihiro, Gary. *Cane Fires: The Anti-Japanese Movement in Hawaii, 1865–1945.* Philadelphia: Temple University Press, 1991.

——. *The Columbia Guide to Asian American History.* New York: Columbia University Press, 2001.

Omi, Michael, and Howard Winant. *Racial Formation in the United States from the 1960s to the 1990s.* New York: Taylor and Francis, 1986.

Palumbo-Liu, David. *Asian/American: Historical Crossings of a Racial Frontier.* Stanford: Stanford University Press, 1999.

Panikkar, K.N. *Culture, Ideology, Hegemony: Intellectuals and Social Consciousness in Colonial India.* New Delhi: Tulika Press, 1995.

——. "In Defence of 'Old' History." *Economic and Political Weekly* 29, 40 (October 1, 1994): 2595–97.

Parnaby, Andrew, and Gregory S. Kealey. "The Origins of Political Policing in Canada: Class, Law, and the Burden of Empire." *Osgoode Hall Law Journal* 41, 2–3 (2003): 211–39.

Pernick, M.S. "Eugenics and Public Health in American History." *American Journal of Public Health* 87, 11 (November 1997): 1767–72. http://dx.doi.org/10.2105/AJPH.87.11.1767.

Perras, Galen Roger. *Stepping Stones to Nowhere: The Aleutian Islands, Alaska, and American Military Strategy, 1867–1945.* Vancouver: UBC Press, 2003.

Popplewell, Richard James. *Intelligence and Imperial Defence: British Intelligence and Defence of the Empire, 1904–1924.* London: Routledge, 1995.

Price, John. "'Orienting' the Empire: Mackenzie King and the Aftermath of the 1907 Race Riots." *BC Studies* 156 (Winter 2007–8): 53–81.

——. *Orienting Canada: Race, Empire, and the Transpacific.* Vancouver: University of British Columbia Press, 2011.

Proceedings of the Asiatic Exclusion League, 1907–1913. San Francisco: Organized Labor Print, 1908. (Reprinted: New York: Arno Press, 1977).

Pula, J.S. "American Immigration Policy and the Dillingham Commission." *Polish American Studies* 37, 1 (Spring 1980): 5–31.

R.L.H. Jr. "Aliens: Naturalization: Who is a White Person?" *California Law Review* 11, 5 (November, 1921): 353.

Razack, Sherene. *Race, Space, and the Law: Unmapping a White Settler Society.* Toronto: Between the Lines, 2002.

——. "Saving the Empire: The Politics of Immigrant Tuberculosis in Canada." *McGill Journal of Medicine* 11, 2 (2008): 199–203.

Ring, Natalie J. *The Problem South: Region, Empire, and the New Liberal State, 1880–1930.* Athens: University of Georgia Press, 2012.

Roberts, Barbara Ann. *Whence They Came: Deportations from Canada, 1900–1935.* Ottawa: University of Ottawa Press, 1988.

Robertson, Craig. *The Passport in America: The History of a Document.* Oxford: Oxford University Press, 2010.

Roediger, David. *Toward the Abolition of Whiteness.* London: Verso, 1994.

——. *The Wages of Whiteness: Race and the Making of the American Working Class.* 2nd ed. London: Verso, 2007.

Ross, Edward A. "The Causes of Race Superiority." *Annals of the American Academy of Political and Social Science* 18, 1 (July 1901): 67–89. http://dx.doi.org/10.1177/000271620101800104.

Roy, Patricia. *A White Man's Province: British Columbia Politicians and Chinese and Japanese Immigrants, 1858–1914.* Vancouver: UBC Press, 1989.

Rushton, J. Philippe. *Race, Evolution, and Behavior: A Life History Perspective.* New Brunswick: Rutgers University Press, 1994.

Ryder, Bruce. "Racism and the Constitution: The Constitutional Fate of British Columbia Anti-Asian Immigration Legislation, 1884–1909." *Osgoode Hall Law Journal* 29, 3 (Fall 1991): 619–76.

Said, Edward. *Orientalism.* New York: Vintage Books, 1979.

Sandmeyer, Elmer Clarence. *The Anti-Chinese Movement in California.* Champaign: University of Illinois Press, 1939.

Saxton, Alexander. *The Indispensable Enemy: Labor and the Anti-Chinese Movement in California.* Berkeley: University of California Press, 1971.

Saywell, J.T., and P. Stevens, eds. *Lord Minto's Canadian Papers,* vol. 1. Toronto: Champlain Society, 1981.

Scheffauer, Herman. "Tide of Turbans." *The Forum* [New York] 43 (June 1910): 616–18.

Schrag, Peter. *Not Fit for Our Society: Immigration and Nativism.* Berkeley: University of California Press, 2010.

Schultz, W.H. "Remedies for Animal Parasites: A Study of the Relative Efficiency and Danger of Thymol as Compared with Certain Other Remedies Proposed for Hookworm Disease." *Journal of the American Medical Association* 57, 14 (September 30, 1911): 1102–6. http://dx.doi.org/10.1001/jama.1911.04260090324003.

Schwantes, Carlos A. *Radical Heritage: Labor, Socialism, and Reform in Washington and British Columbia, 1885–1917.* Seattle: University of Washington Press, 1979.

Scott, W.D. "The Immigration By Races" (1914). In *A Country Nourished on Self-Doubt: Documents in Post-Confederation Canadian History.* 3rd ed., ed. Thomas Thorner and Thor Frohn –Nielson, 73–87. Toronto: University of Toronto Press, 2010.

Sears, Alan. "Immigration Controls as Social Policy: The Case of Canadian Medical Inspection 1900–1920." *Studies in Political Economy* 33 (Autumn 1990): 91–112.

Shah, Hernan. "Race, Nation, and Citizenship: Asian Indians and the Idea of Whiteness in the U.S. Press, 1906–1926." *Howard Journal of Communications* 10, 4 (1999): 249–67. http://dx.doi.org/10.1080/106461799246744.

Shah, Nayan. *Contagious Divides: Epidemics and Race in San Francisco's Chinatown.* Berkeley: University of California Press, 2001.

——. *Stranger Intimacy: Contesting Race, Sexuality, and the Law in the American West.* Berkeley: University of California Press, 2011.

Simpson, W.J. *Report on the Causes and Continuance of Plague in Hongkong [sic] and Suggestions as to Remedial Measures.* London: Colonial Office, 1903.

Singh, Jane. "The Gadar Party: Political Expression in an Immigrant Community." In *Asian American Studies: A Reader,* ed. Jean Wu and Min Song, 36–47. New Brunswick: Rutgers University Press, 2000.

Singh, M. Gundar, ed. *Amrik Vich Hindustanee* [Indians in America]. Vancouver: M.G. Singh, 1976.

Siu, Paul C.P. "The Sojourner." *American Journal of Sociology* 58, 1 (July 1952): 34–44.

Snow, Jennifer. "The Civilization of White Men: The Race of the Hindu in *United States v. Bhagat Singh Thind.*" In *Race, Nation, and Religion in the Americas,* ed. Henry Goldschmidt and Elizabeth McAlister, 259–81. Oxford: Oxford University Press, 2004. http://dx.doi.org/10.1093/0195149181.003.0011.

Sproule-Jones, Megan. "Crusading for the Forgotten: Dr. Peter Bryce, Public Health, and Prairie Native Residential Schools." *Canadian Bulletin of Medical History* 13 (1996): 199–224.

Stanley, Timothy. *Contesting White Supremacy: School Segregation, Anti-Racism, and the Making of Chinese Canadians.* Vancouver: UBC Press, 2011.

Stern, Alexandra Minna. *Eugenic Nation: Faults and Frontiers of Better Breeding in Modern America.* Berkeley: University of California Press, 2005.

Stevens, H.H. *The Oriental Problem, Dealing with Canada as Affected by the Immigration of Japanese, Hindu, and Chinese.* Vancouver: H.H. Stevens, 1912.

Stoler, Ann Laura. Rethinking Colonial Categories: European Communities and The Boundaries of Rule." *Comparative Studies in Society and History* 31, 1 (1989): 134–61. http://dx.doi.org/10.1017/S0010417500015693.

Stout, Arthur B. *Chinese Immigration and the Physiological Causes of the Decay of a Nation.* San Francisco: Agnew and Deffebach, 1862.

Street, Richard. *Beasts of the Field: A Narrative History of California Farmworkers, 1769–1913.* Stanford: Stanford University Press, 2004.

Swanson, Maynard. "The Sanitation Syndrome: Bubonic Plague and Urban Native Policy in the Cape Colony, 1900–9." *Journal of African History* 18, 3 (1977): 387–410. http://dx.doi.org/10.1017/S0021853700027328.

Swarts, G.T., "The Havana Meeting of the American Public Health Association," *Journal of the American Public Health Association* 1, 12 (Dec 1911): 895–96.

Thomas, W.I. "The Mind of Woman and the Lower Races." *American Journal of Sociology* 12, 4 (January 1907): 435–40. http://dx.doi.org/10.1086/211517.

Thorner, Thomas, and Thor Frohn-Nielson, eds. *A Country Nourished on Self-Doubt: Documents in Post-Confederation Canadian History.* 3rd ed. Toronto: University of Toronto Press, 2010.

Tichenor, Daniel. *Dividing Lines: The Politics of Immigration Control in America.* Princeton: Princeton University Press, 2002.

Todd, Frank. *Eradicating Plague from San Francisco.* San Francisco: Murdock, 1909.

Tomes, Nancy J. "American Attitudes toward the Germ Theory of Disease: Phyllis Allen Richmond Revisited." *Journal of the History of Medicine* 52 (January 1997): 17–50.

Trauner, J.B. "The Chinese as Medical Scapegoats in San Francisco, 1870–1905." *California History* 57, 1 (Spring 1978): 70–87. http://dx.doi.org/10.2307/25157817.

United States [Government of]. *Annual Reports of the Commissioner of Immigration, for Years Ending June 30, 1903–1915.* Washington: US GPO, 1910–15.

——. Congress Act, March 3, 1891, 51 Cong. 2nd Sess, 26 Stat. 1084.

——. *Restriction of Immigration Hearings Before the Committee on Immigration and Naturalization,* House of Representatives, 63rd Cong., 2nd Sess., HR 6060, Pt. 1, December 6 and 7, 1913 (Washington: US GPO, 1913).

——.Senate. *Reports of the Immigration Commission in 25 Parts* [Includes *Abstracts of Reports*]. [Senate Document 633] Washington: US GPO, 1911.

United States v. Bhagat Singh Thind, 261 US 204 [1923].

Valverde, Mariana. *Age of Light, Soap, and Water: Moral Reform in English Canada, 1885–1925.* 2nd ed. Toronto: University of Toronto Press, 2008.

Vancouver [City of]. *Annual Reports of the Health Department of Vancouver for Years Ending December 31, 1906–24.* Vancouver: 1924.

Victoria Friends of the Hindus. "Summary of the Hindu Question and Its Results in B.C., Presented to the Empire as a Whole." Westminster: Friends of the Hindus, 1911.

Wallace, Isabel. "*Komagata Maru* Revisited." In *Interpreting Canada's Past: A Post-Confederation Reader,* 5th ed., ed. Michael Ducharme, Damien-Claude Belanger, and J.M. Bumsted. New York: Oxford University Press.

——. "Review of Hugh Johnston, *Voyage of the Komagata Maru,*" *Canadian Historical Review* 96, 1 (March 2015): 128–30.

Ward, Peter. *White Canada Forever: Popular Attitudes and Public Policy Towards Orientals in British Columbia.* 3rd ed. Kingston and Montreal: McGill–Queen's University Press, 2002.

Webber, Roger. *Communicable Disease Epidemiology and Control.* 3rd ed. Oxford: CABI International, 2009.

Williams, J. Barclay, and Saint Nihal Singh. "Canada's New Immigrant: The Hindu." *Canadian Magazine* XXVIII (February 28, 1907): 383–91.

Woodsworth, J.S. *Strangers within Our Gates, Or, Coming Canadians.* Toronto: University of Toronto Press, 1909.

Worboys, Michael. *Spreading Germs: Disease Theories and Medical Practice in Britain, 1865–1900.* Cambridge: Cambridge University Press, 2000.

Yew, Elizabeth. "Medical Inspection of Immigrants at Ellis Island, 1891–1924." *Bulletin of the New York Academy of Medicine* 56 (1980): 488–510.

Yoell, A.E., "The Hindoo Question in California, February 1908." In *Proceedings of the Asiatic Exclusion League (AEL), 1907–1913* (reprint). New York: Arno Press, 1977, 8–9.

Index

Note: "(i)" after a page number indicates an illustration; "(f)" after a page number indicates a figure; "(t)" after a page number indicates a table; "South Asians" and "Indians" used interchangeably throughout to reduce repetition

Aboriginal peoples (of North America), 112–13, 193, 199*n*2
acts (and orders-in-council, except continuous journey provision): of *British Columbia*, 1892 Health Act, 54; of *California*, Webb-Haney act (alien land act), 150, 178, 181–82, 235*n*40; of *Canada*, 1869 Immigration Act, 15; Dominion Elections Act, 170–71; 1887 Quarantine provision, 15; 1891 Immigration Act, 38, 207*n*97; 1906 Immigration Act, 16; 1907 Immigration Act, 38; 1907 Plague Act, 54; 1917 Immigration Act, 147, 154–58, 161–62, 177, 189, 192–93; 1921 Immigration Act, 178, 235*n*38; 1924 Immigration Act (Johnson-Reed Act), (Asian Exclusion Act under), 177–78, 189–90, 235*n*38; 1930 amendment to Immigration Act, 138; PC 1908–926 (later removed and reissued as PC 23), 3, 212*n*1, 214*n*10, 228*n*47, 229*n*67; PC 1912–2218, 137; PC 1913–2462, 138, 140; PC 1930–2215, 228*n*47; 2010 Amendment of Immigrant and Refugee Protection Act, 194; *of the United States of America*, 1882 Immigration Act, 38, 78. *See also* continuous journey; human smuggling; Immigration Act of 1917; Immigration Act of 1924; landownership; Natal acts; voting rights

African Canadians and African Americans, 43, 102, 138, 152, 175–76, 219*n*83, 223n43
agency (human). *See* immigrant subjectivity
Ainsworth, Frank: opposition to H.H. North at Angel Island, 86, 91, 97. *See also* Angel Island; North, H.H.
alcoholism: and Indians, 128, 133, 139, 156, 166–67. *See also* drug addiction; South Asian immigrants, immorality
American Federation of Labor (AFL), 5. *See also* unions of the Pacific coast
American west. *See* British Columbia (BC); California; Oregon; Portland, OR; San Francisco, CA; Seattle, WA; Vancouver, BC; Victoria, BC; Washington State
American-ness: European immigrants and, 235*n*35; South Asian immigrants and, 84. *See also* eugenics movement; nativism; United States of America (USA); whiteness
anemia: and South Asians, 45, 120
Angel Island (immigration station, San Francisco), 5, 219*n*78; adoption of bacteriology at, 97; Asian vs non-Asian experiences at, 85; bonds for appealed cases at, 221*n*28, 223*n*41; California criticisms of medical inspection procedures at, 88–89; case of Ottam Singh and hookworm testing, 221n27; general entry and exit statistics of, 84; hookworm discovery

Taylor, Louis D., 21, 25, 54; on climate argument, 70
teleological accounts of history, 6–7, 200nn14–15; G.W.F. Hegel's defence of, 7. *See also* theory
theories on methodology: Kevin Kenny on international vs. cross-national methodologies on migration, 7–8; K.N. Panikkar's "middle ground" approach to interpreting history and, 6–7
theory (social). *See* colonial theory; medicalized nativism; Orientalism; race theory; sick immigrant paradigm; transnational
Thind, Bhagat Singh. *See* naturalization
Thoburn, James Mills, 1, 47–48, 199n1, 209n203
trachoma, 16, 78, 212n60; and Asian immigrants in BC, 16, 35; as "Class A" excludable disease, 207n97; cost for treatment for at Angel Island, 91; and *Komagata Maru* incident, 229n61; and Public Health Service, 77; and South Asians arriving at BC, 35, 61–62; and South Asians arriving at San Francisco, 82–84, 89, 92
Trades and Labour Congress (TLC), 5, 207n1; Vancouver chapter, 20, 27–28; Victoria chapter, 22, 24–25
transnational (North American): protest against South Asians, 5; South Asian migration and community ties, 5. *See also* theories on methodology
transshipment. *See* continuous journey
tropical (or fatal) miasmas (theory of), 13; Linda Nash and, 13, 99; as reverse of climate argument, 13, 70; susceptibility to as a sign of whiteness, 99. *See also* climate argument
tropical diseases. *See* diseases (contagious); tropical miasmas; typhoid fever
Trudeau, Justin: *Komagata Maru* apology by, 194, 237n9. *See also* Canada; *Komagata Maru* incident
tuberculosis, 23, 180, 187; BC Royal Commission on Labour testimony on, 133; and Canadian immigration, 31,

33, 42; connection with South Asians in BC, 4, 9, 23, 32–35, 45, 58–60, 70–71, 75, 203n47, 205n78, 206n83; "cure" for, 62; E. Blake Robertson's association of South Asians with, 34, 139–40; and family reunification, 139; F.C. Blair's association of South Asians with, 128; G.L. Milne's association of South Asians with, 125; Immigration Branch instructions on screening Indians for, 34; included as reason for PHS rejections, 38, 76, 79(t), 87; "poor physique" as evidence of past infection or susceptibility to, 87; and Public Health Service, 77; South Asian deaths and, 169–70; South Asians deported from Canada for having, 75; SS *Komagata Maru* passengers and, 146; W.L.M. King's association of South Asians with, 139–40
turban (Sikh), 1, 82, 98, 199n2; as foreign apparel, 69, 73; and hygiene, 89, 91; mistakenly associated with Hinduism, 91; used for lung protection, 23. *See also* Sikhism
typhoid fever, 49; and healthy carriers, 49, 100; and South Asians, 23, 102

Underhill, Frederick T., 20–21; and bubonic plague inspections, 54–55; and Eburne cannery venture, 32
unions of the Pacific coast, 1, 50; concerns over Asian participation in the workforce, 14; and "Hindu disease" thesis, 37, 48–49, 83–84, 92; labour vote and, 20; perspectives of on South Asian immigration, 227n28; South Asian sexuality and, 80
United Kingdom (UK): Parliamentary responses to continuous journey order, 68; Parliamentary responses to South Asian immigration to North America, 35, 206n84. *See also* British Empire; Colonial Office
United States of America (USA): American observations on treatment of Indians within the British Empire, 86; Congress of, including Representatives and Senators, 10,